THE

ARTIST'S

COMPLETE

HEALTH

AND SAFETY

GUIDE

Monona Rossol

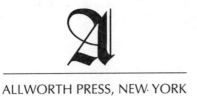

ALLWORTH PRESS, NEW YORK

Published by Allworth Press, an imprint of Allworth Communications, Inc., 10 East 23rd Street, New York, NY 10010.

Distributor to the trade in the United States and Canada:
North Light Books, an imprint of F&W Publications, Inc.
1507 Dana Avenue, Cincinnati, OH 45207.
To order additional copies of this book, call toll-free 1-800-289-0963.

Book Design by Douglas Design Associates, New York.

Library of Congress Catalog Card Number: 90-80002

ISBN: 0-927629-10-0

This book was written to provide the most current and accurate information about health and safety hazards in the arts and about applicable laws and regulations. However, the author and publisher can take no responsibility for any harm or damage that might be caused by the use or misuse of any information contained herein. It is not the purpose of this book to provide medical diagnosis, suggest health treatment, or provide legal or regulatory counseling. Readers should seek advice from physicians, safety professionals, industrial hygienists, environmental health specialists, and attorneys concerning specific problems.

Dedication

To John S. Fairlie and the vast Fairlie clan to which I belong.

Acknowledgements

There are so many professional friends and colleagues I would like to thank, but the list is far too long. Instead I will mention only a crucial few. First, always, is Jack Holzhueter who labored long to "learn" me to write. Next, my thanks to Ted Rickard at the Ontario College of the Arts for his help on the Canadian regulations, to Tad Crawford who knows how to spur a writer along without puncturing the ego, and to Denise O'Sullivan for keeping me sane at the Copy Factory.

My deep gratitude goes also to the Board of ACTS (Arts, Crafts and Theater Safety), Susan Shaw, Eric Gertner, and Nina Yahr, for sharing their expertise and encouragement. And to Tom Arminio who gave me the idea of starting ACTS and served on its Board until his death in 1988.

CONTENTS

SECTION I	The Regulated Art World

CHAPTER

SECTION II	Artist's Raw Materials

SECTION III	Precautions for Individual Media

SECTION IV	Teaching Art

List of Tables

List of Figures

PREFACE

T he idea for this book can be traced back to the University of Wisconsin where I earned a BS in chemistry. I was working and teaching in the chemistry department when I decided to enter the graduate art program. As I went back and forth between the chemistry and art schools, it occurred to me that many of the same acids and other chemicals were used in both places.

As a research chemist I defended myself against chemicals with goggles, gloves, fume hoods, and other safety equipment. My art colleagues and I, on the other hand, saw these same chemicals as art materials that were to be used lovingly and intimately. As I look back at our work practices now, I think we must have confused "exposure to art" with "exposure to art materials."

My first writings on art hazards were graduate school seminar and term papers in the early 60's. They were not well-received. My classmates and teachers told me bluntly that this kind of information interfered with their creativity. Unfortunately, illness and death also interfere with creativity, so I have persisted. This book is the result of that persistence.

The book's subject is necessarily technical and you may find you have questions or need additional information. For this reason, I have made arrangements for readers to be able to reach me at:

> Arts, Crafts and Theater Safety (ACTS)
> 181 Thompson Street, #23
> New York, NY l0012.

ACTS is a not-for-profit corporation dedicated to providing a variety of health and safety services for artists. I already answer thousands of requests for information at ACTS every year and would be pleased to hear from you.

Monona Rossol, M.S., M.F.A., Industrial Hygienist.

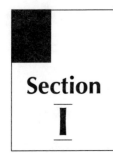

Section

I

The Regulated Art World

CHAPTER 1

INDUSTRIAL HYGIENE FOR THE ARTS

As artists and teachers, most of us believe our creative work must be free, uninhibited, and independent. Actually, it is encumbered by a host of laws and regulations.

For example, fire, health, and safety laws affect how we must design our studios and what we can teach in our classrooms. And environmental protection laws limit the kinds of art materials available to us, as well as how we must store, use and dispose of them. These laws apply to us because many materials used in art contain substances which now are known to be both toxic and hazardous to the environment. By using these materials improperly, we risk our health and pollute our world just as industry does. While we each may use much smaller amounts of chemicals than industry, there are so many of us.

Today, these laws are becoming more restrictive. They not only apply to professional and industrial materials, but to many common household and hobby products. Art materials packaged for consumer use, in particular, now are regulated under a special amendment to the Toxic Substances Control Act (see page 43).

Either we can see these new laws as impositions and resist them at every turn, or we can accept change and do our share in protecting ourselves and the environment. But whether we resist or not, progressively stricter regulation and enforcement is inevitable.

Schools and universities should be in the forefront of this movement. They could encourage teachers and students to explore safer media, find substitutes for toxic materials, and research and develop alternatives to hazardous processes.

Schools that teach art also must develop curricula which include formal health and safety training. This kind of training is already mandated by law for all employed teachers using toxic art materials (see page 19-20) and it should be made available to students and self-employed artists as well.

This health and safety training for artists, teachers, students, and all users of art materials should consist of basic industrial hygiene which has been adapted for the arts.

INDUSTRIAL HYGIENE FOR THE ARTS

Industrial hygiene is the science of protecting workers' health through control of the work environment. As an artist-turned-industrial hygienist, I have spent more than a dozen years specializing in protecting artists from their environments—and themselves.

To be honest, I would not describe this work as a "glamorous career in the arts." However, my work enables me to visit each year between 80 and 100 schools, universities, museums, commercial studios, theaters, and other sites in the United States, Canada, Australia, and England. I have also been involved in developing state and federal art materials regulations, testifying as an expert witness in art-related lawsuits, and counseling literally thousands of artists, teachers, administrators, and the like.

This book is an attempt to share the prospective I have developed through these experiences and to provide a training reference to help us comply with applicable health and safety laws and regulations.

THE CARROTS (INDUCEMENT)

One of the most humbling aspects of my first few years in industrial hygiene was observing how steadfastly both artists and administrators ignored my advice. I talked enthusiastically about health and safety programs, ventilation, respiratory protection, and so on. While I was talking, there would be interest, motivation, and good intentions. But before my vocal cords cooled, people would be back to business as usual.

It wasn't that people didn't want to be safer and healthier— they did. It wasn't that they didn't understand the technical information—they did.

It wasn't even that the precautions would cost too much—they often didn't. The failure to institute proper health and safety procedures usually boiled down, in the main, to inertia and old habits.

These are formidable foes. We are all infected terminally with the desire to do the familiar—even if we know it is not in our best interest. There is an exquisite pain associated with the effort of hauling habits out of our spinal cord reflexes and putting them back into our brains to be thought through again. Confronting this resistance taught me that there is no industrial hygienist clever enough, no lecturer interesting enough, no argument convincing enough to make us change the way we make art. The lectures and training only make us feel a little more guilty as we routinely bet little bits of our life on risky familiar activities.

THE STICKS (ENFORCEMENT)

If lectures and training will not change our habits, force, in the form of our own governmental agencies, and the courts, will. Enforcement is necessary and beneficial, despite the bitter complaints we hear about excessive jury awards and restrictive Occupational Safety and Health Administration (OSHA) rules.

And certainly, enforcement works. One lawsuit improves safety practices in an entire school district overnight. One hefty OSHA fine causes shop managers for a hundred miles around to put the guards back on the saws.

Personally, I have found that juries and judges usually are fair. And complaints about the cost of complying with regulations merely reflect our difficulty in facing the fact that for far too many years we have spent far too little on health and safety.

In this case the law and the lawsuit are not our enemies. They reflect our own collective (not always perfect) wisdom in the form of our governmental servants and a jury of our peers. If you doubt this, try this exercise: imagine yourself defending your work practices, reporting your accident, or describing conditions in your studio or classroom to OSHA or a jury.

LAWS PROTECTING ART WORKERS

Both the United States and Canada have very complex regulations governing the relationship between employer and employee. However, whether the regulations are called the Occupational Safety and Health

Act (OSHAct in the United States) or Occupational Health and Safety Act (OHSAct in Canada), their main purpose is very simple—to protect workers.

The OSHAct general duty clause reads in part that the "employer shall furnish...employment and a place of employment which are free from recognized hazards." The Canadian OHSAct requires employers and supervisors to "take every precaution reasonable in the circumstances for the protection of a worker."

These brief general statements serve as the foundation for complex regulatory structures. The Acts include rules about chemical exposures, noise, ladder safety, machinery guarding, and a host of subjects. And many of these rules apply to schools, art-related businesses, etc.

All of us should be aware of these rules. In my opinion, even high schools should not graduate students who are unacquainted with their rights in the workplace. If you also are not versed in these regulations, first call your nearest department of labor and obtain a copy. Although the Acts are not reader-friendly, become as familiar with them as possible.

THE RIGHT-TO-KNOW

Certain recently instituted regulations are proving particularly useful in pressing us to upgrade our health and safety practices. These are the so-called "right-to-know" laws.

United States right-to-know laws were first passed by a number of states. Then a similar federal regulation called the OSHA Hazard Communication Standard was instituted. The result is that *all* employees in the United States now are covered by one or the other (sometimes both) of these laws. Even federal workers, so long exempt from OSHA regulations, come under this rule. There is a similar history in Canada with the resulting passage of the federal Workplace Hazardous Materials Information System (WHMIS).

For the most part, all these laws require employers to provide written hazard communication programs, give workers access to complete inventories and data sheets for all potentially hazardous chemicals in the workplace, and require formal training of all employees who potentially are exposed to toxic chemicals.

Even an ordinary office worker comes under the rule if he or she works long hours with an ozone-producing copy machine. That worker must be told of the effects of ozone, shown what kind of ventilation is necessary to reduce it to acceptable limits, given access to a data sheet describing details of the toner's hazardous ingredients, instructed formally about what to do if the toner spills, and so on.'

How much more, then, should the law be applied to art teachers, craftspeople, or artists who use hazardous paints, dyes, solvents, metals, and so on.

Yet many schools and art-related businesses still do not comply with the new laws. This is partly due to a peculiar common belief that the laws do not apply to art—that art is somehow "special." Actually, producing art should more correctly be considered a "light industry" which uses toxic substances to create a product. This also is how government inspectors see artmaking.

Today, OSHA gives more citations for hazard communication violations than for any other rule infraction. Some art schools, businesses, and institutions have been cited. (I have participated in program development and training in cited schools and businesses. To illustrate that all workplaces are covered: a Broadway theater company was cited and I trained the actors and technicians between matinee and evening performances.)

WHO'S COVERED?

*Essentially, all employees** in the United States are covered by state, or federal hazard communication (right-to-know) laws. *All employees* in Canada are covered by the Workplace Hazardous Materials Information System (WHMIS). *All employers* in workplaces where hazardous materials are present, therefore, are required to develop programs and train their employees. (The employer is the person or entity that takes the deductions out of the paycheck.)

Self-employed artists/teachers are *not* covered, but may be affected by the laws. For example, if you work as an independent contractor working or teaching at a site where there are employees, all the products and materials you bring onto the premises must conform to the employer's hazard communication or Workplace Hazardous Materials Information System program labeling requirements. Your use of these products also must conform.

Teachers in the United States have a unique hazard communication obligation arising from the fact that they can be held liable for any harm classroom activities cause their students. To protect their liability, teach-

---

*A few state and municipal employees in states that do not have an accepted state OSHA plan are still exempt.

ers should formally transmit to students hazard communication training about the dangers of classroom materials and processes. They also must enforce the safety rules and act as good examples of proper precautions.

(Precautionary training need not be done by elementary school teachers since they should not use materials for which training would be required.)

Complying with the Hazard Communication Standard and Workplace Hazardous Materials Information System

1. To comply, first find out which law applies to you. Call your local department of labor and ask them to tell you whether you must comply with a state/provincial or federal right-to-know.

2. Ask for a copy of the law which applies to you. Also ask for explanatory materials. Some of the government agencies have prepared well-written guidelines to take you through compliance step by step.

General Requirements—Hazard Communication Standard and Workplace Hazardous Materials Information System

There are small differences between the United States and Canadian laws. For example, the definition of "hazardous" varies, and the Canadian law requires information in French. However, the two laws require employers to take similar steps toward compliance:

1. *Inventory all workplace chemicals.* Remember, even products such as bleach and cleaning materials may qualify as hazardous products. List everything. (This is an excellent time to cut down paper work by trimming your inventory. Dispose of old, unneeded or seldom-used products.)

2. *Identify hazardous products in your inventory.* Apply the definition of "hazardous" in the right-to-know law which applies to you.

3. *Assemble Material Safety Data Sheets (MSDSs) on all hazardous products.* Write to manufacturers, distributors, and importers of all products on hand for MSDSs. Require MSDSs as a condition of purchase for all new materials.

4. *Check all product labels to be sure they comply with the law's labeling requirements.* Products which do not comply must be eliminated or relabeled.

5. *Prepare and apply proper labels to all containers into which chemicals have been transferred.* (Chemicals in unlabeled containers that are used up within one shift need not be labeled.)

6. *Consult Material Safety Data Sheets to identify all operations which use or generate hazardous materials.* Be aware that nonhazardous materials when chemically reacted, heated, or burned may produce toxic emissions.

7. *Make all lists of hazardous materials, Material Safety Data Sheets, and other required written materials available to employees.* (The OSHA Hazard Communication Standard also requires a written Hazard Communication program which details all procedures.)

8. *Implement a training program* (see Training below).

9. *Check to see if you are responsible for additional state and provincial requirements.* In the United States, the Supreme Court recently upheld (July 3, 1989) the right of states to enforce certain amendments to the federal right-to-know law.

TRAINING

Since both laws are in effect, all employees in both the United States and Canada already should have received right-to-know training. Additional training should take place whenever new employees are hired or new materials or processes introduced. Some state laws require yearly training as well.

The amount of time the training should take is not specified. This is because the law intends the training requirements to be performance oriented--that is, the employees must be given whatever information they need to understand the hazards of their specific jobs and how to work safely. Often short quizzes are used to verify that the employees have understood the presentation.

Training for artists and art teachers usually can be accomplished in a full day. The information which must be communicated includes:

1. *The details of the hazard communication program* that the employer is conducting including an explanation of the labeling system, the Material Safety Data Sheets and how employees can obtain and use hazard information.

2. *The physical and health hazards of the chemicals in the work area.* This should include an explanation of physical hazards such as fire and explosions, and health hazards such as how the chemical enters the body and the effects of exposure.

3. *How employees can protect themselves.* This should include information on safe work practices, emergency procedures, use of personal protective equipment that the employer provides, and explanation of the ventilation system and other engineering controls that reduce exposure.

4. *How the employer and employees can detect the presence of hazardous chemicals in the work area.* This should include training about environmental and medical monitoring conducted by the employer, use of monitoring devices, the visual appearance and odor of chemicals, and any other detection or warning methods.

This book can be used to address points 2 through 4 above, providing employers, employees, and teachers with formal training materials. The lists of precautions as the ends of chapters on specific media can be used as shop safety inspection checklists.

CHAPTER

2

HEALTH HAZARDS AND THE BODY

Art and craft workers need to understand how chemicals in their materials affect them, in order to protect their health and to meet the requirements of new occupational and environmental laws. Studying the hazards of art and craft materials is difficult because they contain so many different toxic chemicals. For example, many toxic metals, including highly toxic ones such as lead and cadmium, are still found in traditional paint and ink pigments, ceramic glazes, metal enamels, and in alloys used in sculpture, stained glass, jewelry, and other crafts. In addition, new synthetic dyes and pigments, plastics, organic chemical solvents, and a host of materials may be used.

Each of these chemicals affects the body in its own unique way. The study of these effects is called toxicology.

BASIC CONCEPTS

DOSE. Chemical toxicity is dependent on the dose—that is the amount of the chemical which enters the body. Each chemical produces harm at a different dose. Highly toxic chemicals cause serious damage in very small amounts. Moderately and slightly toxic substances are toxic at relatively higher doses. Even substances considered nontoxic can be harmful if the exposure is great enough.

TIME. Chemical toxicity is also dependent on the length of time over which exposures occur. The effects of short and long periods of exposure differ.

SHORT-TERM OR ACUTE EFFECTS. Acute illnesses are caused by large doses of toxic substances delivered in a short period of time. The symptoms usually occur during or shortly after exposure and last a short time. Depending on the dose, the outcome can vary from complete recovery, through recovery with some level of disability, to—at worst—death. Acute illnesses are the easiest to diagnose because their cause and effect are easily linked. For example, exposure to turpentine while painting can cause effects from lightheadedness to more severe effects such as headache, nausea, and loss of coordination. At even higher doses, unconsciousness and death could result.

LONG-TERM OR CHRONIC EFFECTS. These effects are caused by repeated low-dose exposures over many months or years. They are the most difficult to diagnose. Usually the symptoms are hardly noticeable until permanent damage has occurred. Symptoms appear very slowly, may vary from person to person, and may mimic other illnesses. For instance, chronic exposure to turpentine during a lifetime of painting may produce dermatitis in some individuals, chronic liver or kidney effects in other, and nervous system damage in still others.

EFFECTS BETWEEN ACUTE AND CHRONIC. There are also other effects between acute and chronic such as "sub-acute" effects produced over weeks or months at doses below those which produce acute effects. Such in between effects also are difficult to diagnose.

CUMULATIVE/NONCUMULATIVE TOXINS. Every chemical is eliminated from the body at a different rate. Cumulative toxins, such as lead, are substances which are eliminated slowly. Repeated exposure will cause them to accumulate in the body.

Noncumulative toxins, like alcohol and other solvents, leave the body very quickly. Medical tests can detect their presence only for a short time after exposure. Although they leave the body, the damage they cause may be permanent and accumulate over time.

THE TOTAL BODY BURDEN is the total amount of a chemical present in the body from all sources. For example, we all have body burdens of lead from air, water, and food contamination. Working with lead-containing art materials can add to this body burden.

MULTIPLE EXPOSURES. We are carrying body burdens of many chemicals and are often exposed to more than one chemical at a time. Sometimes these chemicals interact in the body.

- *Additive Exposures.* Exposure to two chemicals is considered additive when one chemical contributes to or adds to the toxic effects of the other. This can occur when both chemicals affect the body in similar ways. Working with paint thinner and drinking alcohol is an example.

- *Synergistic Exposures.* These effects occur when two chemicals produce an effect greater than the total effects of each alone. Alcohol and barbiturates or smoking and asbestos are common examples.

CANCER. Occupational cancers are a special type of chronic illness. Chemicals which cause cancer are called carcinogens. Examples include asbestos and benzidine dyes and pigments. Unlike ordinary toxic substances, the effects of carcinogens are not strictly dependent on dose. No level of exposure is considered safe. However, the lower the dose, the lower the risk of developing cancer. For this reason, exposure to carcinogens should be avoided altogether or kept as low as possible.

Occupational cancers typically occur ten to forty years after exposure. This period of time, during which there are no symptoms, is referred to as a latency period. Latency usually makes diagnosis of occupational cancers very difficult.

MUTAGENICITY. Mutations (and cancer) can be caused by chemicals which alter the genetic blue print (DNA) of cells. Once altered, such cells usually die. Those few that survive will replicate themselves in a new form.

Any body cell (muscle, skin, etc.) can mutate. However, when the effected cell is the human egg or sperm cell, mutagenicity can affect future generations. Most pregnancies resulting from mutated sperm and eggs will result in spontaneous termination of the pregnancy (reabsorption, miscarriage, etc.). In other cases, inherited abnormalities may result in the offspring.

Only a handful of chemicals, pesticides, and drugs have been studied sufficiently to prove they are human mutagens. Such proof requires that thousands of exposed individuals be studied for many decades. Since this is not practical, chemicals are considered "suspect human mutagens" if they cause mutation in bacteria or animals. Some chemicals found in arts and crafts have been shown to be suspect mutagens, including a number of pigments, synthetic dyes, and solvents. (See Tables 5 and 6, Common Solvents & Their Hazards and Pigments used in Paints & Inks, pages 89 and 102.) Both men and women should avoid exposure to suspect mutagens, since both may be affected.

TERATOGENICITY. Chemicals that affect fetal organ development—that is, cause birth defects—are called teratogens. They are hazardous primarily during the first trimester. Two proven human teratogens include the drug, Thalidomide, and grain alcohol. Chemicals which are known to cause birth defects in animals are considered "suspect teratogens." Among these are many solvents, lead, and other metals.

FETAL TOXICITY. Toxic chemicals can affect the growth and development of the fetus at any stage of development.

ALLERGENICITY. Allergies are adverse reactions of the body's immune system. Common symptoms may include dermatitis, hay fever effects, and asthma. Although a particular person can be allergic to almost anything, certain chemicals produce allergic responses in large numbers of people. Such chemicals are called "sensitizers." Some strong sensitizers include epoxy adhesives, chrome compounds, batik dyes, and many wood dusts.

The longer people work with a sensitizing chemical the greater the probability they will become allergic to it. Once developed, allergies tend to last a lifetime and symptoms may increase in severity with continued exposure. A few people even become highly sensitized—that is, develop life-threatening reactions to exceedingly small doses. This effect is caused by bee venom in some people, but industrial chemicals have produced similar effects—including death.

HOW CHEMICALS ENTER THE BODY (Routes of Entry)

In order to cause damage, toxic materials must enter the body. Entry can occur in the following ways:

SKIN CONTACT. The skin's barrier of waxes, oils, and dead cells can be destroyed by chemicals such as acids, caustics, solvents, and the like.

Once the skin's defenses are breached, some of these chemicals can damage the skin itself, the tissues beneath the skin, or even enter the blood, where they can be transported throughout the body causing damage to other organs.

Cuts, abrasions, burns, rashes, and other violations of the skin's barrier can allow chemicals to penetrate into the blood and be transported throughout the body. There are also many chemicals that can—without your knowing it—enter the blood through undamaged skin. Among these are benzene and wood alcohol.

INHALATION. Inhaled substances are capable of damaging the respiratory system acutely or chronically at any location—from the nose and sinuses, to the lungs. Examples of substances which can cause chronic and acute respiratory damage include acid gases and fumes from heating or burning plastics.

Some toxic substances are absorbed by the lungs and are transported via the blood to other organs. For example, lead in solder fumes may be carried via the blood to damage the brain and kidneys.

INGESTION. You can accidently ingest toxic materials by eating, smoking, or drinking while working, pointing brushes with your lips, touching soiled hands to your mouth, biting your nails, and similar habits. The lung's mucous also traps dusts and removes them by transporting them to your esophagus where they are swallowed.

Accidental ingestions occur when people pour chemicals into paper cups or glasses and later mistake them for beverages. Some of these accidents have even killed children who were allowed in the studio.

WHO IS AT RISK?

EVERYBODY is susceptible to occupational exposures. How they are affected will depend on the nature of the chemical, its route of entry, the degree of exposure, and, in some cases, the susceptibility of the exposed person. For example, most people's lungs will be affected equally by exposure to similar concentrations of strong acid vapors. However, someone who already has bronchitis or emphysema may be even more seriously harmed.

HIGH RISK INDIVIDUALS. Certain segments of the population—particularly the disabled, the chronically ill (especially those with preexisting damage of organs such as the liver or lungs), pregnant women and the fetus, children, and elderly—are at especially high risk from certain art activities. For example, the hearing-impaired may risk further damage to their already defective hearing if they engage in woodworking activities that employ noisy machinery. The retarded should not be exposed to chemicals which are known to adversely affect mental acuity and behavior, such as lead and chemical solvents.

People taking certain medications are sometimes at higher risk. For example, medications (and recreational drugs) which are narcotic may potentiate the effects of solvents and metals which also are narcotic (affect the brain).

OCCUPATIONAL ILLNESSES

Any organ in the body can be affected by an occupational illness. Some occupational illnesses include the following:

SKIN DISEASES. Two types of dermatitis are among the most common occupational skin diseases.

1. Primary irritant contact dermatitis. This is a nonallergic skin reaction from exposure to irritating substances. Exposure to irritants account for 80 percent of the cases of occupational contact dermatitis. There are two major types of irritants:

- mild irritants which require repeated and/or prolonged exposure. Included in this category are soaps, detergents, and many solvents.

- strong irritants which require only short exposures to cause damage. Substances included in this category are strong acids, alkalis, and peroxides.

2. Allergic contact dermatitis (sometimes called hyper-sensitivity dermatitis) is a delayed allergic skin reaction occurring when sensitized individuals are exposed to allergens. Common allergens include epoxy adhesives, chrome and nickel compounds, and many woods.

Other occupational skin diseases include infections and skin cancer. Working with cuts, abrasions, or other kinds of skin damage may lead to infections. Lamp black pigments and ultraviolet radiation are associated with skin cancer.

EYE DISEASES. Irritating, caustic, and acid chemicals can damage the eye severely. Infrared (from glowing hot kilns) or ultraviolet light (e.g., from welding) can cause eye damage. A few chemicals, such as methanol and hexane, also can damage the eyesight when inhaled or ingested.

RESPIRATORY SYSTEM DISEASES. Any irritating airborne chemical can be potentially hazardous to the respiratory system. Damage can range from minor irritation to life-threatening chemical pneumonia, depending on how irritating the substance and how much is inhaled. Exposures to smaller amounts of irritants over years can cause chronic respiratory damage such as chronic bronchitis or emphysema.

Often the first symptom of respiratory irritation is an increased susceptibility to colds and respiratory infections. This is commonly seen among artists exposed to the small amounts of ammonia and formaldehyde released by acrylic paints.

Another factor affecting respiratory damage is the irritant's solubility in liquid and mucous. Highly soluble irritants, such as hydrochloric acid gas, produce immediate symptoms in the upper respiratory tract. These warning symptoms usually cause people to take action to avoid further exposure. Less soluble irritants such as ozone or nitric acid (from acid etching) cause delayed damage to the lower respiratory tract. In cases of heavy exposure, pulmonary edema may occur as much as twelve hours after exposure.

Some types of soluble chemicals, including lead and solvents, are absorbed by the lungs, pass into the blood stream and are transported to other organs in the body. Insoluble particles, on the other hand, may remain in the lungs for life if they are deposited deeply in the air sacs (alveoli). Some of these insoluble particles such as asbestos and silica can cause lung scarring diseases (fibroses) such as asbestosis and silicosis, and/ or lung cancer.

Allergic diseases such as asthma, alveolitis, and hypersensitivity pneumonia may result from exposure to sensitizing chemicals. Smokers are at greater risk from lung cancer and almost all other diseases of lungs. Smoking inhibits the lungs' natural clearing mechanisms, leaving toxic particles in them longer and allowing them to do more damage.

HEART AND BLOOD DISEASES. Many solvents at high doses can alter heart rhythms (arrhythmia) and even cause a heart attack. Deaths related to this phenomenon have been noted among both industrial workers, and glue-sniffers whose level of exposure to solvents were very high.

Benzene, still found as a contaminant in some solvents and gasoline, can cause aplastic anemia (decreased bone marrow production of all blood cells) and leukemia.

NERVOUS SYSTEM DISEASES. Metals like lead and mercury are known to cause nervous system damage. The early symptoms of exposure often are psychological disturbances and depression.

Almost all solvents can affect the nervous system. Symptoms can vary from mild narcosis (lightheadedness, headache, dizziness) to coma and death at high doses. People exposed to small amounts of solvent daily for years often exhibit the symptoms of chronic nervous system damage such as short-term memory loss, mental confusion, sleep disturbances, hand-eye coordination difficulties, and depression.

Some chemicals such as n-hexane (found in rubber cements, some aerosol sprays, etc.) are particularly damaging to the nervous system and chronic exposure can result in a disease similar to multiple sclerosis.

LIVER DISEASES. Hepatitis can be caused by chemicals as well as by disease organisms. Some toxic metals and nearly all solvents, including grain alcohol, can damage the liver if the dose is high enough. Liver cancer is caused by chemicals such as carbon tetrachloride.

KIDNEY DISEASES. Kidney damage is also caused by many metals and solvents. Lead and chlorinated hydrocarbon solvents such as trichloroethylene are particularly damaging. Heat stress and accidents (damaged blood and muscle cell debris block kidney tubules) are also causes of kidney damage.

BLADDER DISEASES. Benzidine-derived pigments and dyes are documented causes of bladder cancer.

REPRODUCTIVE EFFECTS. Chemicals can affect any stage of reproduction: sexual performance, the menstrual cycle, sperm generation, all stages in organ formation and fetal growth, the health of the woman during pregnancy, and the newborn infant through chemicals secreted in breast milk. More is being learned each day regarding such effects. Prudence dictates that both men and women planning families exercise care when working with art and craft materials containing toxic chemicals. (See also the section above on mutagenicity and teratogenicity.)

CHAPTER 3 | CHEMICAL HEALTH HAZARDS AND THEIR CONTROL

H ealth-damaging chemicals can enter our body by inhalation, skin contact, and ingestion. Exposure by skin contact usually can be prevented by wearing gloves, using tools to handle materials, and the like. Ingestion can be prevented by good work habits and by not eating, smoking, or drinking in the workplace. Precautions against inhalation are more complex.

INHALATION HAZARDS

To prevent inhalation of airborne chemicals, it is first necessary to understand the nature of airborne contaminants such as gases, vapors, mists, fumes, and dust.

GASES. Scientists define gas as "a formless fluid" that can "expand to fill the space that contains it." We can picture this fluid as many molecules moving rapidly and randomly in space.

Air, for example, is a mixture of different gases—that is different kinds of molecules. Even though each different gas has a different molecular weight, the heavier gases will never settle out because the rapid molecular movement will cause them to remain mixed. In other words, once gases are mixed, they tend to stay mixed.

In almost all cases, gases created during art-making are mixed with air as they are released. This means that they also will not settle, but instead will "expand into the space that contains them." In most cases the gas will diffuse evenly throughout the space—the room—in time.

When the gas escapes from the room or is exhausted from the room by ventilation, expansion of the gas continues theoretically forever. It is this expansion, for example, that causes spray can propellants to reach the stratospheric ozone layer.

Under certain conditions, gases will not freely mix with air. For example, carbon dioxide gas from dry ice will form a foggy layer at ground level because the cold gas is denser and heavier than air (the molecules are closer together). In another instance, gases may layer out or take a long time to mix with air in locations where there is little air movement—such as in storage areas.

Gases vary greatly in toxicity. They can be irritating, acidic, caustic, poisonous, and so on. Some gases also have dangerous physical properties such as flammability or reactivity. Toxic gases which may be encountered in art making include: hydrochloric acid gas from etching and pickling solutions; ozone and nitrogen oxides from welding; and sulfur dioxide and acetic acid gases from photographic developing baths.

Some gases are not toxic. An inert gas such as argon used in inert gas welding is an example. Such gases are dangerous only when present in such large quantities that they reduce the amount of oxygen in the air to levels insufficient to support life. These gases are called asphyxiants.

VAPORS. Vapors are the gaseous form of liquids. For example, water vapor is created when water evaporates—that is, releases water molecules into the air. Once released into the air, vapors behave like gases and expand into space. However, at high concentrations they will recondense into liquids. This is what happens when it rains.

There is a common misconception that substances do not vaporize until they reach their "vaporization point"—that is their boiling point. Although greater amounts of vapor are produced at higher temperatures, most materials begin to vaporize as soon as they are liquid.

Even some solids convert to a vapor form at room temperature. Solids that do this are said to "sublime." Mothballs are an example of a chemical solid which sublimes.

Vapors, like gases, may vary greatly in toxicity, flammability and reactivity. Among the most common toxic vapors created in art work are organic chemical vapors from solvents such as turpentine, mineral spirits, and lacquer thinners.

MISTS. Mists are tiny liquid droplets in the air. Any liquid, water, oil, or solvent can be misted or aerosolized. The finer the size of the droplet, the more deeply the mist can be inhaled. Some mists, such as paint spray mists, also contain solid material. Paint mist can float on air currents for a time. Then the liquid portion of the droplet will vaporize—convert to a vapor—and the solid part of the paint will settle as a dust.

A mist of a substance is more toxic than the vapor of the same substance at the same concentration. This results from the fact that when inhaled, the droplets deliver the mist in little concentrated spots to the respiratory systems tissues. Vapors, on the other hand, are more evenly distributed in the respiratory tract.

FUMES. Laymen commonly use this term to mean any kind of emission from chemical processes. In this book, however, only the scientific definition will be used.

Technically, fumes are very tiny particles usually created in high heat operations such as welding, soldering, or foundry work. They are formed when hot vapors cool rapidly and condense into fine particles. For example, lead fumes are created during soldering. When solder melts, some lead vaporizes. The vapor immediately reacts with oxygen in the air and condenses into tiny lead oxide fume particles.

Fume particles are so small (0.01 to 0.5 microns in diameter)* that they tend to remain airborne for long periods of time. Eventually, however, they will settle to contaminate dust in the workplace, in the ventilation ducts, in your hair or clothing, or wherever air currents carry them. Although fume particles are too small to be seen by the naked eye, they sometimes can be perceived as a bluish haze rising like cigarette smoke from soldering or welding operations.

Fuming tends to increase the toxicity of a substance because the small particle size enables it to be inhaled deeply into the lungs and because it presents more surface area to lung fluids (is more soluble).

In addition to many metals, some organic chemicals, plastics, and silica will fume. Smoke from burning organic materials may also contain fumes.

---

*A micron is a metric system unit of measurement equaling one millionth of a meter. There are about 25,640 microns in an inch. Respirable fume and dust particles are in the range of 0.01 to 10 microns in diameter. Such particles are too small to be seen by the naked eye.

DUSTS. Dusts are formed when solid materials are broken down into small particles by natural or mechanical forces. Natural wind and weathering produces dusts from rocks. Sanding and sawing are examples of mechanical forces which produce dusts.

The finer the dust, the deeper it can be inhaled into the lung and the more toxic it will be. Respirable dusts—those which can be inhaled deeply into the lungs—are too small to be seen with the naked eye (0.5 to 10 microns in diameter).

SMOKE. Smoke is formed from burning organic matter. Burning wood and hot wire-cutting plastics are two smoke-producing activities. Smoke is usually a mixture of many gases, vapors, and fumes. For example, cigarette smoke contains over four thousand chemicals, including carbon monoxide gas, benzene vapor, and fume-sized particles of tar.

EXPOSURE STANDARDS

Exposure to airborne chemicals in the workplace is regulated in the United States and Canada. The United States limits are called OSHA Permissible Exposure Limits (PELs). The Canadian limits are called Occupational Exposure Limits (OELs).

Although the levels at which various chemicals are regulated may differ occasionally, both countries' regulations are based on a concept called the Threshold Limit Value (TLV). The Permissible Exposure Limit and Occupational Exposure Limit for most substances are identical to the Threshold Limit Value.

Threshold Limit Values are airborne substance standards set by the American Conference of Governmental Industrial Hygienists (ACGIH). Copies of the Threshold Limit Values can be obtained from the ACGIH. (see address in footnote). Threshold Limit Values are designed to protect the majority of healthy adult workers from adverse effects. There are three types:

1. *Threshold Limit Value-Time Weighted Average.* Threshold Limit Value-Time Weighted Averages are airborne concentrations of substances averaged over eight hours. They are meant to protect from adverse effects those workers who are exposed to substances at this concentration over the normal eight-hour day and a forty-hour work week.

FOOTNOTE
ACGIH, 6500 Glenway Ave., Bldg. D-7, Cincinnati, OH 45211-4438; 513/661-7881.

2. *Threshold Limit Value-Short Term Exposure Limit.* Threshold Limit Value-Short-Term Exposure Limits are fifteen minute average concentrations that should not be exceeded at any time during a work day.

3. *Threshold Limit Value-Ceiling.* Threshold Limit Value-Ceilings are concentrations that should not be exceeded during any part of the workday exposure.

Threshold Limit Values should not be considered absolute guarantees of protection. Threshold Limit Values previously thought adequate have repeatedly been revised as medical tests have become more sophisticated, and as long-term exposure studies reveal chronic diseases previously undetected.

At best, Threshold Limit Values are meant to protect most, but not all, healthy adult workers. They do not apply to children, people with chronic illnesses, and other high risk individuals.

Threshold Limit Value-Time Weighted Averages also do not apply to people who work longer than eight hours a day. This is especially true of people who live and work in the same environment, such as artists whose studios are at home. In these cases, very high exposures have been noted, since the artist is likely to be exposed to contaminants twenty-four hours a day. With no respite during which the body can detoxify, even low concentrations of contaminants become significant.

Expensive and complicated air-sampling and analysis are usually required to prove that Threshold Limit Values are exceeded. For this reason, Threshold Limit Values are primarily useful to artists as proof that a substance is considered toxic, and that measures should be taken to limit exposure to substances with Threshold Limit Values.

Artists should also be aware that many substances known to be toxic have no Threshold Limit Values. In some cases the reason is that there is insufficient data to quantify the risk from exposure.

When additional factors, such as evaporation rate, are considered, artists also can use Threshold Limit Values to compare the toxicity of various chemicals. Table 1 lists the Threshold Limit Value-Time Weighted Averages of some common air contaminants. In general, the smaller the Threshold Limit Value, the more toxic the substance. Gases and vapors with Threshold Limit Value-Time Weighted Averages 100 parts per million (ppm) or lower can be considered highly toxic. Dusts whose Threshold Limit Value-Time Weighted Averages are set at ten milligrams per cubic meter (mg/m³) are considered only nuisance dusts. Particulates with

Threshold Limit Value-Time Weighted Averages smaller than 10 mg/m^3 are more toxic.

TABLE 1	Threshold Limit Value-Time Weighted Averages* of Common Substances

Gas or Vapor	ppm**
ethanol (grain alcohol)	1000
acetone	750
VM & P naphtha (paint thinner)	300
turpentine	100
toluene and xylene	100
n-hexane (common in rubber cement thinner)	50
ammonia	25
formaldehyde	1
acrolein (created when wax is burned/overheated)	.1
MDI and TDI (from urethane casting/foaming)	.005

Fume or Dust	mg/m^3**
calcium carbonate (marble dust, whiting)	10
aluminum:	
aluminum oxide (abrasives)	10
metal dust	10
fume	5
manganese:	
metal	5
fume	1
graphite (synthetic and natural)	2
silica:	
amorphous (unfired diatomaeous earth, silica gel)	10
crystalline (quartz, sand, flint, etc.)	.1
calcined/fired (cristobalite, tridymite)	.05
beryllium (metal and compounds)	.002

* Threshold Limit Value-Time Weighted Averages taken from 1989-90 ACGIH list.
** ppm=parts per million, mg/m^3=milligrams per cubic meter.

CHAPTER 4 | *PHYSICAL HAZARDS AND THEIR CONTROL*

P hysical phenomena such as noise, vibration, various kinds of light, and heat also can be damaging to the body. There are Threshold Limit Values for these phenomenon similar to those for chemical exposures.

NOISE

Artists perform many noise-producing tasks. Working with electrical tools, hammering on hard surfaces, or even playing loud music can produce ear-damaging sound.

Whether caused by music or machinery, noise-induced hearing loss is permanent and untreatable. Signs of over exposure may include a temporary ringing in the ears or difficulty in hearing for a while after work. Except for these minor symptoms, there are no obvious signs or pain to warn artists that their hearing is being damaged. Noise may also cause increased blood pressure and stress-related illnesses.

Threshold Limit Values for noise vary with the length of time of exposure and with the intensity of the noise (sound pressure) measured in decibels (dB). (See Table 2 and Figure 1, page 36.) Decibels are nonlinear, logarithmic functions, so a doubling of noise increases the sound level by only 3 dB. For example, if one table saw produces 105 dB, turning on another equally noisy saw adds only 3 dB to the sound level for a total of 108 dB.

Conversely, an increase of 3 dB corresponds to a doubling of the sound intensity. So, 108 dB is not "just a little over 105 dB," it is twice as intense and does twice as much damage. To illustrate this point, see Fig. 2.

TABLE 2	Threshold Limit Values for Noise

Duration per Day Hours	Sound Level dBA
16	80
8	85
4	90
2	95
1	100
1/2	105
1/4	110
1/8	115 *

Sound level in decibels are measured on a sound level meter, conforming as a minimum to the requirements of the American National Standard Specification for Sound Level Meters, SI.4(1971) Type S2A, and set to use the A-weight network with slow meter response.

* No exposure should be allowed to continuous or intermittent in excess of 115 dBA.

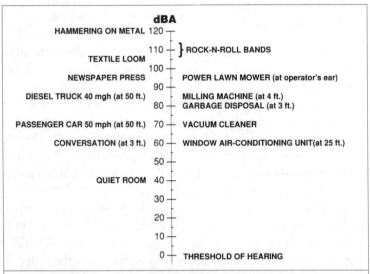

Fig 1. Typical A-weighted noise levels in decibels (dBA)*

Artists should evaluate the noise-levels produced by their work. As a rule of thumb, if you must raise your voice to be heard by someone only two feet away, you probably need hearing protection. If you are not sure about the amount of noise in your workplace, you may want to call in an industrial hygienist to measure it.

To protect yourself from noise, use ear plugs. Ear plugs, particularly the foam type, provide the best and cheapest protection. Package labels on ear plugs list their attenuation or noise reduction ratings (NRR).

Intensity of Noise	dB
10,000,000,000,000	130
1,000,000,000,000	120
10,000,000,000	100
1,000,000,000	90
100,000,000	80
10,000,000	70
1,000,000	60
100,000	50
10,000	40
1,000	30
100	20
10	10
0	0

Fig.2

For example, those with a 25 dB NRR would reduce the noise level at most frequencies by about 25 dB.

Ear muffs are more expensive and not always more effective. However, muffs can be designed to attenuate specific frequencies.

Engineering methods for reducing noise include installing muffling and damping devices on machinery or mounting machines on vibration-absorbing rubber pads. When selecting new equipment, try to choose those whose manufacturers provide decibel ratings. Select machines with low dB ratings if they are available, or at least listen to equipment before purchasing.

Artists working in noisy environments also should get baseline hearing tests and yearly reexaminations to monitor any change in hearing.

VIBRATION

Hand-held tools also transfer harmful vibration to the user. It may be noticed as a tingling of the hands and arms that usually disappears within an hour. Some people, however, risk a more permanent condition known as "white hand," "dead fingers," or Raynaud's syndrome. This disease, more correctly called Vibration Syndrome, may progress in stages from intermittent tingling, numbness, and white fingertips to pain, ulcerations, and gangrene.

Recommendations to avoid this condition include using tools with low amplitudes of vibration, keeping tools in good condition, taking ten-minute work breaks for every hour of continuous exposure, maintaining normal workplace temperatures (cold weather aggravates the condition), and not grasping tools harder than needed for safe use.

IONIZING RADIATION

Radiation is either ionizing or nonionizing. Ionizing radiation can cause harmful biological effects. Sources of ionizing radiation include X-rays and radioactive metals such as uranium. Artists rarely encounter these forms of radiation unless they work with uranium-containing glass, glaze chemicals, or metal enamels (e.g., Thompson's Burnt Orange # 153 and Forsythia # 108), or work with radioactive minerals of various types. Uranium should be replaced with safer ingredients.

Conservators of art use ionizing radiation when they X-ray paintings or artifacts. They should follow all guidelines which apply to medical and dental X-ray use.

NONIONIZING RADIATION

LIGHT. Natural light contains a wide spectrum of visible, ultraviolet, and infrared rays. Artificial light contains a more limited array of light waves. It is well known that ultraviolet rays can damage the skin and eyes, and even cause skin cancer. Both sunlight and unshielded fluorescent lights have been implicated in causing cancer.

Inadequate lighting, glare, and shadow-producing direct lighting can cause eye strain and accidents. Use accepted lighting guidelines to plan lighting, especially for close work. Good diffuse overhead lighting combined with direct light on the task is a good solution for many situations.

ULTRAVIOLET (UV) AND INFRARED (IR) RADIATION. Ultraviolet sources include sunlight, welding, and carbon arc lamps. Infrared is produced whenever metals or ceramic materials are heated until they glow. Ultraviolet is well-known for causing eye damage and even skin cancer in welders and others exposed to it. Infrared radiation also can damage the eye and has produced Infrared cataracts in potters and enamelists after many years of looking into their kilns. Protective goggles should be worn whenever these types of radiation are present. Standards for appropriately shaded protective goggles can be obtained from the American National Standards Institute (see figures 4 and 5, Chapter 6).

VIDEO DISPLAY TERMINALS. Video display terminals emit a number of kinds of radiation including low level pulsed electromagnetic radiation. This kind of radiation is emitted from all electrical appliances and was thought to be harmless for many years. Now clusters of abnormal pregnancies in some workers using video display terminals and increased cancer rates in children living near power lines have cast suspicion on it. However, at this time there is no conclusive evidence that these affects are due to radiation.

To be on the safe side, pregnant Canadian government workers have been given the right to transfer from video display terminal jobs without loss of pay. Similar rights are being legislated for pregnant workers in other provinces and states.

Some new video display terminal models are being designed to shield users from all types of radiation suspected to be hazardous. When these are perfected, they may be recommended for use by pregnant women.

In addition to radiation, video display terminals are associated with eye strain, overuse injuries (see below), and stress. Artists using video display terminals should plan lighting and desk and chair arrangement carefully. Be sure your vision is checked frequently and get regular physical examinations. Take frequent work breaks.

RADIATION THRESHOLD LIMIT VALUES: There are Threshold Limit Values for the forms of ionizing and nonionizing radiation discussed above. In addition, there are Threshold Limit Values for heat stress, laser radiation, microwaves, and more. All these phenomena can be harmful. Artists exposed to such radiation should obtain appropriate guidelines, codes of practice, and other information about these hazards.

PHYSIOLOGICAL HAZARDS AND THEIR CONTROL

Artists' specialized activities often cause unusual bodily stresses and strains. Potters, glassblowers, and weavers, for example, engage in repetitive actions which cause wear and tear on their muscles and tendons. "Potter's thumb," for instance, is the term some potters have used to describe symptoms which are now associated with the early stages of carpel tunnel syndrome, a debilitating nerve problem.

In response to artists' special needs, a new field called "arts medicine" has been created. Doctors and clinics specializing in arts medicine can be located by consulting your doctor or arts organizations such as ACTS (See Preface) .

OVERUSE INJURIES

Artists doing repetitive tasks such as hand sanding and polishing are at risk from a special type of injuries called Cumulative Trauma Disorders (CTDs). These usually affect tendons, bones, muscles, and nerves of the hands, wrists, arms, and shoulders. Examples include tendonitis, carpal tunnel syndrome, and tennis elbow.

To prevent these injuries, pay careful attention to your body for signs of fatigue, pain, changes in endurance, weakness, and the like. Try using good work habits to resolve early symptoms, including:

- good posture.
- frequent rest breaks.
- alternating tasks or varying the types of work done often.
- warming up muscles before work; moving and stretching muscles during breaks.
- easing back into heavy work schedules rather than expecting to work at full capacity immediately after holidays or periods away from work.
- modifying technique and/or equipment to avoid uncomfortable positions or movements (see Ergonomics below).

If your symptoms do not respond quickly to better work habits, seek medical attention. Early medical intervention will cause the majority of overuse injuries to resolve without expensive treatment or surgery. Delaying treatment can leave you disabled for long periods of time or even for life.

ERGONOMICS. Ergonomics is defined as designing work environments using data from engineering, anatomical, physiological, and psychological sources so that the best use is made of human capabilities.

With these principles in mind, many tools, machines, and much office and shop furniture have been redesigned. This equipment, combined with good posture, reasonable workloads, reduced levels of job stress and noise, good lighting, and other factors can prove useful to many artists.

CHAPTER 5

IDENTIFYING HAZARDOUS MATERIALS

I   Identifying potentially hazards products in the studio or work place can be accomplished most easily by the procedures outlined in the right-to-know laws. These include developing an accurate, chemical inventory, labeling materials properly, and collecting hazard information about each product in the form of material safety data sheets, fact sheets and simular materials.

INVENTORY

The first step in any program to control chemical hazards, is to make a complete inventory of all the products you use. The list also should include all ordinary consumer products—even if your right-to-know law does not require it. This is necessary because artists may use consumer products in greater amounts or in ways which are not typical. For example, a small tube of glue meant to be used a drop at a time may become hazardous when a full tube is used at once.

Be careful to include all soaps, cleansers, and maintenance products. Many of these now are known to contain toxic materials. Consumer art materials often are especially hazardous. In both the United States and Canada, artists' paints are exempt from the consumer paint lead laws and often contain lead, cadmium, and a host of toxic ingredients.

Reduce your inventory by discarding old materials for which ingredient information is no longer available. Throwing things away is often psychologically difficult for artists and teachers who have spent years existing on tight budgets. However, it is a violation of the right-to-know laws to have unlabeled or improperly labeled products, or products whose hazards and ingredients are unknown in the workplace.

READING CONSUMER PRODUCT LABELS

To identify hazardous materials in your inventory, begin by reading product labels. However, do not assume that the label will warn of all the product's potential hazards. The truth is that the hazards of many of the ingredients in consumer products have never been fully studied, especially for chronic hazards.

Evaluating label information is further complicated by the fact that many common art products are imported. By law, these products' labels are supposed to conform to standards in the United States and Canada. However, many improperly labeled products escape scrutiny and turn up in art stores.

Even if the labeling meets standards, the label terminology may be difficult to interpret. The following United States and Canadian label terms illustrate the point:

USE WITH ADEQUATE VENTILATION: Many people think this means a window or door should be kept open while using the product. It actually indicates that the product contains a toxic substance which becomes airborne during the product's use and the ventilation should be sufficient to keep the airborne substance below levels considered acceptable for industrial use (see section on industrial Threshold Limit Values). Sufficient ventilation could vary from an ordinary exhaust fan to a specially designed local exhaust system depending on the amount of the material and how it is used.

In order to plan such ventilation, you must know exactly what substance the product gives off and at what rate. Ironically, this is often precisely the information the manufacturer excludes from the label.

NONTOXIC. Under the provisions of the United States Federal Hazardous Substances Act and the Canadian Federal Hazardous Products Act, toxic warnings are required only on products capable of causing acute (sudden onset) hazards. Products which can cause long-term hazards such as cancer, birth defects, allergies, chronic illnesses, and cumulative poisoning legally may be labeled "nontoxic."

To illustrate how grossly inadequate this labeling is, powdered asbestos could legally be labeled "nontoxic" under these laws. This is because the laws identify hazardous products by short term tests which expose animals through skin and eye contact, inhalation, and ingestion. Two weeks after exposure, the animals are examined for harm. Since asbestos causes only long term damage (cancer, asbestosis), the animals will be unharmed in this period of time.

Seven states passed laws to provide better labeling for art materials. Then in October of 1989, the United States Federal Hazardous Substances Act was amended to provide special labeling for art materials. It will provide chronic hazard labels for art materials and will allow the Consumer Product Safety Commission (CPSC) to ban all materials which are required to carry either acute or chronic warnings from grade six and under.

The new amendment will not be in effect until about 1992 because the CPSC must first develop the chronic labeling standards, after which manufacturers will have another year to label their products. Plans are being made to provide similar labeling in Canada.

VOLUNTARY STANDARD SEALS. For many years, a voluntary labeling program has been used by some manufacturers in the United States and Canada. Instituted by the Arts and Crafts Materials Institute (ACMI),* this program's labels can be identified by seals.

The "CP" (Certified Product) and "AP" (Approved Product) seals indicate that these products are considered safe for children according to the ACMI's toxicological evaluation guidelines. The "HL" seal (Health Label) indicates the product has been reviewed by the ACMI. If the product is judged to have chronic hazards the label will carry appropriate warnings.

The quality of the ACMI's voluntary program has varied over the years, however, for almost fifty years it was the only program in existence. The program now is compatible with most of the standards of the new mandatory federal art materials labeling law and it is hoped that all art materials soon will be labeled in accordance with ACMI or other equally stringent standards.

---

*Previously called the Crayon, Watercolor and Crafts Institute.

LABELS FOR INDUSTRIAL / PROFESSIONAL USE ONLY.

Products carrying this label are not supposed to be readily available to general consumers and should never be used by children or untrained adults.

Rules for the types of information and warning symbols which conform to your right-to-know law can be obtained from your local department of labor. This label warns workers that they should be skilled in the use of the product and should have a Material Safety Data Sheet (see next section) as a guide to safe use of the product.

MATERIAL SAFETY DATA SHEETS

WHAT ARE THEY? Material Safety Data Sheets are forms which provide information on a product's hazards, and the precautions required for its safe use in the working environment. Material Safety Data Sheets are usually filled out by the product's maker and the quality of the information varies depending on the diligence and cooperativeness of the individual manufacturer. However, manufacturers are responsible to their respective government agencies for the accuracy of information they provide.

The Material Safety Data Sheets are essential starting points for the development of a data base for health and safety programs. They should not be considered complete sources of information on their own.

WHO NEEDS THEM? The Hazard Communications Standard, WHMIS, and right-to-know laws require that Material Safety Data Sheets be made available to all those who use or could be exposed to potentially hazardous products in the workplace. This would include not only the products' users, but those working near the material, those storing or distributing the material (in case of breakage), and anyone exposed to airborne emissions from the products use, and so on.

All employers and administrators are required by the new laws to obtain Material Safety Data Sheets and make them available to all employees. Art teachers, who are employees, must have access to Material Safety Data Sheets and should in turn make them available to all students old enough to understand them. Self-employed artists should also obtain Material Safety Data Sheets for their protection as well.

In addition, all employers and administrators are responsible for training employees to interpret and use Material Safety Data Sheet information (see TRAINING, pages 19-20).

HOW ARE THEY OBTAINED? Material Safety Data Sheets can be obtained by writing to manufacturers, distributors, or importers of the product. Schools, businesses, and institutions can require Material Safety Data Sheets as a condition of purchase. If makers or suppliers do not respond to requests for Material Safety Data Sheets, send copies of your requests and other pertinent information to the agency responsible for enforcing your federal or local right-to-know law. These agencies usually get very good results.

Products for which there are no Material Safety Data Sheets or incomplete Material Safety Data Sheets must be removed from the workplace and replaced with products for which better information is available.

WHERE SHOULD THEY BE KEPT? Material Safety Data Sheets should be filed or displayed where the products are used and stored. For schools, experience has shown that the best procedure is to have a central file for all Material Safety Data Sheets and also to have smaller files in each classroom, shop, or work area which contains copies of the Material Safety Data Sheets for products used at that location.

WHAT DO THEY LOOK LIKE? To begin with, the words "Material Safety Data Sheet" must be at the top. Some manufacturers resist sending Material Safety Data Sheets, sending instead sheets labeled "Product Data Sheet," "Hazard Data Sheet," or other improper titles. These information sheets do not satisfy the laws' requirements.

Although Material Safety Data Sheets must contain the same basic information, the actual sheets may look very different. For example, some are computer generated and some are government forms. Figure 3 (pages 49 and 50) is a copy of the most recent United States Material Safety Data Sheet form (the OSHA 174 form). The Canadian forms require similar information (see Figure 3A, pages 51 and 52); one important difference being that they require the chemicals' odor threshold (OT) when known. This is a practical piece of information. For example if the Odor Threshold is higher than the Threshold Limit Value, workers know they are overexposed if they can smell the substance.

INFORMATION REQUIRED ON MATERIAL SAFETY DATA SHEETS. All of the information on the form in Figures 3 and 3A (pages 49-52) should be on a Material Safety Data Sheet. In general, Material Safety Data Sheets should identify the product chemically (with the exception of trade secret products), identify any toxic ingredients, list its physical properties, its fire and explosion data, its acute and chronic health hazards, its reactivity (conditions which could cause the product to react or decompose dangerously), tell how to clean up large spills and dispose of the material, identify the types of first aid and protective equipment needed to use it safely, and discuss any special hazards the product might have.

HOW TO READ MATERIAL SAFETY DATA SHEETS. It would take a small book to explain how to read a Material Safety Data Sheet and define all the terms you are likely to encounter. Fortunately there already are many small books and pamphlets on this subject. Your local department of labor, the American Lung Association, and many other organizations publish such items. You should obtain some of these materials and append them to your written right-to-know program to be used as training aids. (See Appendix 1, Your Right-To-Know Library, page 319.)

There are some common problems which are associated with art materials Material Safety Data Sheets, however, that should be addressed here. (Remember that some Material Safety Data Sheets are not divided into the sections below, but all the information should be present somewhere in the Material Safety Data Sheet.)

Section I — THE MATERIAL SAFETY DATA SHEET must have the art material manufacturer's name, address, and emergency telephone number at the top. It is the company whose name is on the Material Safety Data Sheet that is responsible to you for providing information and help.

Some art materials makers send out other companies' Material Safety Data Sheets. This improper procedure occurs because art materials makers often use other companies raw materials. They buy pigments, oils, solvents, acrylic, clay, and the like from other manufacturers and mix them. Sometimes they do not even mix materials, but simply relabel another manufacturer's materials.

The Material Safety Data Sheet also must be written with the intended use of the product in mind. If the product is to be used in some other way, further information must be obtained. For example, if a product is to be sprayed and the Material Safety Data Sheet only reflects the hazards of the material in liquid form, the Data Sheet is improper for the use intended.

Some suppliers send old, outdated Material Safety Data Sheets. Check the date of preparation. If there is no preparation date (sometimes found at the end of the form) or if the Material Safety Data Sheet is several years old, demand a more recent one. In Canada, three-year-old Material Safety Data Sheets are automatically invalid.

Section II — HAZARDOUS INGREDIENTS.The definition of a "hazardous ingredient" varies in different state, provincial, and federal laws. But the OSHA Hazard Communication Standard definition is most frequently used. OSHA considers as hazardous any chemical which is a physical hazard (flammable, unstable, etc.,) or a health hazard. Health hazard is further defined to mean any "chemical for which there is statistically significant evidence based on at least one study..."

This means that a chemical must be listed if there is even one proper animal study indicating a potential problem. On the other hand, manufacturers may decline to list many chemicals which have never been studied. Some of these also may be health hazards.

Some art materials manufacturers decline to list any of their ingredients, because they claim their products are proprietary or trade secrets. Artists should be aware that there are legal criteria for claiming trade secret status. If you receive an Material Safety Data Sheet for a trade secret product, call your department of labor to find out if these criteria were met. For example, in many states, a trade secret product must be registered with the state health department or Department of Labor.

Uninformative Material Safety Data Sheets with most of the blanks left empty may be sent. Insist that Material Safety Data Sheets be complete. Even when the product is not very hazardous, the blanks should be filled with information showing that this is the case.

Proper identification of an ingredient should include: chemical name, chemical family, synonyms, and common name(s). Good Material Safety Data Sheets also include the "CAS" number. "CAS" stands for the Chemical Abstracts Service, an organization that indexes information about chemicals. The CAS number enables users to look up information about the chemical in many sources.

Exposure limits should also be listed if they exist. (for example, ACGIH-Threshold Limit Values, OSHA-Permissible Exposure Limits, and Canadian Occupational Exposure Limits; see page 32). Sometimes manufacturers will also list their own recommended limits if no others exist for the material.

The percentage of each ingredient in materials that are mixtures is optional, but good manufacturers usually supply these.

Section III — PHYSICAL/CHEMICAL CHARACTERISTICS. Boiling point, evaporation rate, and other properties of the material are listed here. The description of appearance and odor can be compared to the look and smell of your product to verify that you have the right Material Safety Data Sheet.

Section IV — FIRE AND EXPLOSION HAZARD DATA. Flash point and other data are listed here along with information about the proper fire extinguisher to use and any special fire hazard properties of the material. This section should be consulted when planning emergency procedures.

Section V — REACTIVITY DATA. Artists who experiment with their media should pay special attention to the section on reactivity. This section describes how stable the material is, under what conditions it can react dangerously, and materials with which it is incompatible. If you don't understand this section, do not experiment.

Section VI — HEALTH HAZARD DATA. Toxicological information about the product is summarized here. You may need to use one of the resources in Appendix 1 to look up some of the terminology or abbreviations. Remember that this data is only a summary. Further investigation is often needed.

Cancer information which should be included on United States Material Safety Data Sheets includes whether the material is considered a cancer agent by either the National Toxicology Program (NTP), the International Agency for Research on Cancer (IARC), or OSHA. If any of these agencies consider the material to be carcinogenic, treat it as such.

Section VII — PRECAUTIONS FOR SAFE HANDLING AND USE. Use the information in this section to plan storing and handling of the material. Waste disposal information is usually not detailed because so many different local, state, provincial, and federal regulations exist. Check regulations that apply to your location.

Section VIII — CONTROL MEASURES. Proper respiratory protection, ventilation, and other precautions should be described here. Consult the section in this book on ventilation and respiratory protection for more detailed information.

Material Safety Data Sheet
May be used to comply with
OSHA's Hazard Communication Standard.
29 CFR 1910.1200. Standard must be
consulted for specific requirements.

U.S. Department of Labor
Occupational Safety and Health Administration
(Non-Mandatory Form)
Form Approved
OMB No. 1218-0072

IDENTITY *(As Used on Label and List)*

Note: Blank spaces are not permitted. If any item is not applicable, or no information is available, the space must be marked to indicate that.

Section I

Manufacturer's Name	Emergency Telephone Number
Address *(Number, Street, City, State, and ZIP Code)*	Telephone Number for Information
	Date Prepared
	Signature of Preparer *(optional)*

Section II — Hazardous Ingredients/Identity Information

Hazardous Components (Specific Chemical Identity; Common Name(s))	OSHA PEL	ACGIH TLV	Other Limits Recommended	% *(optional)*

Section III — Physical/Chemical Characteristics

Boiling Point		Specific Gravity (H_2O = 1)	
Vapor Pressure (mm Hg.)		Melting Point	
Vapor Density (AIR = 1)		Evaporation Rate (Butyl Acetate = 1)	
Solubility in Water			
Appearance and Odor			

Section IV — Fire and Explosion Hazard Data

Flash Point (Method Used)	Flammable Limits	LEL	UEL
Extinguishing Media			
Special Fire Fighting Procedures			
Unusual Fire and Explosion Hazards			

(Reproduce locally)   OSHA 174, Sept. 1985

Fig. 3. Material Safety Data Sheet (U.S.)

Section V — Reactivity Data

Stability	Unstable		Conditions to Avoid
	Stable		

Incompatibility (*Materials to Avoid*)

Hazardous Decomposition or Byproducts

Hazardous Polymerization	May Occur		Conditions to Avoid
	Will Not Occur		

Section VI — Health Hazard Data

Route(s) of Entry:	Inhalation?	Skin?	Ingestion?

Health Hazards (*Acute and Chronic*)

Carcinogenicity:	NTP?	IARC Monographs?	OSHA Regulated?

Signs and Symptoms of Exposure

Medical Conditions
Generally Aggravated by Exposure

Emergency and First Aid Procedures

Section VII — Precautions for Safe Handling and Use

Steps to Be Taken in Case Material Is Released or Spilled

Waste Disposal Method

Precautions to Be Taken in Handling and Storing

Other Precautions

Section VIII — Control Measures

Respiratory Protection (*Specify Type*)

Ventilation	Local Exhaust		Special	
	Mechanical (*General*)		Other	

Protective Gloves		Eye Protection

Other Protective Clothing or Equipment

Work/Hygienic Practices

Page 2   ☆ U S G P O 1986-491-529/45775

Fig. 3. (Continued)

Minimum Information Required on Canadian Material Safety Data Sheets for Controlled Products

Hazardous Ingredient Information

   I. Chemical identity and concentration
      a) of the product (if the product is a pure substance);
      b) of each controlled ingredient (if the product is a mixture);
      c) of any ingredient that the supplier/employer has reason to believe may be harmful; and
      d) of any ingredient whose toxic properties are unknown.
   2. The products CAS, UN and/or NA registration numbers.
      a) CAS=Chemical Abstracts Service Registration Number.
      b) UN=number assigned to hazardous materials in transit by the United Nations.
      c) NA=number assigned by Transport Canada and the United States Department of Transportation and for which a UN number has not been assigned.
   3. The LD^{50} and LC^{50} of the ingredient(s).
      a) LD^{50}=the dose (usually by ingestion) which kills half of the test animals in standard acute toxicity tests.
      a) LC^{50}=the airborne concentration which when inhaled kills half of the test animals in standard acute toxicity tests.

Preparation Information

   1. The name and telephone number of the group, department or person responsible for preparing the Material Safety Data Sheet.
   2. The date the Material Safety Data Sheet was prepared.

Product Information

   1. The name, address, and emergency telephone number of the product's manufacturer and, if different, the supplier.
   2. The product identifier (brand name, code or trade name, etc.)
   3. The use of the product.

Physical Data

   Physical state (gas, liquid, solid), odor and appearance, odor thresh old (level in parts per million at which the odor becomes notice-able), specific gravity, vapor pressure, vapor density, evaporation rate, boiling point, freezing point, pH (degree of acidity or alkalinity), and co-efficient of water/oil distribution.

Fig. 3A

Fire and Explosion Hazards

> Conditions under which the substance becomes a flammable hazard, means of extinguishing a fire caused by the substance, flash point, upper flammable limit, lower flammable limit, auto-ignition temperature, hazardous combustion products, explosion data including sensitivity to mechanical impact and to static discharge.

Reactivity Data

1. Conditions under which the product is chemically unstable.
2. Name(s) of any substance with which the product is chemically unstable (will react hazardously).
3. Conditions of reactivity.
4. Hazardous decomposition products.

Toxicological Data

1. Route of entry (skin contact, inhalation, ingestion, eye contact).
2. Acute effects.
3. Chronic effects.
4. Exposure limits (Occupational Exposure Limits, Threshold Limit Values, etc.).
5. Irritancy.
6. Sensitization potential (ability to cause allergies).
7. Carcinogenicity.
8. Reproductive toxicity.
9. Teratogenicity (ability to cause birth defects).
10. Mutagenicity (ability to cause mutation).
11. Synergistic effects (names of substances which may enhance toxic effects).

Preventative Measures

1. Personal protective equipment needed.
2. Specific engineering controls required (e.g. ventilation).
3. Spill or leak procedures.
4. Waste disposal methods.
5. Handling procedures and equipment.
6. Storage requirements.
7. Special shipping information.

First Aid Measures

> Specific first aid measures in event of skin/eye contact, inhalation or ingestion.

Fig. 3A. (Continued)

CHAPTER

6

GENERAL PRECAUTIONS

I n addition to specific precautions such as ventilation and respiratory protection, there are several general precautions which should be used in most situations.

SUBSTITUTION

The most effective precaution, of course, is substituting safe materials for more hazardous ones. Material Safety Data Sheets and labels can be used to compare products for toxicity and to identify the safest one. General rules for substitution include the following:

1. Always choose water-based or latex paints, inks, and other products over solvent-containing ones whenever possible. Solvents are among the most hazardous chemicals used by artists. For this reason, acrylic or water colors are much safer to use than oils and enamels, which are thinned with turpentine or paint thinner.

2. If solvents must be used, Threshold Limit Values, evaporation rates, and other data on Material Safety Data Sheets can be used to choose the least toxic ones. (See also Chapter 9, Solvents, page 87, for additional guidelines.)

3. Choose products which do not create dusts and mists. Avoid materi-

als in powdered form or aerosol products whenever possible to avoid inhalation hazards.

4. Avoid products containing known cancer-causing chemicals whenever possible, since there is no safe level of exposure.

PERSONAL HYGIENE

One of the simplest and most neglected methods of avoiding exposure to toxic substances is to practice good hygiene in the workplace. Industrial experience has taught that tiny amounts of toxic substances left on the skin, or brought home on clothing can affect even the workers' families. Some basic hygiene rules include the following:

I. Do not eat, smoke, or drink in studios, shops, or other environments where there are toxic materials. Dust, after all, settles in coffee cups, vapors can be absorbed by sandwiches, and hands can transfer substances to food and cigarettes. Smoking is especially hazardous because some substances inhaled through a cigarette can be converted by the heat to more hazardous forms.

2. Wear special work clothes and remove them after work. If possible, leave them in the workshop and wash them frequently and separately from other clothing. If the workplace is dusty, wear some form of hair covering (hair is a good dust collector). And for safety as well as hygiene, do not wear loose clothing, scarves or ties, or jewelry. Tie back long hair.

3. Wash hands carefully after work, before eating, using the bathroom, and applying make-up.

STORAGE OF MATERIALS

Many accidents, spills, and fires can be avoided by following rules for safe storage and handling of materials.

I. Clearly mark every bottle, box, or gas cylinder as to its contents, its hazards, and the date received and opened. Even containers into which materials are transferred for storage should be so labeled.

2. Use unbreakable containers whenever possible.

3. Apply good bookkeeping rules to chemical storage. Keep a current inventory of all the materials on hand and their locations. Post locations of flammable or highly toxic materials.

4. Maintain records of dates of purchase of materials in order to dispose of chemicals with limited shelf-lives properly. Some chemicals even become explosive with age.

5. Apply good housekeeping rules to chemical storage. Have cleaning supplies and facilities for handling of spills at hand. Never store any material which you are not prepared to control or clean up if it spills. If respiratory protection, gloves, or other personal protective equipment will be needed for cleaning up spills, have these in the studio at all times.

6. Organize storage wisely. For example, do not store large containers on high shelves where they are difficult to retrieve. Never store hazardous chemicals directly on the floor or above shoulder height.

7. Store reactive chemicals separately. Check each product's Material Safety Data Sheet and other technical sources for advice.

8. Keep all containers closed except when using them in order to prevent escape of dust or vapors.

9. Ventilate the storage room. Keep it cool and keep chemicals out of direct sunlight.

10. Do not allow dispensing or mixing of chemicals in or near the storage area.

11. If chemical corrosives or irritants are stored, be prepared with an eye wash station and emergency shower.

12. Storage of flammable chemicals should conform to all state/provincial fire regulations. Contact your local authorities for advice. Store large amounts of flammable solvents in metal flammable storage cabinets or specially designed storage rooms.

13. Have fire protection or extinguishers available which are approved for fires caused by the type of chemicals stored. Train personnel to use this type of extinguisher.

HANDLING/DISPOSAL OF MATERIALS

1. Check labels and Material Safety Data Sheets of your materials and have available the types of face, eye protection, gloves, wash-up facilities, and first aid equipment which are recommended.

2. When accidents occur, wash skin with lots of water and remove contaminated clothing. If eyes are affected, rinse eyes for at least fifteen minutes in an eye wash fountain and get medical advice.

3. Do not use any cleaning methods which raise dust. Wet mop floors or sponge surfaces.

4. Dispose of waste or unwanted materials safely. Check federal and local environmental protection regulations. Sometimes product labels or manufacturers can provide advice. Do not pour solvents down drains. Pour nonpolluting aqueous liquids down the sink one at a time with lots of water. For large amounts of regularly produced wastes, engage a waste disposal service.

5. Clean up spills immediately. If you use flammable or toxic liquids in the shop, stock chemical absorbants or other materials to collect spills, self-closing waste cans, and respiratory protection if needed. Empty waste cans daily.

6. When practical, dispense solvents from self-closing safety cans to reduce evaporation.

7. Do not store flammable or combustible materials near exits or entrances. Keep sources of sparks, flames, UV light, and heat as well as cigarettes away from flammable or combustible materials. (See Chapter 9, Solvents, page 87, for addition rules about flammable liquids.)

8. Have appropriate fire protection or extinguishers handy and train workers to use them.

CHOOSING PROPER PROTECTIVE EQUIPMENT

Many types of protective equipment are on the market. Some general rules for selecting appropriate equipment include:

1. Get expert advice when planning for safety and health. For example, consult an industrial hygienist (either private or governmental) to survey your facilities for hazards and recommend equipment. Some state/provincial government industrial hygiene services are free.

2. Get advice from more than one source when purchasing protective equipment, machinery, etc. Never rely solely on equipment manufacturers or distributors for information.

3. Survey personnel and students' special needs and problems regarding protective equipment. For example, people with dermatitis may need special hand protection.

4. Enforce proper use of protective equipment. Respirators are useless if they are not worn, hearing is not protected by unused ear muffs, etc.

5. Develop programs for regular repair, replacement, and maintenance of protective equipment.

WHERE TO BUY SAFETY SUPPLIES
There are several safety equipment directories available. One is *Best's Safety Directory*. It lists manufacturers and distributors of all types of safety equipment and supplies. Many technical libraries have a copy or it can be purchased for about $ 30.00 from A.M. Best Co., Ambest Road, Oldwick, NJ 08858 or call (201)439-2200.

EYE AND FACE PROTECTION
Suitable face and eye protection in the form of goggles or shields will guard against a variety of hazards, including impact (from chipping, grinding, etc.), radiation (welding, carbon arcs, lasers, etc.), and chemical splash (solvents, acids, etc.).

Only use protective equipment which conforms to American National Standards Institute (ANSI) standards. (See figures 4 and 5.)

AMERICAN NATIONAL STANDARD Z87.1-1989
SELECTION CHART

PROTECTORS

	ASSESSMENT SEE NOTE (1)	PROTECTOR TYPE	PROTECTORS	LIMITATIONS	NOT RECOMMENDED
IMPACT — Chipping, grinding, machining, masonry work, riveting, and sanding.	Flying fragments, objects, large chips, particles, sand, dirt, etc.	B,C,D, E,F,G, H,I,J, K,L,N	Spectacles, goggles faceshields. SEE NOTES (1) (3) (5) (6) (10). For severe exposure add N	Protective devices do not provide unlimited protection. SEE NOTE (7)	Protectors that do not provide protection from side exposure. SEE NOTE (10). Filter or tinted lenses that restrict light transmittance, unless it is determined that a glare hazard exists. Refer to OPTICAL RADIATION.
HEAT — Furnace operations, pouring, casting, hot dipping, gas cutting, and welding.	Hot sparks	B,C,D, E,F,G, H,I,J, K,L,*N	Faceshields, goggles, spectacles *For severe exposure add N	Spectacles, cup and cover type goggles do not provide unlimited facial protection.	Protectors that do not provide protection from side exposure.
	Splash from molten metals	*N	SEE NOTE (2) (3) *Faceshields worn over goggles H,K	SEE NOTE (2)	
	High temperature exposure	N	Screen faceshields. Reflective faceshields. SEE NOTE (2) (3)	SEE NOTE (3)	
CHEMICAL — Acid and chemicals handling, degreasing, plating	Splash	G,H,K	Goggles, eyecup and cover types *For severe exposure, add N	Ventilation should be adequate but well protected from splash entry	Spectacles, welding helmets, handshields
		*N	SEE NOTE (2) (3)		
	Irritating mists	G	Special purpose goggles	SEE NOTE (3)	

Fig. 4. ANSI Protection Standards

These materials (Fig. 4 and 5) are reproduced with permission from American National Standard "Practice for Occupational and Educational Eye and Face Protection," Z87.1-1989, copyright 1989 by the American National Standards Institute. Copies of this standard may be purchased from the American National Standards Institute at 1430 Broadway, New York, NY 10018.

ASSESSMENT	Operation	Hazard	Protectors	Typical Filter Lens Shade	Protectors (9)	Information
DUST	Woodworking, buffing, general dusty conditions.	Nuisance dust	G,H,K	Goggles, eyecup and cover types		Atmospheric conditions and the restricted ventilation of the protector can cause lenses to fog. Frequent cleaning may be required.
OPTICAL RADIATION				SEE NOTE (9)		Protectors that do not provide protection from optical radiation. SEE NOTE (4)
	WELDING: Electric Arc		O,P,Q	10-14	Welding Helmets or Welding Shields	Protection from optical radiation is directly related to filter lens density. SEE NOTE (4). Select the darkest shade that allows adequate task performance.
	WELDING: Gas		J,K,L, M,N,O, P,Q	4-8	Welding Goggles or Welding Faceshield	SEE NOTE (9)
	CUTTING			3-6		
	TORCH BRAZING			3-4		SEE NOTE (3)
	TORCH SOLDERING		B,C,D, E,F,N	1.5-3	Spectacles or Welding Faceshield	
GLARE			A,B	Spectacle SEE NOTE (9) (10)		Shaded or Special Purpose lenses, as suitable. SEE NOTE (8)

16

Fig. 4. ANSI Protection Standards (Continued)

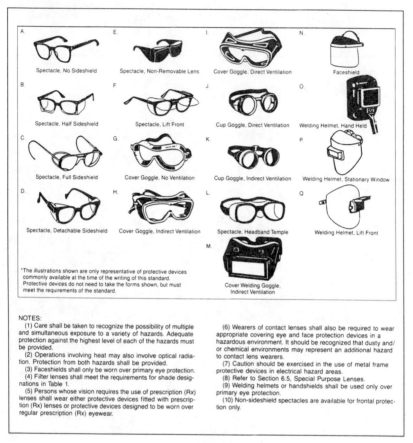

Fig. 5. Eye Protection Products

These standards are recognized in both the United States and Canada. Approved items will be labeled with the numbers of the standards with which they comply. Be certain to choose equipment appropriate to the hazard. A common mistake is to see chemical splash goggles used for protection against grind-wheel particles.

If you use any materials which can damage the eyes, an eye wash fountain should be a fixture in your shop. The fountain should be able to deliver at least fifteen minutes of water flow. Small eye wash bottles are not satisfactory for this purpose and also may become contaminated with bacteria.

Fountains should be activated by a foot pedal, lever or other mechanism which requires only a single movement to turn on the water and keep it running. Fountains should be flushed by running the water a few minutes once a week to keep fresh, clean water in the line.

Ordinary glasses are not proper eye protection. Do not wear contact lenses in shops where irritating liquids such as acids or solvents are used or where dusts are present.

SKIN PROTECTION

Satisfactory chemical-resistant gloves have been developed for almost any use imaginable. They can be purchased in any length up to shoulder length, and in any thickness from paper thin to very thick, and in many types of plastic and rubber to resist almost every kind of material. Surgical or ordinary household gloves should not be expected to stand up to solvents, acids, and other strong chemicals.

Find a glove supplier who provides information (usually in the form of a chart) which indicates how long each type of glove material can be in contact with a chemical before it is 1) degraded and 2) permeated. Degradation occurs when the glove deteriorates from the chemical's attack. Permeation occurs when molecules of the chemical squirm through the glove material. Permeated gloves often appear unchanged and the wearer may be unaware they are being exposed to the chemical.

Many artists are unaware that even common solvents like acetone, glycol ether, and xylene can penetrate certain chemical gloves in minutes and begin damaging and/or penetrating the skin.

Manufacturers' catalogues often provide access to proper gloves for other purposes, such as protection from heat, radiation, and abrasion. Asbestos gloves should not be used and substitutes for them are available.

For protection from occasional splashes or very light exposure to chemicals, you may use special creams called "barrier creams." Some of these creams protect skin from solvents and oils, others from acids, and so on. Choose the right cream and use it exactly as directed.

Do not use harsh hand soap. Waterless skin cleaners are useful if their ingredients do not include solvents or other harsh chemicals. Never wash your hands with solvents. Some people find that rubbing baby oil (mineral oil) on the skin and then washing with soap and water will remove many paints and inks. Using a barrier cream should enable you to wash off paints with soap and water. After cleaning your skin, apply a good hand lotion to replace any lost skin oils.

Hands are not the only part of the body for which skin protection has been developed. Aprons, leggings, leather or plastic clothing, shoes, and myriad special protective products are available. Remember, your skin's protective barrier is your first defense against many hazardous agents.

MEDICAL SURVEILLANCE

Artist should keep in mind that there are no tests for some types of chemical exposures, and there are no treatments for many kinds of bodily damage from workplace chemical and physical agents. Medical monitoring is never a replacement for preventing exposure to toxic substances.

Medical monitoring, however, can be a valuable tool in early recognition and prevention of occupational illnesses. Such tests can serve three purposes: 1) to identify preexisting disorders so artists can avoid media that would put them at great risk; 2) to detect early changes in performance before serious damage occurs; 3) and to detect damage that has already occurred and which may be permanent.

Examples of some types of useful medical tests might include regular (in some cases yearly) lung function tests for artists exposed to clay, stone, or wood dust, etching acid vapors, or who intend to wear a respirator (see chapter on Respiratory Protection). Artists using lead materials also should have blood tests for lead at least once a year. There are blood or urine tests for several other toxic metals as well.

Choosing the right tests and interpreting the results can be done best by doctors who are Board Certified in Occupational Medicine or Toxicology, or who have experience with occupational health problems. Such doctors may be found by contacting your state or provincial health departments or artists' advocacy organizations such as ACTS (see Preface).

Only consult physicians who explain the results of medical tests in meaningful terms so you can be an active participants in your own health care.

CHAPTER

7 | *VENTILATION*

Providing proper ventilation is the single most important method of protecting artists from hazardous airborne substances. There are two basic kinds of ventilation: 1) comfort ventilation to keep people in modern buildings comfortable; and 2) industrial ventilation to keep artists and others who work with chemicals healthy.

COMFORT VENTILATION. Comfort ventilation provides sufficient air movement and fresh air to avoid buildup of humidity, heat, and air pollution in buildings. This usually is accomplished by either natural or recirculating ventilation systems.

Natural ventilation takes advantage of rising warm air and prevailing winds to cause the air in buildings to circulate and exchange with outside air in sufficient amounts to provide comfort to those inside the building. Often chimney-like flues are constructed behind walls to draw out warm air. Such systems are found mostly in older buildings where high ceilings and open spaces enhance the system.

Some of these buildings also employ "univents" installed in rooms on outside walls. These units draw in some outside air through louvres in the wall, mix it with room air, and heat and expel the mixture. During the energy crisis, many of these units' access to outside air was cut off to save fuel. In this case, the units provide no ventilation, only heat.

Recirculating ventilation systems use fans or blowers to circulate air from room to room throughout the building. On each recirculating cycle, some fresh air from outside is added and some recirculated air is exhausted. The amount of fresh air added usually varies from 5 to 30 percent, depending on how tightly insulated the building is and the vagaries of the particular ventilation system or its operator. Building engineers who operate ventilation systems often are encouraged to add as little fresh air as possible to reduce heating and cooling costs.

People often feel ill when insufficient amounts of fresh air are added to comfort ventilation systems. They may complain of eye irritation, headaches, nausea, and other symptoms. Taken together, these sometimes are called the "sick building syndrome." The symptoms are apparently caused by the accumulation of body heat, humidity, cigarette smoke, dust, formaldehyde, and other pollutants in the air.

INDUSTRIAL VENTILATION. Processes which produce airborne toxic substances should never be done in environments employing either natural or recirculating comfort ventilation systems. All such processes require industrial ventilation.

There are two types of industrial ventilation: 1) dilution ventilation, and 2) local exhaust ventilation.

Dilution ventilation does exactly what its name implies. It dilutes or mixes contaminated workplace air with large volumes of clean air to reduce the amounts of contaminants to acceptable levels. Then the diluted mixture is exhausted (drawn by fans or other devices) from the workplace. Dilution systems usually consist of fresh air inlets (often having fans and systems for heating or cooling the air), and outlets (exhaust fans).

Although often cheap and easy to install, dilution ventilation has limits. For example, only vapors or gases of low toxicity or very small amounts of moderately toxic vapors or gases are removed sufficiently by dilution ventilation. Never use dilution ventilation to remove dusts, mists, or any highly toxic materials.

For example, dilution ventilation might be used for areas where small amounts of solvent vapors are created, such as when you paint with latex paints (which usually contain 5 to 15 percent solvents). Other good places for dilution ventilation include photographic darkrooms (black and white) and commercial art studios where small amounts of rubber cement and solvent-containing marking pens are used. Successful dilution ventilation also depends on the control and direction of air flow through the workspace. Careful positioning of the air inlets and outlets will assure that air flow moves in the desired direction, that the whole room is ventilated (no dead air spaces), and that expelled air cannot return via an inlet.

In special cases, the exhaust fan can be positioned very close to the work station (see figure 6). In this way it is effective as a local exhaust. Do not use this system with aerosol cans, spray painting, airbrush operations, or with flammable materials unless the fan is explosion proof.

Local exhaust ventilation is the best means by which materials of moderate to high toxicity—gases, vapors, dusts, fumes, etc.—are removed from the work place. Because local exhaust ventilation captures the contaminants at their source rather than after they have escaped into the room air, local exhaust systems remove smaller amounts of air than dilution systems. Table 3, page 70 lists processes which require local exhaust ventilation.

Local exhaust systems consist of a *hood* enclosing or positioned very close to the source of the contamination to draw in the air, *ductwork* to carry away the contaminated air, possibly an *air-cleaner* on some system to filter or purify the air before it is released outside, and a *fan* to pull air through the system. (See figure 7, page 66.)

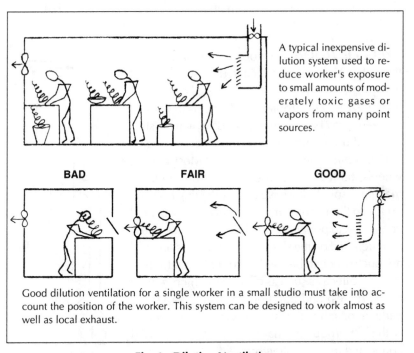

A typical inexpensive dilution system used to reduce worker's exposure to small amounts of moderately toxic gases or vapors from many point sources.

BAD   FAIR   GOOD

Good dilution ventilation for a single worker in a small studio must take into account the position of the worker. This system can be designed to work almost as well as local exhaust.

Fig. 6. Dilution Ventilation

Some of the rules to consider when choosing a local exhaust system include:

a. Enclose the process as much as possible by putting the hood close to the source or surrounding the process as completely as possible with the hood. The more the process is enclosed, the better the system will work.

b. Make sure the air flow is great enough to capture the contaminant. Keep in mind that dusts are heavy particles and require higher velocity air flow for capture than lighter vapors and gases.

c. Make sure that contaminated air flows away from your face, not past it.

d. Make sure that the exhausted air cannot re-enter the shop through make-up air inlets, doors, windows, or other openings.

e. Make sure enough make-up air is provided to keep the system operating efficiently.

TYPES OF HOODS. A hood is the structure through which the contaminated air first enters the system. Hoods can vary from small dust collecting types built around grind wheels to walk-in-sized spray booths. Some hoods which artists may find useful include the following:

Dust-collecting systems. (Fig. 8.) Most grind wheels, table saws, and other dust-producing machines sold today have dust collecting hoods built into them. Some machines need only to be connected to portable dust collectors which can be purchased off the shelf. In other cases, stationary ductwork can be used to connect machines to dust collectors such as cyclones (which settle out particles) and bag houses (which capture particles on fabric filters). Artists should not work with dust-producing machines unless they are connected to dust collectors.

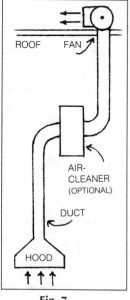

Fig. 7

Spray booths.(Fig. 9.) Spray booths from small table models to walk-in-sized or larger can be purchased or designed to fit the requirements of a particular shop. Some common uses for spray booths include spraying of paints, lacquers, adhesives and other materials, plastic resin casting, paint stripping, and solvent cleaning of silk screens. Since spray paints and other sprays are likely to contain flammable solvents, the spray booth, its ducts and fans, and the area surrounding the booth must be made safe from explosion and fire hazards.

Movable exhaust systems. (Fig. 10.) Also called "elephant trunk" systems, these flexible duct and hood arrangements are designed to remove fumes, gases, and vapors from processes such as welding, soldering, or any small table top processes which use solvents or solvent-containing products. Movable exhausts also can be equipped with pulley systems or mechanical arms designed to move hoods to almost any position.

Canopy hood systems. (Fig.11.) These hoods take advantage of the fact that hot gases rise. They are used over processes such as kilns, hot dye baths, wax and glue pots, stove ranges, and the like. Unfortunately, they often are installed above worktables where they are not only ineffective because the hood is too far from the table, but even dangerous because they draw contaminated air past the worker's face.

Slot hood systems. (Fig. 12.) These systems draw gases and vapors across a work surface, away from the worker. Slot hood systems are good for any kind of bench work, including silk-screen printing, color photo developing, air brushing, and soldering. They are rather expensive to design and build, but provide a shop with surfaces on which many processes can be safely carried out.

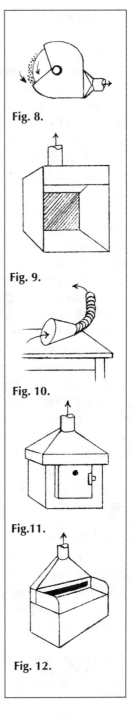

Fig. 8.

Fig. 9.

Fig. 10.

Fig.11.

Fig. 12.

PLANNING VENTILATION

Planning ventilation systems for large schools, studios, and shops usually requires experts for each phase of work. You should carefully apprise these experts of your special needs before they begin their work.

Ideally, you first should choose an industrial hygienist to evaluate shop and house hazards and recommend specific ventilation systems. Next select a professional engineer experienced in industrial ventilation to design both dilution and local exhaust ventilation systems. You may also want to employ a heating, ventilating, and air conditioning (HVAC) engineer to help integrate the new ventilation systems into existing ones, or to upgrade comfort ventilation systems. Once the experts have designed the systems, employ an appropriate contractor to install it. Be particularly careful to choose qualified experts. Engineering and contracting errors can result in very expensive and time-consuming problems.

Planning ventilation for small shops and individual studios is much less complicated. A good reference called *Ventilation: A Practical Guide* (Available from CSA, 5 Beekman St., New York, NY 10038) provides basic ventilation principles and calculations. Mechanically inclined artists should be able to use this manual to design and install simple systems.

Artists should be leery of salesmen who tout products which appear to solve ventilation problems cheaply by purifying contaminated air and returning it to the workplace. Some of these devices, such as the negative ion generator**, are not only useless in most studios, but they actually can be harmful if they also generate irritating ozone gas. Others, such as electrostatic precipitators, are very limited in their uses and at best can be used only as adjuncts to traditional ventilation. For example, they can successfully remove cigarette smoke fume particles, but not the gases and vapors produced by cigarettes.

CHECKING THE SYSTEM. After a ventilation system has been installed, it should be checked to see that it is operating properly. If an engineer, industrial hygienist, or contractor worked on the job, he or she should make the initial check and recommend any changes necessary to meet design specifications. If experts were not consulted, you may decide to consult one at this stage.

**These systems cannot collect gases or vapors. They only remove positive electric charges on some kinds of particles such as pollens and house dust causing them to settle temporarily on surfaces and walls. While this might be helpful to some individuals sensitive to pollens and certain dusts, it is essentially useless against toxic gases, vapors, fumes and dusts.

For example, air flow devices can be used by an expert to measure air velocity and determine how well the system is functioning.

Even without the advice of an expert, some common-sense observations can be made:

1. Can you see the system pulling dusts and mists into it? If not, you might use incense smoke or soap bubbles to check the system visually. When released in the area where the hood should be collecting, the smoke or bubbles should be drawn quickly and completely into the system.

2. Can you smell any gases or vapors? Sometimes placing inexpensive perfume near a hood can demonstrate a system's ability to collect vapors or it can show that exhausted air is returning to the workplace (or some other place where it should not be).

3. Do people working with the system complain of eye, nose, or throat irritation or have other symptoms?

4. Is the fan so noisy and irritating that people would rather endure the pollution than turn it on? Fans should not be loud, and installers should be expected to work on the system until it is satisfactory.

Check ventilation systems periodically to see that they are continuing to work properly. Maintenance schedules for changing filters, cleaning ducts, changing fan belts and the like also should be worked out and kept faithfully.

TABLE 3	Processes and Equipment Requiring Local Exhaust Ventilation

Equipment or Processes which create:

Dusts   abrasive blasting
dry grinding and polishing
dry mixing of clays and glazes
powered carving and chipping of stone, cement, etc.
powered sanding
woodworking machinery

Heat, Fumes, and Other Emissions
burn-out kilns
ceramic and glass paint kilns
firing (all types)
enameling and slumping kilns
glassblowing furnaces
foundry furnaces
hot dye baths
metal melting and casting
paint-removing with torches or heat guns
soldering
welding

Mists   aerosol spraying
air-brushing
power spraying (all types)

Solvent Vapors and/or Gases
acid etching (all types including hydrofluoric)
acid pickling baths
electroplating
paint-removing (solvent methods)
photochemical processes:
      color processing
      toning
      photoetching
      photolithography
plastic resin casting
screen printing:
      printing
      print drying
      screen cleaning

CHAPTER

8 *RESPIRATORY PROTECTION*

Adequate ventilation, not respirators, should be the primary means of controlling airborne toxic substances. United States Occupational Safety and Health Administration (OSHA) regulations restrict use of respiratory protection except: when a hazardous process is used only very occasionally (less than thirty times a year); or while ventilation is being installed, maintained, or repaired; where engineering controls result in only a negligible reduction in exposure; during emergencies; or for entry into atmospheres of unknown composition.

Most Canadian provincial regulations allow more liberal use of respiratory protection.

NIOSH APPROVAL

The National Institute for Occupational Safety and Health (NIOSH) sets standards for respirators, filters, and all respirator parts and components. Both the United States and Canada accept these standards. All approved respirators and components will carry the initials "NIOSH" and an approval number. Only NIOSH-approved products should be used.

TYPES OF RESPIRATORS

It is important to choose precisely the right type of protection for a particular task. Wearing the wrong type of respirator, a surgical mask (which is designed as protection against biological hazards, not chemical ones), or a damp handkerchief, actually may make the situation worse.

There are three basic respirator types: air-supplying, air-purifying, and powered air-purifying.

AIR-SUPPLYING RESPIRATORS bring fresh air to the wearer usually by means of pressurized gas cylinders or air compressors. They are the only respirators which can be used in oxygen-deprived atmospheres. They also are complex and expensive systems requiring special training for those using them.

AIR-PURIFYING RESPIRATORS use the wearer's breath to draw air through filters or chemical cartridges in order to purify it before it is inhaled. Most air-purifying respirators are priced in a range that artists will find practical. These respirators will be covered in detail below.

POWERED AIR-PURIFYING RESPIRATORS provide wearers with air which has been pumped (usually by a small unit attached to the wearer's belt) through filters or cartridges. This filtered air is supplied under slight pressure to a mask or shield over the wearers face. These are usually priced somewhere between the other two types of respirators.

TYPES OF AIR-PURIFYING RESPIRATORS

Artists are most likely to find the following types of air-purifying respirators useful:

1. Disposable or single-use types which often look like paper dust masks and are thrown away after use.

2. Quarter-face types which cover the mouth and nose, only and have replaceable filters and cartridges,

3. Half-face types which cover the mouth, nose, and chin, and have replaceable filters and cartridges, and

4. Full-face types which look like old-fashioned gas masks and have a replaceable canister.

RESPIRATOR PROGRAMS

Learning to select and use respirators properly is not as easy as it looks. For this reason, United States employers are required by OSHA (the Occupational Safety and Health Administration) to institute written programs for all workplaces where respirators are used. At present, Canadian regulations are not as strict, but many regulations for specific chemicals require written respirator programs. Among these substances are several used by artists and conservators including silica, lead, and ethylene oxide.

Written respirator programs should be instituted in schools, universities, businesses, museums, and all institutions whose personnel use respirators. If students are allowed to use respirators, the program should be extended to include them. Although students are not covered under occupational laws, the schools' liability will be jeopardized if students do not receive equal or better protection than staff.

The formal program requirements include fit testing to assure that contaminated air does not leak in, institution of proper procedures for cleaning, disinfecting, and storing, plus provisions for periodic inspection and repair of respirators, and for formal training of people in the use and limitations of respirators. Also included are recommendations for medical screening for users.

Medical tests or questionnaires are needed to identify users who have physical conditions which make wearing respirators dangerous. For example, heart or lung problems may be worsened by the additional breathing stress created by a respirator. Some psychological problems such as claustrophobia also preclude respirator use. Temporary conditions which curtail respirator use include head colds, skin infections, and, in come cases, pregnancy.

FIT TESTING

Fit testing is needed to identify those people who should not wear a respirator because its facepiece will not form a good seal against their skin allowing contaminants to bypass the filters. Respirators originally were designed to fit a large percentage of male caucasian faces. Some people whose faces do not conform to this shape may not find any respirator that will fit. To accommodate women, many companies now make smaller sizes. But some people simply cannot find respirators that fit them.

Other reasons respirators will not fit include the presence of facial hair (such as beards and sideburns or even a few hours growth of facial hair), facial scars, broken nose, missing dentures or very large or small faces. Fit testing should be done annually in order to catch changes in fit or physical condition. For example, losing or gaining about fifteen pounds can alter respirator fit.

FIT TESTING METHODS

There are two types of fit testing, quantitative and qualitative. Quantitative methods involve the use of equipment to measure airborne concentrations both inside and outside the respirator. This is the best method, but it is very expensive.

Qualitative fit testing involves exposing the wearer to an agent which can be detected by odor or taste if it leaks into the respirator. Isoamyl acetate (banana oil) is commonly used to test organic vapor respirators. Irritant smokes (often titanium tetrachloride) and saccharin mists can be used to test fume, dust, and mist filtered respirators and masks.

Fit tests involve placing a hood or plastic tent over the wearer, adding the testing chemical, and having the wearer report any taste or odor while he or she performs a routine series of simple tasks including deep breathing, reading/talking, and moving the head up, down, and from side to side.

Industrial hygienists or trained representatives of respirator manufacturers are usually able to perform fit tests. These people often will train selected personnel to do fit tests so that respirator programs can function without outside help.

Other simpler tests also can be done each time you wear a cartridge respirator. These include a negative pressure test (blocking cartridge air inlets with your hands, inhaling, holding your breath for fifteen to twenty seconds to see if the negative pressure remains in the facepiece), a positive pressure test (blocking the exhalation valve, exhaling gently, and seeing if you can detect air escaping around the facepiece), and a cartridge test (see the next section).

Formal fit testing is especially important when wearing paper masks since positive and negative pressure tests cannot be done.

FILTERS AND CARTRIDGES

When air is drawn through a properly fitted respirator, it passes through either a filter or a chemical material. Filters are designed to trap particles such as dusts or metal fumes (which are fine particles created when metals are melted). Chemical air-purifying materials, on the other hand, trap vapors (such as those created when solvents evaporate) and gases (like ammonia). Different cartridges and filters are designed to trap specific gases, vapors, fumes, dusts, and mists.

No filter or cartridge can remove all of a contaminant from the air. Instead, respirators are capable of reducing the amount of a particular contaminant to an acceptable level as defined by NIOSH standards.

WHEN TO REPLACE THEM

Both filters and chemical cartridges wear out and become ineffective with use. Filters clog progressively until breathing through them becomes difficult and breathing pressure begins to draw more particles through. Spent chemical cartridges, on the other hand, will simply stop collecting the contaminant and allow it to pass through.

Chemical cartridges usually are considered spent after eight hours of use or two weeks after they have been exposed to air, which ever comes first. Chemical cartridges also wear out with time, even if they are not used. For this reason, many brands of cartridges have an expiration date stamped on them.

No filter or cartridge is designed to be effective when contaminants reach very high concentrations. At high concentrations, more contaminants pass through cartridges and filters than is desirable, and they will wear out in a shorter time—sometimes in minutes.

To be sure they are not spent, chemical cartridges should also be tested before each use. For example, a simple test for organic vapor or spray paint cartridges is to pass an open bottle of nail polish or iso-amyl acetate (banana oil) in front of the respirator when you first put it on. If you can detect the odor, replace the cartridge.

CHEMICALS AGAINST WHICH THEY ARE EFFECTIVE

Filters and cartridges are designed only for specific kinds of airborne contaminants. Table 4 lists abbreviations for some of the filters and cartridges which artists might use.

TABLE 4	Respirator Cartridges and Filters

Cartrige or Filter Use and (Abreviation)

ACID GAS   Acid gases rising from bleaches, etching and
(AG)   pickling baths, photochemicals, etc.

AMMONIA   Ammonia from diazo copiers, cleaners, etc.
(NH_3)

ORGANIC VAPOR   Vapors from evaporating solvents,
(OV)   solvent-containing products, etc.

FORMALDEHYDE   Formaldehyde from plywood, formalin, urea
(CH_2O or FOR)   formaldehyde glues, etc.

PAINT, LACQUER,   Sprays and aerosols from solvent-containing
& ENAMEL MIST (PLE)*   paints and other products.

PESTICIDES   Pesticide sprays and dusts.
(PEST)

ASBESTOS   Air-supplied respirators are needed.
(A)

DUSTS   Toxic and fibrosis-producing dusts (e.g. silica)
(D)   having a Threshold Limit Value of not less than
     0.05 milligrams per cubic meter (mg/m^3).

MISTS   Water-based mists having a Threshold Limit
(M)   Value of not less than 0.05 mg/m^3.

FUMES   Fumes (e.g. metal fumes) having a Threshold
(F)   Limit Value of not less than 0.05 mg/m^3.

HIGH EFFICIENCY   Dusts, mists, and fumes of highly toxic materi-
(H)   als with Threshold Limit Values of 0.05 mg/m^3
     or less such as lead, and radionuclides.

* PLE cartridges are organic vapor cartridges preceded by a spray mist prefilter to keep mists from soaking into and saturating the chemical cartridge.

WHEN THEY SHOULD NOT BE USED

Never use air-purifying respirators in oxygen-deficient atmospheres such as when gas is released in a confined space or in fire-fighting. They also should not be used for protection from cancer-causing substances since they merely reduce rather than eliminate toxic exposure.

In addition, NIOSH does not approve air-purifying respirators for use against chemicals which are of an extremely hazardous nature, or lack sufficient warning properties (smell or taste), are highly irritating, or are not effectively captured by filter or cartridge materials. Included among these are hot or burning wax vapors (acrolein and other hazardous decomposition products), carbon monoxide, methyl (wood) alcohol, isocyanates (from foaming or casting polyurethane), nitric acid, ozone, methyl ethyl ketone peroxide (used to harden polyester resins), and phosgene gas (created when chlorinated hydrocarbon solvents come into contact with heat or flame).

CHOOSING A RESPIRATOR

It is important that you know precisely what contaminant is in the air and its physical form (gas, vapor, particle, fume) before you choose filters and cartridges. (See Table 3, page 70.)

The amount of a substance in the air is also a factor affecting respirator choice. Single-use dust masks and some quarter-faced respirators are only good for low airborne concentrations of up to five times the Threshold Limit Value for the substance. Higher concentrations will require the use of those half- or full-faced respirators which are approved for concentrations up to ten times the Threshold Limit Value. Full-faced respirators also should be used when the contaminant concentration is up to 100 times the Threshold Limit Value and/or is an eye hazard or irritant.

Heavily contaminated atmospheres cannot be safely handled by air-purifying respirators at all. In this case, air-supplying respirators are needed.

Obviously it is a complicated procedure to estimate or measure airborne concentrations in order to choose a proper respirator. Such decisions will require expert advice. Consult an industrial hygienist or a technical expert associated with a reputable respirator manufacturer.

RESPIRATOR CARE

At the end of a work period, clean the respirator and store it out of sunlight in a sealable plastic bag. Respirators never should be hung on hooks in the open or left on counters in the shop. Cartridges left out will continue to capture contaminants from the air. They also should be stored in sealable plastic bags.

If a respirator is shared, it should be cleaned and disinfected between users. Most respirator manufacturers provide educational materials which describe proper break-down and cleaning procedures. Inspect respirators carefully and periodically for wear and damage.

WHERE TO BUY RESPIRATORS

Schools and businesses can easily contact their safety equipment suppliers for advice about good local sources. However, individual artists may find it more difficult.

Begin by talking to some of the safety equipment suppliers in the yellow pages of your telephone book. If this route proves unproductive, consult *Best's Safety Directory* (see page 57) or call some of the companies listed in Figure 13. Ask if they have a distributor near you.

Be sure to explain that you need a company which provides fit-testing, expert advice on matching the respirator to the hazard, and other technical services. These services are more important than the cost of the respirator.

Respiratory Protection Suppliers

American Optical Corp.
14 Mechanic St., Southbridge, MA 01550. 1-800-225-7768.

Direct Safety Co.
7815 S. 46th St., Phoenix, AZ 85044. 1-602-968-7009.

Glendale Protective Technologies, Inc.,
130 Crossways Park Drive, Woodbury, NY 11797. 1-516-921-5800.

Industrial Safety & Security,
1390 Neubrecht Rd., Lima, OH 45801. 1-800-537-9721.

Lab Safety Supply Co.
P.O. Box 1368, Janesville, WI 53547. 1-800-356-0783.

Mine Safety Appliances Co.
P.O. Box 425, Pittsburgh, PA 15230. 1-800-MSA-2222.

North Safety Equipment
2000 Plainfield Pike, Cranston, RI 02920. 1-401-943-4400.

Racal Airstream, Inc.
7309A Grove Rd., Fredrick, MD 21701. 1-800-682-9500.

Scott Aviation
2225 Erie St., Lancaster, NY 14086. 1-716-863-5100.

Standard Glove and Safety Equipment Corp.
34300 Lakeland Blvd., Eastlake, OH 44094. 1-800-223-1434.

SURVIVAIR, Div. of Comasec, Inc.,
3001 S. Susan St., Santa Ana, CA 92704. 1-800-821-7236.

U.S. Safety,
1535 Walnut, P.O. Box 417237, Kansas City, MO 64108.
1-800-821-5218.

Wilson Safety Products
P.O. Box 622, Second & Washington Sts., Reading, PA 19603.
1-215-376-6161.

3M Co., Occupational Health and Safety Products Div.,
3M Center/Bldg. 220-3E-04, St. Paul, MN 55144. 1-800-328-1667.

Inclusion of a company on this list does not constitute endorsement of their products.

Fig. 13

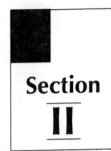

Section

II

Artist's Raw Materials

CHAPTER 9
SOLVENTS

Y ears ago, many art schools and universities taught highly technical courses on art materials. In these courses students learned about the chemical and physical nature of their materials, how to control their materials' properties to produce desired effects, and how to experiment with materials intelligently rather than accidently. Back then they knew that even effects achieved by accident must be understood if they are to be repeated and exploited.

Not only should these technical courses be revived and updated, but detailed information on the hazards of our raw materials should be added to them. This information could be organized by the chemical nature of the material. For instance, most of the hazardous chemicals in art materials can be organized in five groups of related materials. These are 1) solvents, 2) pigments and dyes, 3) metals and their compounds, 4) minerals, frits, and glass, and 5) plastics.

The following sections of this book will cover these groups materials in depth and provide information to be used as references for subsequent chapters on individual media.

SOLVENTS

Solvents are used in almost every kind of art material. They are found in many paints, varnishes, inks, and their thinners; in most aerosol spray products; in some leather and textile dyes; in ceramic lustre glazes, felt tip pens, glues and adhesives, some photographic chemicals, and much more.

WHAT ARE SOLVENTS?

The term "solvents" refers to liquid organic chemicals used to dissolve solid materials. Examples of solvents are turpentine, acetone, kerosene, and lacquer thinner. Solvents are used widely because they dissolve materials like resins and plastics, and because they evaporate quickly and cleanly.

SOLVENT TOXICITY

All solvents are toxic. They are hazardous in both their liquid and vapor state. There are no "safe" solvents.

In general, solvents can irritate and damage the skin, eyes, and respiratory tract, cause a narcotic effect on the nervous system, and damage internal organs such as the liver and kidneys. These kinds of damage can be acute (from single heavy exposures) or chronic (from repeated low dose exposures over months or years). In addition, some solvents are especially hazardous to specific organs or can cause specific diseases such as cancer.

SKIN DISEASE. All solvents can dissolve the skin's protective barrier of oils, drying and chapping the skin and causing a kind of dermatitis. In addition, some solvents can cause severe burning and irritation of the skin. Others may cause no symptoms, but may penetrate the skin, enter the bloodstream, travel through the body and damage other organs.

IRRITATION OF THE EYES AND RESPIRATORY TRACT. All solvent vapors can irritate and damage the sensitive membranes of the eyes, nose, and throat. Inhaled deeply, solvent vapors also can damage lungs. The airborne concentration at which irritation occurs varies from solvent to solvent. Often workers are unaware of solvents' effects at low concentrations. Their only symptoms may be increased frequency of colds and respiratory infections. Years of such exposure could lead to chronic lung diseases such as chronic bronchitis.

At higher concentrations symptoms are more severe and may include nose bleeds, running eyes, and sore throat. Inhaling very high concentrations or aspirating liquid solvents may lead to severe disorders including chemical pneumonia and death. Liquid solvents splashed in the eyes can cause severe eye damage.

EFFECT ON THE NERVOUS SYSTEM. All solvents can affect the brain or central nervous system (CNS) causing "narcosis." Immediate symptoms of this effect on the CNS may include dizziness, irritability, headaches, fatigue, and nausea. At progressively higher doses, the symptoms may proceed from drunkenness to unconsciousness and death. Years of chronic exposure to solvents can cause permanent CNS damage resulting in memory loss, apathy, depression, insomnia, and other psychological problems which are hard to distinguish from problems caused by everyday living.

Solvents also may damage the peripheral nervous system (PNS) which is the system of nerves leading from the spinal cord to the arms and legs. The symptoms caused by this PNS damage are numbness and tingling in the extremities, weakness, and paralysis. Some solvents such as *n*-hexane (found in rubber cement and many spray products) can cause a combination of CNS and PNS effects resulting in a disease with symptoms similar to multiple sclerosis.

DAMAGE TO INTERNAL ORGANS. There is considerable variation in the kinds and degrees of damage different solvents can do to internal organs. Many solvents can damage the liver and kidney as these organs attempt to detoxify and eliminate the solvents from the body. One solvent, carbon tetrachloride, has such a devastating effect on the liver, especially in combination with alcohol ingestion, that many deaths have resulted from its use. Many solvents also can alter heart rhythm, even causing heart attacks or sudden cardiac arrest at high doses. Methylene chloride, a solvent often found in spray-can products and plastics adhesives, is especially capable of damaging the heart because it also metabolizes (breaks down) in the bloodstream to form heart-stressing carbon monoxide.

Some solvents also are known to cause cancer in humans or animals. Benzene can cause leukemia. Carbon tetrachloride can cause liver cancer. Many experts suspect that all chlorinated solvents (those with "chloro" or "chloride" in their names) may be carcinogens. For example, methylene chloride is now considered a suspect carcinogen since it causes cancer in animals.

REPRODUCTIVE HAZARDS AND BIRTH DEFECTS. The reproductive effects of solvents are not well researched. Those studies which do exist show there is reason for concern. For example, Scandinavian studies show higher rates of miscarriages, birth defects, and other problems among workers who were exposed to solvents on their jobs. Also, two types of solvents—the glycol ethers or cellosolves (which are found in many photographic chemicals, liquid cleaning products, some paints and inks, and aerosol sprays) and the glycidyl ethers (found in epoxy resin products)—atrophy animals' testicles and cause birth defects.

In addition, recent studies of one of the least toxic solvents—grain alcohol—have shown that babies born to drinking mothers may be of low birth weight, have varying degrees of mental retardation, and suffer from other abnormalities. Cautious doctors counsel both men and women planning pregnancies to avoid both drinking alcohol and solvent exposure.

EXPLOSION AND FIRE HAZARDS. Solvents have two properties which especially influence their capacity to cause fires and explosions—evaporation rates and flashpoints. In general, the higher a solvent's evaporation rate (see definition in footnote to Table 5.) the faster it evaporates and the more readily it can create explosive or flammable air/vapor mixtures.

In addition, some solvents are more flammable than others, that is, they have a lower flash point (the temperature at which vapors can ignite in the presence of a spark or flame). Materials with flashpoints at around room temperature or lower are particularly dangerous.

The chlorinated hydrocarbons (see Chemical Classes, below) are usually not flammable and have no flash points. However, some can react explosively on contact with certain metals and heating or burning them creates highly toxic decomposition products including phosgene gas. Hazardous amounts of these toxic gases can be created even by working with chlorinated solvents in a room where a pilot light is burning.

Clearly, all solvents should be isolated from sources of heat, sparks, flame, and static electricity.

CHEMICAL CLASSES OF SOLVENTS. All solvents fall into various classes of chemicals. A class is a group of chemicals with similar molecular structures and chemical properties. Important classes of solvents are aliphatic, aromatic, and chlorinated hydrocarbons, alcohols, esters, and ketones. Table 5 shows various solvents and their properties by class.

RULES FOR CHOOSING SAFER SOLVENTS
(If solvents must be used, choose the least toxic ones.)

1. Compare Threshold Limit Values. The higher the Threshold Limit Value, the less toxic it is. (See definitions of Threshold Limit Values, page 32-33.)

2. Compare evaporation rates. The more slowly a solvent evaporates, the less vapor it creates when used, and the less hazardous it is to work with. In fact, some very toxic solvents which evaporate very slowly may not be as hazardous to use as less toxic ones that evaporates very quickly.

3. Compare flash points and evaporation rates. The higher the flashpoint, the lower its fire and explosion hazard. The more slowly it evaporates the less flammable vapor it creates. Chlorinated solvents with no flash points, however, should not be considered safe. (See Explosion and Fire Hazards section above for details.)

4. Compare toxic effects. Although all solvents are toxic, some may be especially dangerous to you. For example, if you have heart problems, it makes sense to avoid solvents known for their toxic effects on the heart.

5. Compare within classes. Often solvents in the same chemical class can be substituted for each other. Due to their similar chemical structures, many will dissolve the same materials or work the same way.

RULES FOR SOLVENT USE

1. *Try to find replacements for solvent-containing products.* New and improved water-based products are being developed. Keep abreast of developments in new materials.

2. *Use the least toxic solvent possible.* Use Table 5 to select the safest solvent in each class. Consult Material Safety Data Sheets on the products you use and choose those containing the least toxic solvents.

3. *Comply with hazard communication laws* (see pages 18-20). Make a complete inventory of solvents and label all containers, even small ones. Collect Material Safety Data Sheets on all solvents, and file them where all users have access to them. Formally train all potentially exposed persons.

4. *Avoid breathing vapors.* Use solvents in areas where local exhaust ventilation is available. (Dilution ventilation should only be used when very small amounts of solvents or solvent-containing products are used.) Use self-closing waste cans for solvent-soaked rags, keep containers closed when not in use, and design work practices to reduce solvent evaporation. Keep a respirator with organic cartridges or an emergency air-supplying respirator at hand in case of spills or ventilation failure.

5. *Avoid skin contact.* Wear gloves for heavy solvent exposure and use barrier creams for incidental light exposures. Wash off splashes immediately with water and mild soap. Never clean hands with solvents or solvent-containing hand-cleaners. If solvents in amounts larger than a pint are used at one time, or if large spills are possible, have an emergency shower installed.

6. *Protect eyes from solvents.* Wear approved chemical splash goggles whenever solvents are poured or if there is a chance a splash may occur. Do not wear contact lenses, even under goggles. Install an eye wash fountain or other approved source of water which provides at least fifteen minutes flow. Prominently post emergency procedures (usually near telephone) for obtaining emergency medical advice and treatment if necessary.

7. *Protect against fire, explosion, and decomposition hazards.* Follow all local and federal codes for use, handling, ventilation, and storage. Never smoke or permit heat, flames, or sparks near solvents. Install sprinkler system or other proper fire-suppression system. Be sure fire extinguishers are approved for solvent and grease fires. Store amounts larger than a gallon in approved flammable storage cabinets (this recommendation exceeds requirements). Do not use heat and/or ultraviolet light sources near chlorinated hydrocarbons. Local exhaust ventilation fans for solvent vapors must be explosion-proof. Ground containers from which solvents are dispensed.

8. *Be prepared for spills.* Check all applicable local and federal regulations regarding release of solvent liquids and vapors. If spills of large amounts are likely, use chemical solvent absorbers sold by most major chemical supply houses. Special traps to keep solvent spills out of sewers may be required by law. Release of large amounts of liquid or vapor of certain solvents must be reported to environmental protection authorities.

9. *Dispose of solvents in accordance with local or federal regulations.*

TABLE 5	**Common Solvents and their Hazards**

How To Use This Table

COLUMN 1 —SOLVENT CLASS designates the chemical group into which solvents fall. Under each class heading are listed individual solvents and their common synonyms. Try to use the safest solvent in each class.

COLUMN 2 —Threshold Limit Value-Time Weighted Average (TLV-TWA). These are the ACGIH (American Conference of Governmental Industrial Hygienists) eight-hour time-weighted Threshold Limit Values for 1990-1991. All the Threshold Limit Value-Time Weighted Averages are in parts per million (ppm). (See pages 32-33 for definitions.)

COLUMN 3 —ODOR THRESHOLD (OT) in parts per million (ppm). Often they are given as a range of amounts which normal people can detect. Solvents whose odor cannot be detected until the concentration is above the Threshold Limit Value are particularly hazardous.

COLUMN 4 —FLASH POINT (FP) in degrees Fahrenheit (F°). The FP is the lowest temperature at which a flammable solvent gives off sufficient vapor to form an ignitable mixture with air near its surface. Some petroleum solvents exhibit a range of flash points. The lower the flash point, the more flammable the solvent.

COLUMN 5 —EVAPORATION RATE (ER) categorized as FAST, MEDIUM OR SLOW. See footnote at end of chart for precise definition.

COLUMN 6 —COMMENTS about the particular toxic effects of the solvent. Symptoms listed here are in addition to the general solvent hazards common to all solvents such as skin damage, narcosis, etc. (See this chapter.)

SOLVENT CLASS	TLV-TWA ppm	OT ppm	FP F°	ER	COMMENTS
ALCOHOLS					one of the safer classes
ethyl alcohol, ethanol, grain alcohol, denatured alcohol.	1000	5-10	55	MED.	Least toxic in class. Denatured alcohol contains some toxic additives
methyl alcohol, methanol, wood alcohol	200	160-6000	52	FAST	High dose or chronic exposures can cause blindness. Skin absorbs.
isopropyl alcohol, propanol, rubbing alcohol	400	15-300	53	MED	One of the least toxic in class. Long-term hazards not fully studied.
isoamyl alcohol, 3-methyl-1-butanol, fusel oil	100	.01-35	109	SLOW	Irritation begins at the Threshold Limit Value.

ALIPHATIC HYDROCARBONS

many of these are actually mixtures of chemicals derived from petroleum

gasoline	300	0.3	-45	FAST	Do not use. Extremely flammable. Usually contains benzene and organic lead compounds which skin absorbs.
n-hexane, normal hexane, commercial hexanes (55% n-hexane)	50	65-250	-7	FAST	Do not use. Potently toxic to nervous system. Causes disease similar to multiple sclerosis. Extremely flammable. Substitute heptane.
n-heptane, normal heptane, heptanes (mixture of isomers)	400	0.5-330	25	FAST	One of the least toxic in class. Good substitute for hexane and other fast-drying solvents.
kerosene	none	unk	100-150	VERY SLOW	Aspiration known to cause lung hemorrhage and chemical pneumonia.
mineral spirits, Stoddard solvent and similar petroleum fractions	100	1-30	>100-	SLOW	Some fractions contain significant amounts of aromatic hydrocarbons.

SOLVENT CLASS	TLV-TWA ppm	OT ppm	FP F°	ER	COMMENTS
VM & P naphtha, benzine, paint thinner	300	1-40	20-40	MED.	One of the least toxic in class. Good substitute for turps. "Odorless" paint thinner has toxic aromatic hydrocarbons removed.
AROMATIC HYDROCARBONS					a hazardous class, try to avoid.
benzene, benzol	1	0.1-120	12	MED.	Do not use. A cancer agent. Causes leukemia. Skin absorbs.
ethyl benzene, ethyl benzol, phenyl ethane	100	0.1-2.5	59	SLOW	Eye irritation begins at the Threshold Limit Value.
styrene, vinyl benzene, phenyl ethylene	50	.001-60	90	SLOW	Try to avoid. Suspect cancer agent. Skin absorbs.
toluene, toluol, methyl benzene, phenyl methane	100	.02-70	40	MED.	Highly narcotic. Causes liver and kidney damage.

	100	.08-40	81-90	SLOW	
xylene, xylol, dimethyl benzene	100	.08-40	81-90	SLOW	Highly narcotic. Causes liver and kidney damage. Stomach pain often reported by those exposed.

CHLORINATED HYDROCARBONS

Experts suspect all common members of class may cause cancer. Avoid.

carbon tetrachloride	5	2-700	*	FAST	Do not use. Cancer agent. Severe liver damage and death result when combined with alcohol. Skin absorbs.
chloroform	10	50-300	*	FAST	Do not use. Suspect cancer agent.
methylene chloride, dichloromethane	50	160-230	*	FAST	Avoid. Suspect cancer agent. Metabolizes to form carbon monoxide in blood. Stresses heart, causes irregular heart beat.
1,1,1-trichloroethane, methyl chloroform	350	16-715	*	FAST	Causes irregular heart beat, heart arrest. Cancer studies underway.
trichloroethylene	50	0.5-165	*	MED.	Suspect cancer agent. Causes irregular heart beat.

* these solvents do not have typical flash points. They dissociate with heat or ultraviolet radiation to form toxic gases such as phosgene.

SOLVENT CLASS	TLV-TWA ppm	OT ppm	FP F°	ER	COMMENTS
perchloroethylene, tetrachloroethylene, perc	50	2-47	*	MED.	Suspect cancer agent. Irregular heart beat, liver damage, flushing after alcohol consumption.
ESTERS/ACETATES					One of least toxic classes
methyl acetate	200	0.2 42	14	FAST	
ethyl acetate	400	.01-50	24	FAST	Least toxic in class.
isoamyl acetate, banana oil	100	.001-1	64	MED.	Use for respirator fit testing.
ETHERS					Do not use. Extremely flammable. Forms explosive peroxides with air.
GLYCOL ETHERS (CELLOSOLVES) and their acetates					Try to avoid, especially if planning a family
cellosolve, 2-ethoxyethanol, ethyl cellosolve, ethylene glycol monoethyl ether	5	1.3-2.7	110	SLOW	Reproductive hazard for both men and women. Affects blood. Skin absorbs.

methyl cellosolve, 2-methoxyethanol, ethylene glycol monomethyl ether	5	0.4-2.3	102	SLOW	Same as above. Skin absorbs.
butyl cellosolve, 2-butoxyethanol, ethylene glycol monobutyl ether	25	0.1-0.5	141	SLOW	Same as above except not as well studied and may be less toxic. Skin absorbs.
di- and tri-ethylene and propylene glycol ethers and their acetates					There are many more members of this class whose hazards are not well-studied. Experts suspects many are reproductive hazards.

KETONES

					Toxicity of this class varies widely.
acetone, dimethyl ketone, 2-propanone	750	0.1-690	-4	FAST	Highly flammable. Least toxic in the class.
methyl ethyl ketone, (MEK), 2-butanone	200	0.3-85	16	FAST	
methyl butyl ketone, (MBK)	5	.07-.09	77	MED.	Do not use. Causes permanent nerve damage.
methyl isobutyl ketone, (MIBK)	50	.01-16	64	MED.	

SOLVENT CLASS	TLV-TWA ppm	OT ppm	FP F°	ER	COMMENTS
MISCELLANEOUS					
dimethyl formamide (DMF)	10	0.1-100	136	SLOW	Avoid if possible. Skin absorbs.
limonene, d-limonene, citrus oil, citrus turps,menthadiene, cyclohexene	none	unk.	unk.	VERY SLOW	Acutely toxic to rats by ingestion. Pleasant citrus odor has caused children to ingest it. No data on toxicity by inhalation. A natural pesticide. Probably safer than turpentine.
morpholine	20	.01-1	100	SLOW	Avoid if possible. Skin absorbs.
turpentine	100	50-200	95	SLOW	Causes allergies, e.g., dermatitis, asthma, kidney and bladder damage. Substitute: odorless paint thinner.

Footnote: The EVAPORATION RATE is the ratio of time required to evaporate a measured volume of a solvent to the time required to evaporate an equal volume of a reference solvent (usually butyl acetate or ethyl ether) under identical condition of temperature, pressure, air movement, etc. Your Material Safety Data Sheets may not list ERs as FAST, MEDIUM and SLOW, but may provide the rate. In this case you must check to see which reference solvent is used and compare the rate to the following:

WHEN ETHYL ETHER   = 1.0
    < 3.0   = FAST
    3.0-9.0 = MEDIUM
    > 9.0   = SLOW

WHEN BUTYL ACETATE   = 1.0
    > 3.0   = FAST
    0.8-3.0 = MEDIUM
    < 0.8   = SLOW

CHAPTER

10 *PIGMENTS AND DYES*

C olor is the basic element of many arts. And in most arts, color is obtained through the use of pigments and dyes.

WHAT ARE PIGMENTS AND DYES?

The origins of pigments and dyes are lost in antiquity, although we know that both sprang from common natural products such as berries, roots, minerals, and insects. When mauve, the first synthetic dye, was discovered in 1856, it catalyzed the development of the whole organic chemical industry. Since then a host of synthetic chemical dyes and pigments have been created.

Often the distinction between pigments and dyes is based on usage and physical properties rather than on chemical constitution. The principle characteristic of a pigment which distinguishes it from a dye is that it is substantially insoluble in the medium in which it is used. In fact, there are numerous instances in which the same chemical product serves as either a dye or a pigment. Thus it is often difficult to understand how various types of colorants are classified.

PIGMENT AND DYE CLASSIFICATION

Companies selling paints, inks, pigments and dyes list colors in many ways, sometimes using traditional names (Prussian blue, Mars brown etc.), simple colors (white, red, etc.), and sometimes fanciful names designed to attract customers (peacock blue). As a result, it is almost impossible to know the actual color chemicals to which these names refer.

One answer to this identification problem is to prevail upon dye and paint manufacturers and distributors to reveal their products' internationally accepted Color Index (C. I.) names and/or numbers. All but a handful of commercial pigments and dyes are assigned these identifying names and/or numbers. Many responsible manufacturers of fine arts products already provide this service for customers.

Another way to identify some dyes and pigments is by their Chemical Abstracts Service numbers (see page 47). However, not all pigments and dye have Chemical Abstracts Service numbers.

PIGMENTS AND THEIR HAZARDS

The hazards of pigments have been known since 1713 when Ramazzini described illnesses associated with pigment grinding and painting. Many of the pigments used then are still among the several hundred pigments found in art and craft products today. Table 6 lists composition, Color Index name and number, and hazard information for about 140 artists pigments. Most of the pigments you use should be listed somewhere in this table.

All of the artists' pigments in Table 6 also can be classified either as inorganic or organic chemicals.

INORGANIC PIGMENTS come from the earth (ochres, for example), or they are manufactured from metals or minerals (like lead white or cerulean blue). These pigments have been used for many years and their toxic effects are fairly well known. The lead-containing colors are especially toxic and have a long history of causing poisoning. For this reason they are banned in consumer wall paints. But artists' paints and inks, boat paints, automobile paints, and metal priming paints may still employ them.

ORGANIC PIGMENTS are either from natural sources such as Alizarin crimson from madder root, or they are synthesized from organic chemicals. Examples of synthetic pigments include phthalo blue and the fluorescent colors.

There are hundreds of organic pigments used in art materials. Most of the natural organic pigments are not particularly toxic. Only a small percentage of the synthetic pigments have been studied for toxicity or long-term hazards. Of those which have been studied, some have been shown to be toxic, some are not toxic, and some cause cancer in animals. Some synthetic pigments also are hazardous because they contain highly toxic impurities such as cancer-causing PCBs. (These impurities, polychlorinated biphenyls, are unwanted side-products created during manufacture.)

Some pigments are related to the chemical "benzidine" which is known to cause bladder cancer. Benzidine pigments and dyes may also cause this disease. Recent epidemiological studies of artist painters and industrial painters found elevated incidence of diseases, especially bladder cancer.[1]

DYES AND THEIR HAZARDS

NATURAL DYES. Some natural organic dyes such as indigo and various plant and animal extracts are still in use today. Although some natural dyes are hazardous, there are many plant and vegetable materials which are safe enough even for children to use. However, craft dyes sold today usually are synthetic chemical dyes.

SYNTHETIC DYES. The very first synthetic dyes were made from a chemical called aniline which was derived from coal tar. Some manufacturers still call their dyes "aniline" or "coal tar" dyes. However, highly toxic aniline has been replaced for the most part with safer chemicals in the manufacture of this type of dye (azine type). Still, the term "aniline" is used by some dye-sellers to refer to all dyes with some similar (azine) components, and by others to refer to all types of synthetic dyes (even nonazine types). As it is used by dye-sellers today, the term "aniline" is not very meaningful. It is more useful to refer to dyes by their class.

DYE CLASSES. Chemically, dyes can be separated into classes. Each class reacts with certain fibers in certain ways. For example, "direct dyes" are used for cotton, linen, and rayon, and they usually need to be applied using hot water baths containing salt to react properly with the fabrics.

1. Miller, Barry A., Silverman, D.T., Hoover, R.N., Blair, A. "Cancer Risk among Artistic Painters." *American Journal of Industrial Medicine*, 1986; 9:281-287. See also Miller, Barry A., and Blair, Aaron. "Cancer Risks Among Artists." Submitted for publication to *Leonardo (Journal of the International Society for the Arts, Sciences and Technology)*, New York, 1989; and "Occupational Risks of Bladder Cancer in the United States: 1. White Men," *Journal of the National Cancer Institute*, Vol. 81, No. 19, Oct. 4, 1989.

Dyes in the same class usually have some hazards in common, but in addition they may—and usually do—possess some individual hazards. This is because dyes in the same class bind themselves to fibers in the same way chemically, so the hazards related to the fiber-binding part of the dye molecule are similar within each class of dye. But the rest of the molecule may vary from dye to dye and its effects on health may vary correspondingly. Table 7 lists the hazards of some classes of dyes.

DYE HAZARDS. Industrial experience has demonstrated tragically that many dyes can harm those who use them. Some can damage the blood's ability to carry oxygen (methemoglobinemia), others cause severe allergies, produce birth defects, and so on.

One group of dyes (those related to the chemical benzidine) have been shown to cause bladder cancer (see Organic Pigments above). In order to help you avoid using these dyes, a complete list of benzidine-congener dyes by their Color Index is provided in Table 8.

The hazards of most dyes, however, are unknown because only a few of the several thousand commercial dyes have been tested for long-term effects.

Food dyes, however, have been more thoroughly tested. It is interesting that of nearly 200 food dyes available in 1960, only ninety are still considered safe enough for food, drugs, or cosmetics. Prudence dictates handling all dyes cautiously.

EXPOSURE TO PIGMENTS AND DYES

Pigments or dyes are easier to use safely once they are mixed with water or oil as in paints and inks. Artists should try to avoid using pigments and dyes in the raw, powdered state because their dusts can be inhaled or they can contaminate hands and clothing. Examples of artists who may be exposed in this way include art conservators and painters who mix their own paints and textile dyers who buy dye powders and mix them into baths.

Rules for Working with Raw Pigments and Dyes

1. Try to use techniques which employ premixed paints and liquid dyes.

2. Identify your pigments and dyes. Only use materials for which Material Safety Data Sheets are available. Avoid purchasing materials from

companies which do not also provide Chemical Abstract Service numbers and/or Color Index names and numbers.

3. Never use techniques which raise dust such as sprinkling dry colors onto textiles or paper.

4. Weigh out, slurry, mix, or handle pigments and dyes only in local exhaust ventilation or in a glove box (see figure 14).

5. Avoid skin contact with pigments and dyes by wearing gloves or using barrier creams. Should skin stains occur, never use bleach or solvents to remove them. (Bleaches are especially hazardous because they may break complex colorant molecules in the skin into more toxic components.)

6. Wear protective clothing including a full length smock, shoes, and hair covering (if needed). Leave these garments in the studio to avoid bringing dusts home. Wash clothes frequently and separately from other clothes.

7. Clean the studio properly. Work on easy-to-clean surfaces and wipe up spills immediately. Wet mop or sponge surfaces and floors. Do not sweep.

8. Practice good hygiene and do not eat, smoke, or drink in the studio.

9. Keep containers of pigments and dyes closed at all times when not using them.

10. If lead-containing pigments are used, blood tests for lead should be done regularly (at least once a year).

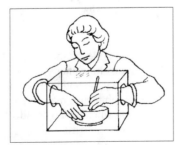

Fig. 14. Glove Box for Controlling Dust from Powdered Materials

TABLE 6	**Pigments Used in Paints and Inks**

Note: This table is not a complete list of all paint and ink pigments, but covers the more common ones. The lists of common names is also far from complete. Most pigments and dyes have dozens of names and often these names apply to more than one pigment.

COLOR INDEX NAME NUMBER COMMON NAMES	INGREDIENTS	TOXIC PROPERTIES
BLACK PIGMENTS (P.BLACK)		
P.BLACK 6 and 7 77266 carbon black channel black lampblack	carbon	Considered carcinogenic due to contamination with cancer-causing impurities.
P.BLACK 8 (two types) 77268 birch black blue black soft black vegetable black vine black willow black	carbon (50-90%) and minerals	No significant hazards
mineral black black chalk Davy's grey	carbon(15-85%) and silicates or iron oxides	No significant hazards.
P.BLACK 9 77267 animal black bone black Frankfurt black ivory black	carbon from charred animal bones	No significant hazards.
P.BLACK 10 77265 graphite plumbago stove black	graphite	Synthetic graphite can cause black lung after years of heavy inhalation. Natural graphite also may contain free silica which could cause silicosis.

P.BLACK 11
77499
    black iron oxide
    magnetic oxide
    mineral black
    natural black
	iron oxide (Fe_3O_4)
	some ores contain
	manganese and
	other impurities
		No significant hazards unless
		contaminated with toxic
		impurities. Often mixed
		with P.BLACK 14.

P.BLACK 14 77728 manganese black	manganese di-oxide	See manganese in Table 10.
P. BLACK 19 77017	grey hydrated aluminum silicate	No significant hazards.

P.BLACK 26
77494
    manganese ferrite
    black
	manganese and
	iron spinel*
		See manganese in Table 10.

P.BLACK 27
77502
    iron cobalt
    chromite black
	iron, cobalt,
	and chrome
	spinel*
		See cobalt, chrome in Table
		10.

P.BLACK 28
77428
    copper chromite
    black
	copper and
	chrome spinel*
		See copper, chrome in Table
		10.

P.BLACK 29 77498 iron cobalt black	iron and cobalt spinel*	See cobalt in Table 10.

77050 (no name)
    antimony black
    black lead
	a black form of
	antimony sulfide
	(Sb_2S_3)
		See antimony in Table 10.
		See sulfides in Table 11.

NATURAL BLACK 3 75290 logwood	hematoxylin from wood	Large amounts could poison.

SOLVENT BLACK 7
    acid black 2
    nigrosine black
	a nigrosine dye	Commonly contain nitro-
		benzene and other impuri-
		ties. May cause allergies
		and dermatitis.

*spinels are natural or synthetic oxides used as both pigments and ceramic colorants. Most are vary stable at high temperatures. Their solubility in body fluids has not been well studied.

104

BLUE PIGMENTS (P.BLUE)

P.BLUE 1 42595:2 Victoria pure blue B	organic chemical pigment	Low acute toxicity. Related chemically to a carcinogenic dye.
P.BLUE 2 44045:2 Victoria blue B	organic chemical pigment	Unknown. Chemically related to a carcinogenic dye.
P.BLUE 3 42140:1 Peacock blue R	organic chemical pigment	Unknown. Chemically related to a carcinogenic dye.
P.BLUE 10 44040:2 Victoria Blue	organic chemical pigment	Unknown. Chemically related to a carcinogenic dye.

P.BLUE 15
74160
  phthalo blue
  thalo blue
  monastral blue
  Vulco fast blue
  Winsor blue
	copper phthalo-cyanine	Always contaminated with small amounts of PCBs (poly chlorinated biphenyls) and 3,3-dichlorobenzidine which cause cancer and birth defects.

P. BLUE 16 74100	metal-free phthalo-cyanine	See above.
P.BLUE 17:1 74200:1 74180:1	sulfonated phthalocyanine	Same as above.
P.BLUE 21 and 22 69835 & 69810 indanthrene blues	complex insoluble anthraquinone vat dyes	Low acute toxicity. Anthraquinone and related chemicals currently being studied for long term hazards.

P. BLUE 24
42090:1
  brilliant blue
  erioglaucine blue
  peacock blue
	barium precipitate (lake) of an organic chemical dye.	Closely related to a dye that causes cancer in animals. See barium in Table 10.

P.BLUE 27 77510	ferric ferrocyanide	Only slightly toxic, but can emit highly toxic hydrogen

Berlin blue bronze blue Brunswick blue celestial blue Chinese blue iron blue lacquer blue Milori blue Paris blue paste blue Prussian blue steel blue toning blue Turnbull's blue		cyanide gas if exposed to hot acid, high heat, or strong ultraviolet light.

P.BLUE 28
77346
  cobalt blue
  cobalt green
  cobalt ultramarine
  Thenard's blue
	cobaltous aluminate of varying composition (blue to green)	See cobalt in Table 10.

P.BLUE 27 /28 mixture
77510, 77520, 77346
  Antwerp blue
  cyanine blue
  Leitch's blue
	cobaltous aluminate Prussian blue and/ or alumina (77520) mixtures.	Only slightly toxic, but can emit highly toxic hydrogen cyanide gas when exposed to hot acid, high heat or strong ultraviolet light.

P.BLUE 29
77007
  ultramarine blue
  ultramarine green
  ultramarine violet
	artifical minerals of sodium, aluminum and silica. Color range: blue, green, and violet.	No significant hazards.

P.BLUE 30
77420
  azurite
  blue malachite
  copper blue
  mountain blue
	azurite, a natural copper-containing mineral	See copper in Table 10.

P.BLUE 31
77437
  blue frit
  Egyptian blue
  Pompeian blue
	copper-calcium-silicate	See copper in Table 10.

P.BLUE 32
77365
  smalt
  Saxon blue
	potassium-cobaltous silicates of varying composition	See cobalt in Table 10.

P.BLUE 33 77112 manganese blue	barium and manganese salts	See barium and manganese in Table 10.

P.BLUE 34
77450
  copper blue
  covellite
	cupric sulfide	Irritating to skin and eyes. Highly toxic by ingestion. Can emit highly toxic hydrogen sulfide gas if exposed to high heat or acid. Also see copper in Table 10.

P.BLUE 35 77346 cerulean blue	artificial mineral of cobalt, tin, and calcium sulfate	See cobalt in Table 10.

P. BLUE 36
77343
  cerulean blue
  chromium
	oxides of cobalt and chrome	See cobalt and chrome in Table 10.

P.BLUE 60,64,65 69800, 69825, 59800 indanthrene blues	complex insoluble anthraquinone vat dyes.	Acute toxicity varies. Anthraquinone and related chemicals are being studied for long term hazards.

BROWN PIGMENTS (P.BROWN)

P.BROWN 5
15800:2
  BON browns
  arylide browns
	azo organic pigment	Unknown.

P.BROWN 6 & 7
77491,77492
  Caledonian brown
  Cyprus umber
  burnt & raw sienna
  burnt & raw umber
  burnt ochre
  metallic brown
  mineral brown
  Turkey umber
	variety of natural and synthetic iron oxides; may contain toxic impurities.	No significant hazards unless manganese or other toxic impurities present.

P.BROWN 9
77430
  Cassel's earth
  Cologne earth
  Ruben's brown
  Vandyke brown
	treated Cassel
	earth containing
	80-90 % organic
	matter plus iron,
	alumina and silica
		No significant hazards.

NATURAL BROWN 9 (2 types) no number assigned 1) sepia	cuttle fish ink, (melanin, calcium carbonate,& other misc. chemicals)	No significant hazards.
2) sepia	mixture of burnt sienna and lampblack	See P.BROWN 6 and P.BLACK 6.

GREEN PIGMENTS (P.GREEN)

P.GREEN 1,2,3, & 4
42040:1, 49005:1,
41100:1, 42000:2
  brilliant green
  aniline green
  malachite green
  emerald green
  fast green
  (many other names)
	insoluble precipi-
	tates of organic
	dyes
		Low acute toxicity expected
		on the basis of tests on PG 1.
		Long term hazards unknown.
		Closely related to dye which
		causes cancer in animals. If
		precipitated with barium,
		they can be highly toxic by
		ingestion. See barium in
		Table 10.

P.GREEN 4
42000:1
  brilliant green
  (many other names)
	hydrochloride of
	pigment 4 above
		Same as above.

P.GREEN 7
74260
  Monastral green
  phthalo green
  thalo green
  Segnale light green G
  Winsor green
	polychloro copper
	phthalocyanine
		Always contaminated with
		small amts of PCBs, etc. See
		P.BLUE 15.

P.GREEN 8 l0006	nitroso green	Low acute toxicity. Chronic hazards not well studied.
P.GREEN 10 12775 nickel azo green	chloroaniline/ nickel complex	Related to cancer-causing dyes. See also nickel in Table 10.

P.GREEN 12 10020:1 naphthol green B	barium precipitate of dye (Acid Green)	Low acute toxicity. Acid Green dye causes cancer in animals.

P.GREEN 15
77520 and 77600,
77601 or 77603
  chrome green
  bronze green
  Brunswick green
  cinnabar green
  Prussian green
  Victoria green
	mixture of PY 34 (lead chromate and P.BLUE 27)	See P.BLUE 27 above; lead and chrome in Table 10.

P.GREEN 17
77288
  chrome oxide green
  emerald green
  emerald oxide
  Emeraude green
	chrome oxide	See chrome in Table 10.

P.GREEN 18
77289
  Emerald oxide of chromium
  emeraude green
  Guignet's green
  oxide of chromium, transparent
  Viridian
	hydrated chrome oxide	See chrome in Table 10.

(permanent green deep is PG 18 reacted with barium sulfate)		

P.GREEN 19
77335
  cobalt green
  Rinnman's green
  Saxony green
  zinc green
	calcined cobalt, zinc, and alumina	See cobalt and zinc in Table 10.

P.GREEN 20 no number verdigris	copper dibasic acetate	See copper in Table 10.

P.GREEN 21
77410
  emerald green
  English green
	cupric aceto-arsenite	See arsenic and copper in Table 10.

Paris green Schweinfurt green Veronese green		
P.GREEN 22 77412 Sheele's green	same as above (historically cupric arsenite)	See Pigment Green 21.

P.GREEN 23
77009
  green earth
  burnt green earth
  Verona green
  Veronese brown
	hydrous iron, mag-
	nesium, aluminum,
	and potassium
	silicates. A variety of
	minerals, e.g.,
	glauconite &
	celedonite.
		No significant hazards for
		most of the minerals. Some
		forms of celedonite are in
		needle/fibrous form.

P.GREEN 24 77013 ultramarine green	mineral of sodium, aluminum, silica and sulfur	No significant hazards. See P.BLUE 29.

P.GREEN 36
74160
  yellow green
  Prussian green
	chlorinated and
	brominated phthalo-
	cyanine (also may
	be mix of P.BLUE 15
	and P.GREEN 7).
		See P. BLUE 15.

P. GREEN 36 (old usage) no number assigned Prussian green	mixture of gamboge (a yellow tree resin) and various pigments.	Unknown. Not used much today.
HOOKER'S GREEN	now mixtures of various pigments	Hazards depend on pig- ments used.

ORANGE PIGMENTS (P.ORANGE)

P.ORANGE 1, 2, & 5
11725, 21060, 12075
  hansa orange
  dinitro- or ortho-
    aniline orange
	insoluble azo dyes	Low acute toxicity. Long
		term hazards generally un-
		studied. PO 5 is a suspect
		carcinogen and mutagen.

P.ORANGE 13
21110
  benzidine orange
  Segnale light
    orange PG
	insoluble azo dye	May cause cancer, particu-
		larly bladder cancer

P.ORANGE 17 & 17:1 15510:1, 15510:2 Persian orange	barium precipitate (lake) of an azo dye	Low acute toxicity. Long term hazards unknown. See barium in Table 10.
P.ORANGE 20 77202, 77199 cadmium orange cadmium yellow	cadmium sulfide and cadmium selenide, other cadmium salts	Highly toxic by ingestion. Can emit highly toxic hydrogen sulfide gas if exposed to high heat or acid. Also see cadmium and selenium in Table10.

P.ORANGE 20:1
77202:1
   cadmium barium
    orange
	cadmium sulfide,
	cadmium
	sulfoselenide,
	and barium
	sulfate
		Same as above. See also
		barium in Table 10.

P.ORANGE 21
77601
   chrome orange
   American vermillion
   Chinese red
   chrome red
   Persian red
   Victoria red
	basic lead
	chromate
		See lead and chrome in
		Table 10.

P. ORANGE 21:1 see above	basic lead chrom- on a silicate base	See lead and chrome in Table 10.
P.ORANGE 23 77201 mercadmium colors	cadmium sulfide/ mercuric complex. Varies from orange to red (see P. Red 113).	Highly toxic by ingestion. Can emit toxic hydrogen sulfide gas if exposed to high heat or acid. Also see copper in Table 10.

P. ORANGE 45
   golden orange-
    yellow
   orange paste
	basic lead chrom-
	ate of a different
	particle size than
	P. ORANGE 21.
		See P. ORANGE 21.

P.ORANGE 48 & 49
no number assigned
   quinacridine gold
   quinacridine deep
    gold
	insoluble dye	Unknown.

P. ORANGE 60
no number assigned
  benzimidazolone
  orange HGL
	complex organic
	chemical
		Unknown.

P.ORANGE 62
11775
  benzimidazolone
  orange H5G
	complex organic
	chemical
		Unknown.

See also P.RED 101, Mars orange.

See also P.RED 104, Molybdate orange.

There are other organic chemical orange pigments, most of whose hazards are unknown.

RED PIGMENTS (NATURAL RED & P.RED)

NATURAL RED 3 75460 crimson	kermesic acid from coccus ilici insect	Unknown. Not in much use today.

NATURAL RED 4
75470
  crimson
  carmine
	carminic acid from
	coccus cacti insect.
	Carmine is laked
	with aluminum or
	calcium.
		Unknown. Not in much use today.

NATURAL RED 6, 8-12 75330 alizarin	alizarin or rubie- rythric acid from certain plant roots.	Low acute toxicity. See also P. RED 83.
P.RED 1 12070 para red	insoluble azo dye	Ingestion can cause cyanosis (ties blood hemoglobin in methemoglobin complex). A suspect carcinogen and mutagen.

P.RED 2,5,7,9,10,14,17,
22,23,63,112,119,146,
148,170,188,63:1,63:2
  arylide reds
  arylamide reds
  BON reds
  naphthol reds
	azo organic pigments	Those tested show low acute icity. Long term hazards generally unknown.

P.RED 3 12120 　hansa red 　segnale light red 　toluidine red	insoluble azo dye	Ingestion can cause cyanosis (ties blood hemoglobin in methemoglobin complex). Long term hazards being studied.
P.RED 4 12085 　aniline red 　permanent red 　D & C Red 36	chlorinated-p-nitroaniline (monazo class)	Low acute toxicity. Approved for drugs and cosmetics except around the eyes. May be weakly carcinogenic. May contain cancer-causing impurities.
P.RED 8,12 12335,12385 　segnale reds	insoluble monazo dyes	Low acute toxicity. Long term hazards unknown.
P.RED 38 & 41 21120, 21200 　pyrazolone reds 　& maroons	azo organic pigment	Low acute toxicity. Long term hazards unknown.
P.RED 48,48:1,2,3&4, 52:1&2 15865,15865:1,2,3&4, 15860:1&2 　BON reds, maroons 　arylamide reds 　segnale reds	calcium, barium and manganese salts of beta-hydroxy-naphthanoic acid azo dyes	Low acute toxicity. Long term hazards unknown. See barium and manganese in Table 10.
P.RED 49,49:1&2 15630,15630:1&2 　lithol reds 　segnale reds	sodium, barium, & calcium salts of a soluble azo pigment	Caused allergies when used in cosmetics. A suspect carcinogen. Some grades contain significant amounts of soluble barium—see Table 10. May also be contaminated with beta-naphthylamine which is a bladder carcinogen.
P.RED 53 15585:1&2 　red lake C	metal salt precipitate of an azo dye	Some grades contain significant amounts of soluble barium—seeTable 10.
P.RED 57,57:1&2, 59 15850, 15850:1&2 　lithol rubines 　segnale rubines	calcium salt of soluble azo dye	Low acute toxicity. Long term hazards unknown.

P.RED 60
16105, 16105:1
  acid red
  acid scarlet
  helio red
  permanent red
  pigment scarlet
  scarlet lake
	barium precipitate
	of azo dye, or an
	insoluble azo dye
		Low acute toxicity. A suspect
		carcinogen.

P.RED 81
45160:1
  day-glo red
  fluorescent red
  rhodamine red
	complex organic
	chemical containing
	tunsten, molybdenum
	and phosphorus.
		Low acute toxicity. Long
		term hazards not well stud
		ied. Some grades contain
		arsenic—see Table 10.

P.RED 83
58000, 58000:1
  alizarin
  alizarin crimson
  crimson madder
  madder lake
  rose madder
	natural or synthetic
	anthraquinone
	(1,2-dihydroxy-
	anthraquinone)
		Low acute toxicity. Long
		term hazards of anthraqui-
		none are being studied. May
		cause allergies.

P.RED 90
45380:1
  phloxine toner
  eosine
	eosine	Moderately toxic. Known to
		cause dermatitis when used
		in cosmetics.

P.RED 101
77015,77491,77538
  Indian red
  Mars red
  Mars orange
  red iron oxide
  Tuscan red
	iron oxides	No significant hazards.

P.RED 102
77015,77491,77538
  Persian gulf oxide
  red bole
  red ochre
  natural red chalk
  Spanish oxide
  Venetian red
	iron oxide, silica,
	alumina, lime,
	magnesia, and/or
	calcium sulfate
		No significant hazards. If
		large amounts were inhaled,
		it could cause silicosis.

P. RED 103
77601
  Derby red, Persian
  red, Vienna red,
  Chinese red
  Victoria red
  American vermillion
  chrome cinnabar
  Australian cinnabar
  garnet chrome
	Basic lead chromate.
	Different particle size
	from P. Orange 21
	and 45.
		See lead and chrome in
		Table 10.

P.RED 104
77605
  chrome vermillion
  mineral fire red
  molybdate orange
  moly orange
	lead chromate, lead
	sulfate,and molybdate
		See lead and chrome in
		Table 10.

P.RED 105
77578
  minium
  orange lead
  orange mineral
  red lead
  saturn red
	red lead (Pb_3O_4)	See lead in Table 10.

P.RED 106
77766
  Chinese vermillion
  cinnabar
  English vermillion
  scarlet vermillion
  vermillion
	mercuric sulfide
	(HgS)
		Insoluble form of mercury,
		but can be contaminated
		with soluble mercury salts,
		lead and other impurities.
		See mercury in Table 10.
		See sulfides in Table 11.

P.RED 108
77202
  cadmium red
  cadmium scarlet
  selenium red
	cadmium sulfo-
	selenide (CdS, CdSe)
		Insoluble form of cadmium,
		but commonly contaminated
		with significant amounts of
		soluble cadmium. See cad-
		mium in Table 10.

P.RED 113
77201
  cadmium vermillion
  red
	cadmium sulfide
	and mercuric sulfides
		Significant amounts of sol-
		uble cadmium may be pres-
		ent. See cadmium and mer-
		cury in Table 10.

P.RED 122 73915	complex organic chemical	Low acute toxicity. Long term hazards unknown.
quinacridone red (used to be P.Red 120)		

P.RED 123,149,179, 190
    perylene vermillion
    perylene red
    perylene maroon
    perylene scarlet
	complex organic chemicals	Low acute toxicity. Long term hazards unknown.

P.RED 144,166 no number assigned	azo organic pigment	Low acute toxicity. Long term hazards unknown.
P. RED 168,175,177, 178,188,192,194,207, 242, and others.	complex organic chemicals	There are many organic chemical reds.The hazards of most of these are unknown.

VIOLET PIGMENTS (P.VIOLET)

P.VIOLET 1
45170:1
    dayglow violet
    fluorescent violet
    rhodamine B
	rhodamine pigment	Low acute toxicity. May cause photosensitive dermatitis. A suspected carcinogen.

P.VIOLET 14 77360 cobalt violet	cobalt phosphate and/or cobalt arsenite	Today, PV 14 usually is all cobalt phospate—see cobalt in Table 10. Old PV 14 may contain the arsenite—see arsenic in Table 10.
P.VIOLET 15 77007 ultramarine violet	artificial mineral of sodium, silica, aluminum, and sulfur	No significant hazards. See also P.Blue 29 above.

P.VIOLET 16
77742
    fast violet
    manganese violet
    mineral violet
    Nurnberg violet
    permanent mauve
	manganese ammonium pyrophosphate	See manganese in Table 10.

P.VIOLET 19
46500
    quinacridone red
    and violet
	complex organic chemical	Low acute toxicity. Long term hazards unknown.

P.VIOLET 31 60010	chlorinated iso-violanthranone	Unknown.

isoviolanthranone violet		
P.VIOLET 38 73395	synthetic indigo derivative	Moderately toxic.
P.VIOLET 47 77363 cobalt lithium violet	mineral of cobalt	See cobalt and lithium in Table 10.
VIOLET 48 77352 red-blue borate cobalt-magnesium red-blue	cobalt magnesium borate	See cobalt in Table 10.
P.RED 101 mars violet	a purplish shade of iron oxide	No significant hazards.

WHITE PIGMENTS (P.WHITE)

P.WHITE 1 77597 Cremnitz white flake white silver white white lead ceruse	basic lead carbonate and small amount of barium sulfate or other extenders	See lead in Table 10.
P.WHITE 2 77633 basic sulfate white lead white lead	basic lead sulfate with small amount of zinc oxide	See lead in Table 10.
P.WHITE 4 (2 types) 77947 1) Chinese white permanent white zinc oxide zinc white	zinc oxide	See zinc in Table 10. Commercial pigments may contain small amounts of impurities including lead.
2) Leaded zinc oxide permanent white	zinc oxide and lead sulfate	See lead and zinc in Table 10.
P.WHITE 5 77115	zinc sulfide and barium sulfate	Barium sulfate is insoluble, but some pigments contain

Carlton white Grifith's patent zinc white Jersey Lily white lithopone Orr's zinc white ponolith	co-precipitate	soluble impurities. See zinc and barium in Table 10.

P.WHITE 6
77891
  titanium white
  titanium dioxide
  Titanox
	titanium dioxide, usually from the mineral rutile	No significant hazards.

P.WHITE 7
77975
  zinc sulfide
  zinc white
	zinc sulfide	Highly toxic by ingestion. Exposure to high heat or acid may cause emission of highly toxic hydrogen sulfide gas. See zinc in Table 10.

P.WHITE 10 77099 whitherite	barium carbonate	See barium in Table 10.
P.WHITE 11 77052 antimony white	antimony oxide	See antimony in Table 10.
P.WHITE 16 77625 basic lead silicate	lead silicate	See lead in Table 10.

P.WHITE 18 (2 types)
77220
  chalk
  calcium carbonate
  whiting
	calcium carbonate	No significant hazards.

77713
  magnesium carbonate
  magnesite
	magnesium carbonate	No significant hazards. In gestion of large amounts causes purging.

P.WHITE 19
77004
  aluminum silicate
  bentonite
  wilkinite
  alumina/china clay mixture
	various aluminum silicate clays	No significant hazards.

P.WHITE 20, 26 77019, 77718 mica pumice talc	various potassium silica, alumina and magnesium-containing minerals	Historically asbestos minerals were used. Some minerals may still contain asbestos impurities.
P.WHITE 21,22 77120 barium sulfate barytes blanc fixe heavy spar permanent white	barium sulfate from chemical and mineral sources	May contain soluble barium and other toxic impurities. See barium in Table 10.
P.WHITE 23 77122 gloss white alumina blanc fixe	aluminum hyroxide and barium sulfate	May contain soluble barium and aluminum. See barium and aluminum in Table 10.
P.WHITE 24 77002 aluminum hydrate	aluminum hydrate	No significant hazards.
P.WHITE 25 77231 gypsum alabaster plaster	calcium sulfate	No significant hazards.
P.WHITE 27 77811 quartz silica	silica	Inhalation of large amounts could cause silicosis.

YELLOW PIGMENTS (P.YELLOW)

P.YELLOW1*, 2, 3*, 4, 5, 6, 10, 73, 74, 75, 60, 65, 83, 97, 98 *toluidine yellows hansa yellows arylide yellows	insoluble azo organic pigments	Low acute toxicity expected on basis of tests on PY 1,5, and 74. Long term hazards unknown, but some related to cancer-causing dyes*.
P.YELLOW 12,13,14, 17, 20,55,83,	insoluble azo organic pigments	Low acute toxicity expected. PY 12 found negative on cancer tests. Others untested, but their relationship to blad-

		der cancer-causing benzidine dyes causes concern. Some are contaminated with PCBs (polychlorinated biphenyls) and 3,3-dichlorobenzidine which cause cancer.
P.YELLOW 31 77103 barium chrome barium yellow baryta yellow lemon yellow permanent yellow ultramarine yellow	barium chromate	See barium and chrome in Table 10.
P.YELLOW 32 77839 lemon yellow strontium chrome strontium yellow ultramarine yellow	strontium chromate	See chrome and strontium in Table 10. Most potent carcinogen of all chromium compounds tested.
P.YELLOW 33 77223	calcium chromate	See chrome in Table 10.
P.YELLOW 34 77600*, 77603** chrome yellow chrome lemon primrose yellow	*pure lead chromate or **mixed with lead sulfate	See lead and chrome in Table 10.
P.YELLOW 35,35:1 77117, 77205 cadmium yellow cadmium lithopone yellow primrose cadmium yellow	cadmium sulfide, sometimes precipitated with barium sulfate and zinc sulfide	Usually contains some soluable cadmium. See cadmium in Table 10.
P.YELLOW 36,36:1 77955,77956	zinc/potassium chromate complex	See chrome in Table 10.

P.YELLOW 37,37:1
77199
  aurora yellow
  cadmium yellow
  greenockite
  hawleyite
	pure cadmium
	sulfate or mixed with
	barium sulfate
		Usually contains some soluble cadmium. See cadmium in Table 10.

P.YELLOW 38 77878 mosaic gold	stannic sulfide	Toxic by ingestion. Exposure to acid or high heat may release hihghly toxic hydrogen sulfide gas. See tin in Table 10.

P.YELLOW 39 (3 types)
1) 77085
  arsenic orange
  realgar
  old king's gold
  orpiment
	arsenic trisulfide
	(As_2S_3)
		See arsenic in Table 10. Sulfide may produce highly toxic hydrogen sulfide gas on exposure to acid or high heat.

2) 77086	arsenic trisulfide or P.Yellow 37 mixed with P.White 4	Formerly an arsenic pigment, but replaced by cadmium sulfide pigment
3) 77600 King's yellow	lead chromate	PY 39 also used to refer to chrome yellow. See PY 34 above.

P.YELLOW 40
77357
  aureolin
  cobalt yellow
	potassium cobaltinitrite	Can tie up blood's hemoglobin to cause cyanosis (methemoglobinemia). See also cobalt in Table 10.

P.YELLOW 41
77588,77589
  antimony yellow
  Naples yellow*
	pure lead antimonate
	or mixed with
	zinc and bismuth
	oxides
		See lead and antimony in Table 10.

P.YELLOW 42,43
77492
  ferrite yellow
  Mars yellow
  ochre: domestic,
    French, and
    yellow
  raw sienna
  sienna
  yellow oxides of iron
	hydrated iron oxide
	and other iron
	compounds
		No significant hazards.

P.YELLOW 46
77577
  lead oxide
  litharge
  yellow lead
    monoxide
	lead oxide	See lead in Table 10.

P.YELLOW 53
77788
  sun yellow
  nickel titanium
  yellow
	nickel, antimony,
	titanium complex
		See nickel and antimony in
		Table 10.

P.YELLOW 57 77900 primrose priderite	nickel, barium, titanium complex	See nickel and barium in Table 10.

P.YELLOW 108
68420
  anthrapyrimidine
  yellow
	complex organic
	chemical
		Low acute toxicity. Long term
		hazards unknown.

INDIAN YELLOW NO C.I. NAME	magnesium salt of euxaanthic acid from mango-fed cows' urine	No significant hazards.

*Naples yellow today may be mixture of other less toxic and less expensive pigments.

METALLIC PIGMENTS (P.METAL)

P.METAL 1 77000	powdered aluminum	No significant hazards.
P.METAL 2 (4 types) 77400 1) copper powder	powdered alloy of copper, zinc, aluminum, and tin.	See copper, zinc, aluminum and tin in Table 10.

2) bronze powder or
  copper bronze
  powder
	powdered alloy of
	copper, zinc, and
	iron
		See copper and zinc in Table
		10.

3) dendritic copper	powdered alloy of copper, zinc, and traces of other metals	See above, plus any other metals present.

4) metalic copper	powdered copper	See copper in Table 10.
P.METAL 3 77480 　metallic gold	gold	No significant hazards.
P.METAL 4 77575 　metallic lead	lead	See lead in Table 10.
P.METAL 5 77860	tin	See tin in Table 10.
P.METAL 6 77945	zinc	See zinc in Table 10.

OTHER METAL ALLOYS can be powdered for metallic pigments and their hazards vary with their composition.

TABLE 7	The Hazards of Dyes by Class. Dye Classifications

Using general dye chemistry as the basis for classification, the Color Index lists 14 categories or classes of textile dyes:

1. acid dyes
2. azoic dyes
3. basic dyes
4. direct dyes
5. disperse dyes
6. fiber reactive dyes
7. vat dyes
8. oxidation dyes
9. mordant dyes
10. developed dyes
11. sulfur dyes
12. pigments
13. optical/fluor-
   escent brighteners
14. solvent dyes

The first seven of these classes are those most often used in textile arts. Although each individual dye is unique, some general observations can be made about their toxicity based on their class.

1. ACID DYES can be used to dye acrylics, wool, nylon, and nylon/cotton blends. They are called acid dyes because they are usually applied in acid solutions. The three most important chemical types of acid dyes are azo, anthraquinone, and triarylmethane. They appear in general to be of low acute toxicity, but the long-term hazards of many are unstudied. Some cancer-causing benzidine and food dyes have been identified in this class.

2. AZOIC DYES are used primarily on cellulosic fibers such as cotton, silk, and acetates. Allergic reactions to these dyes have been reported and some are considered carcinogens.

3. BASIC DYES can be applied to wool, silk, and some synthetics. Fluorescent dyes usually belong to this class. Allergic reactions to these dyes have been reported and some are considered carcinogens.

4. DIRECT DYES are applied from salt-containing baths to cellulosic materials such as cotton. These dyes usually present few acute hazards, but many are considered carcinogens. Most of the cancer-causing benzidine dyes are in this class. It is still possible to find benzidine dyes among direct dyes sold for art and craft purposes.

5. DISPERSE DYES are used primarily to dye water-repellant fibers such as polyester, nylon, and acetates. They are called disperse dyes because they disperse or absorb directly (colloidally) into the fiber. Some are applied at high temperatures. While many classes of dyes have caused dermatitis on direct skin contact, only disperse dyes have caused widespread dermatitis from contact with the finished product.

6. FIBER REACTIVE DYES are used most often with cellulosic fibers and wool. They can also be used with silk and nylon. The dyes derive their name from the fact that they form a chemical bond (covalent) with the fiber becoming an integral part of it. They are the fastest growing group of dyes and many are so new that they have not been assigned Color Index numbers. Industrial use has demonstrated the dyes' capacity to produce respiratory allergies and asthma. Their long term hazards are poorly studied. However, one chemical class of fiber reactive dyes (bromacrylamide) were shown to have a high percentage of positive mutagenicity tests in a 1980 study. Researchers suggested that a possible explanation may be that the small molecule size and the high reactivity of these dyes may enable them to react directly with genetic material (DNA). These tests indicate that cancer and birth defect studies should be undertaken.

7. VAT DYES are used primarily for cellulosic fibers, although some are suitable for wool and acetates. Lye or caustic soda are often used either in the bath or as a dye pretreatment. Pretreated vat dye powders are caustic and irritating to handle or inhale. Vat dyes also require an oxidation treatment after they have been applied. Some dyes oxidize in the air, but others require treatment with dichromate salts which cause allergies (see Chromium in Table 10). Some of the dyes themselves also can cause allergies. Certain vat dyes are sold as pigments. Using these is not recommended.

OTHER CLASSIFICATIONS

FOOD DYES are also a separate Color Index group, Most are acid dyes, but many other classes also are represented among Food Dyes. Most dyes in this class were selected in the 1950s because they were thought to be safe. Tests required for food additives have shown that many of these dyes cause cancer or have other toxic effects. Even dyes found safe for use in food may contain highly toxic impurities if they are not carefully manufactured. Art materials sellers who claim that their products contain "food dyes" should be required to tell customers whether the dyes are currently approved for use in food and whether they are "food grade" chemicals.

ALL-PURPOSE or UNION DYES are the common household dyes. These products contain two or more classes of dyes together with salt so that a wide variety of fabrics may be dyed. Only the dye which is specific for the material will be "taken" by the fabric. Until the early 80's, most all-purpose products contained cancer-causing benzidine dyes. Many of the new dyes are anthraquinone dyes whose hazards are not well-studied.

Table 8	Benzidine-Congener Dyes

Benzidine-Based Dyes	C.I. Direct Blue 6
	C.I. Direct Blue 6, Tetrasodium Salt
C.I. Acid Orange 45	C.I. Direct Brown
C.I. Acid Orange 63	C.I. Direct Brown 1
C.I. Acid Red 85	C.I. Direct Brown 1, Disodium Salt
C.I. Acid Red 85, Disodium Salt	C.I. Direct Brown 111
C.I. Acid Red 89	C.I. Direct Brown 154
C.I. Acid Red 97, Disodium Salt	C.I. Direct Brown 154, Disodium Salt
C.I. Acid Yellow 42	C.I. Direct Brown 2
C.I. Acid Yellow 42, Disodium Salt	C.I. Direct Brown 2, Disodium Salt
C.I. Acid Yellow 44	C.I. Direct Brown 31
C.I. Acid Yellow 44, Disodium Salt	C.I. Direct Brown 31, Tetrasodium Salt
C.I. Direct Black 4	C.I. Direct Brown 59
C.I. Direct Black 4, Disodium Salt	C.I. Direct Brown 6
C.I. Direct Black 38	C.I. Direct Brown 6, Disodium Salt
C.I. Direct Blue 158	C.I. Direct Brown 74
C.I. Direct Blue 158, Tetrasodium Salt	C.I. Direct Brown 95
C.I. Direct Blue 2	C.I. Direct Green
C.I. Direct Blue 2, Trisodium Salt	C.I. Direct Green 1

C.I. Direct Green 1, Disodium Salt
C.I. Direct Green 6, Disodium Salt
C.I. Direct Green 8,
C.I. Direct Orange 1
C.I. Direct Orange 8
C.I. Direct Orange 8, Disodium Salt
C.I. Direct Red 1
C.I. Direct Red 1, Disodium Salt
C.I. Direct Red 10
C.I. Direct Red 10, Disodium Salt
C.I. Direct Red 13
C.I. Direct Red 13, Disodium Salt
C.I. Direct Red 28
C.I. Direct Red 28, Disodium Salt
C.I. Direct Red 37, Disodium Salt
C.I. Direct Red 89
C.I. Direct Violet 1
C.I. Direct Violet 1, Disodium Salt
C.I. Direct Violet 22
C.I. Direct Yellow 20
C.I. Mordant Yellow 26
C.I. Mordant Yellow 26, Tetrasodium Salt
*C.I. 22120
*C.I. 22130
C.I. 22145
C.I. 22155
C.I. 22195
*C.I. 22240
*C.I. 22245
*C.I. 22310
*C.I. 22311
C.I. 22345
C.I. 22370
C.I. 22410
C.I. 22480
C.I. 22570
*C.I. 22590
*C.I. 22610
C.I. 22870
C.I. 22880
C.I. 22890
C.I. 22910
C.I. 23900

C.I. 23910
C.I. 24555
C.I. 30045
*C.I. 30120
*C.I. 30140
*C.I. 30145
*C.I. 30235
*C.I. 30245
*C.I. 30280
*C.I. 30295
C.I. 30315
*C.I. 35660
*C.I. 36300

o-Tolidine-Based Dyes

C.I. Acid Red 114
C.I. Acid Red 167
C.I. Azoic Coupling Component 5
C.I. Azoic Orange 3
C.I. Azoic Yellow 1
C.I. Azoic Yellow 2
C.I. Azoic Yellow 3
C.I. Direct Blue 14
C.I. Direct Blue 25
C.I. Direct Blue 25, Tetrasodium Salt
C.I. Direct Blue 26
C.I. Direct Orange 6, Disodium Salt
C.I. Direct Red 2
C.I. Direct Red 2, Disodium Salt
C.I. Direct Red 39
C.I. Direct Red 39, Disodium salt
C.I. Direct Yellow 95
*C.I. 23365
*C.I. 23375
*C.I. 23500
*C.I. 23630
*C.I. 23635
*C.I. 23790
*C.I. 23850
*C.I. 31930
*C.I. 37090
*C.I. 37120

*C.I. 37610

Dianisidine-based Dyes

C.I. Azoic Black 4
C.I. Azoic Blue 2
C.I. Azoic Blue 3
C.I. Azoic Coupling component 3
C.I. Direct Black 114
C.I. Direct Black 91
C.I. Direct Black 91, Trisodium Salt
*#C.I. Direct Black 118
*C.I. Direct Black 167
*C.I. Direct Blue 1
C.I. Direct Blue 1, Tetrasodium Salt
*#C.I. Direct Blue 100
*C.I. Direct Blue 15
C.I. Direct Blue 15, Tetrasodium Salt
*C.I. Direct Blue 22
*#C.I. Direct Blue 151
C.I. Direct Blue 151, Disodium Salt
*C.I. Direct Blue 156
*C.I. Direct Blue 160
*#C.I. Direct Blue 191
*#C.I. Direct Blue 218
*C.I. Direct Blue 269
C.I. Direct Blue 22
C.I. Direct Blue 22, Disodium Salt

*#C.I. Direct Blue 224
C.I. Direct Blue 225
C.I. Direct Blue 229
*#C.I. Direct Blue 267
C.I. Direct Blue 269
*#C.I. Direct Blue 76
*#C.I. Direct Blue 76, Tetrasodium Salt
*#C.I. Direct Blue 77
*C.I. Direct Blue 8
C.I. Direct Blue 8, Disodium Salt
*#C.I. Direct Blue 80
*#C.I. Direct Blue 90
*#C.I. Direct Blue 98
*#C.I. Direct Brown 200
*C.I. Direct Violet 93
*C.I. Direct Yellow 68
*#C.I. 23155
*C.I. 24140
*#C.I. 24175
*C.I. 24280
C.I. 24315
*C.I. 24400
*#C.I. 24401
*C.I. 24410
*#C.I. 24411
*C.I. 30400
*C.I. 37235
*C.I. 37575

*Dyes in production as of 1983.

"Metallized dyes" which have a metal ion added to their chemical structure. Industry claims these dyes are less hazardous. Since NIOSH does not now have enough information to determine whether the commercial grade metallized dyes are safer, the "#" should not be construed as NIOSH support for safety claims.

Credit: Preventing Health Hazards from Exposure to Benzidine-Congener Dyes, U.S. Department of Health and Human Services (NIOSH) Publication No. 83-105.

CHAPTER	*METALS AND*
11	*METAL*
	COMPOUNDS

Sculptors, smiths, jewelrymakers, stained-glass artists, and foundry workers use many metals. Ceramicists, glass blowers, and enamelists also use many metallic oxides and other metal compounds. Even painters and printmakers use inorganic pigments which are metallic compounds and powdered metal pigments (see Table 6, Pigments Used in Paints and Inks, page 102). Artists using these materials need to understand the nature of metals and their toxicology.

ALLOYS

Metals can be blended together into almost any combination. Sometimes nonmetallic elements such as silica and carbon are also blended with metals. These blends are called alloys. Casting metals, solders, welding and brazing rods, and sheet metals are examples of alloys. They are formulated to have certain properties such as a specific melting point, hardness, or color. In fact, almost all metals used in metalworking are alloys.

To assess metalworking hazards, then, it is necessary to know the composition of the alloys. For example, brass is an alloy which often contains lead and arsenic. Brass nonsparking tool metals contain cancer-causing beryllium. Silver solders and brazing rods often contain cadmium, antimony, and sometimes lithium.

Sometimes the common names of the products identify metals in an alloy. Examples include silicon bronze, manganese steel, or nickel silver. Never assume these names identify all the metals in the alloy. Always obtain Material Safety Data Sheets or complete ingredient information on metals.

CORROSION PRODUCTS

Metal oxides and other corrosion products are always found on metal surfaces. You can see the formation of such compounds when metals like lead are polished or cut to expose a clean shiny surface. After a few days, the metal will grow dull as a coating of lead oxide begins to form. Silver tarnishes as black silver sulfide deposits form.

This phenomenon explains why merely touching or handling some metals provides sufficient contamination of the skin to cause systemic damage if the worker transfers these contaminants to the mouth by eating or smoking before washing up.

Larger amounts of metal corrosion products are created if metals are allowed to weather (especially in polluted city air) or come in contact with acids or other chemicals which attack the metal. Cleaning or brushing corroded metal surfaces may be hazardous to workers if dust control is not provided.

The formation of a corrosion product due to contact with air is often called "oxidation." This process also occurs on the surface of particles of metal dusts and fumes.

DUSTS

Bronze powders and metal pigments are finely divided metal dusts. Some of these metal powders are explosion hazards in the presence of a spark or flame. Fireworks always contain metal powders.

Metal dusts also are created when metals are ground, polished, cut, and the like. These dusts can vary in size from large particles which drop immediately to surfaces, to fine respirable particles. In general, the smaller the particle size, the deeper the dust can be inhaled and the more toxic it is liable to be.

When inhaled, some metal dusts, such as lead and zinc, dissolve in a short time and are released into the blood stream. These metals then are free to travel throughout the body.

Other metals, such as cerium or titanium, dissolve very slowly. They will remain in the lungs a long time, perhaps a lifetime. Their effects are on the lungs themselves.

FUMES

Metal fumes are created when metal is heated to its melting point or above. Metal vapors form which oxidize and condense into tiny metal oxide particles (see page 31). Since metal fumes are exceedingly small particles, they can float for hours in the air, can settle as dust throughout a workspace, and when inhaled or ingested, they are likely to be absorbed by the body. Metal fumes are generally more toxic than metal dusts (see aluminum and manganese dust and fume Threshold Limit Values, Table 9, page 131 and Table 1, page 34).

Fumes from melting or cutting scrap or found metal may be a serious hazard if highly toxic metals are present in the alloys. In industry, many deaths from cadmium oxide fume have resulted from melting scrap.

METAL-CONTAINING GASES

Some metals, such as arsenic and antimony, emit highly toxic gases when in contact with acids. For example, this could happen when acid fluxes, cleaners, or patinas are used with arsenic/antimony contaminated metals or solders.

METAL COMPOUNDS

When metals combine with other elements, these other elements can be called "radicals." Common examples of radicals include oxides (O), carbonates (CO_2), and sulfates (SO_4).

OXIDES of metals are formed by corrosion processes or can be found in nature as metal ores. For example, iron oxidizes to form rust, but various iron oxides, from yellow ocher to red and black iron oxides, are found in nature. The toxicity of oxides will depend on the toxicity of the individual metal and how soluble the oxide is in body fluids. The effect of the oxygen molecule is negligible.

OTHER COMPOUNDS When metals combine with elements other than oxygen, these other elements may effect the toxicity of the resulting compound. For example, rust (Fe_2O_3-red iron oxide) is not very toxic, but iron arsenate ($Fe(AsO_4)^2 \bullet 6H_2O$) very toxic because it combines the hazards of iron with those of arsenic.

In some cases, combination with radicals alters the toxicity of a compound because it alters its solubility in body fluids. For example, barium carbonate ($BaCO_3$) is only slightly soluble, but releases enough highly toxic barium to be an effective rat poison. However, highly purified barium sulfate ($BaSO_4$) is so insoluble that we can swallow large amounts of it prior to X-ray studies of the digestive system.

Chemistry handbooks, artists' textbooks, and manufacturers of metallic compounds often claim many metallic compounds are safe because they are insoluble. They may even provide data on the solubility of these materials obtained from tests in solutions of acid.

However, it has been shown that some chemicals that are insoluble in acid solutions may be quite soluble in body fluids such as lung and digestive fluids. This is probably due to the combined actions of acids, bases, enzymes, and other physiological mechanisms. In addition, laboratory solubility tests are usually done on very pure chemicals. The chemicals used in art are often highly impure and contaminated.

For these reasons, it is prudent to consider all compounds containing toxic metals or radicals as potentially toxic. Table 10, Metal and Metal Compounds, page 133, lists the hazards of various metals, oxides and other compounds. Table 11 lists the hazards of common radicals.

EXPOSURE STANDARDS

The American Conference of Governmental Industrial Hygienists (ACGIH) sets Threshold Limit Values (TLVs) for exposure to airborne concentrations of metal dusts and fumes (see pages 32-33). Table 10 also lists these Threshold Limit Values when they are available.

The Threshold Limit Values for metals and metal compounds are usually expressed in milligrams per cubic meter (mg/m^3). Ten mg/m^3 is often referred to as a nuisance dust level. Even nuisance dusts may be harmful in concentrations greater than 10 mg/m^3. Threshold Limit Values which are lower than 10 mg/m^3 indicate the material is more toxic. Table 9 lists examples of Threshold Limit Value-Time Weighted Averages.

TOXICOLOGY OF METALS AND METAL COMPOUNDS

There are certain occupational illnesses which are especially associated with metals and their compounds.

TABLE 9	Examples of Threshold Limit Values For Metals

SUBSTANCE	Threshold Limit Value-Time Weighted Average (mg/m³)
calcium carbonate, whiting	10
aluminum dust	10
aluminum welding fume	5
manganese dust	5
manganese fume	1
tin metal and compounds	2
arsenic	0.2
soluble barium compounds	0.2
mercury compounds	0.1
cadmium fume & dusts	0.05
beryllium & its compounds	0.002

SKIN DISEASES. Handling metals usually does not harm the skin unless the metal is radioactive or unusually toxic. For example, beryllium can produce skin tumors if it penetrates broken skin, and arsenic is corrosive to the skin and causes skin cancer.

Some metals and metallic compounds also cause skin allergies. Many people are so sensitized to certain metals that even wearing metal jewelry will cause a reaction.

METAL FUME FEVER. Fumes of metals such as zinc, copper, magnesium, and iron, can cause metal fume fever. This disease resembles the flu. It usually onsets 2 to 6 hours after exposure and symptoms may include a fever, chills, and body aches. There appears to be no long term damage to the body from episodes of metal fume fever caused by metals of low toxicity. However, when toxic fumes such as cadmium are inhaled, the early symptoms may be similar, but serious consequences or even death may result.

NERVOUS SYSTEM DISEASES. A number of metals are known to affect the brain and other nervous system tissues. For example, lead, mercury, and manganese can cause effects ranging from psychological problems at low doses, to profound retardation and paralysis at higher doses. Chronic manganese exposure can cause a disease similar to Parkinson's disease.

REPRODUCTIVE EFFECTS. A number of metals are known to affect human reproduction at various stages. For example, the ability to impregnate or conceive may be impaired, birth can be complicated, end in miscarriage, or the fetus may be affected. Metals which are known to cause such effects include antimony, arsenic, cadmium, lead, manganese, mercury, and selenium. Many other metals are suspected of causing reproductive effects or are shown to cause them in animals.

RESPIRATORY SYSTEM DISEASES. Respiratory system diseases may be caused by irritation or allergy to metals. Occasionally, lung scarring (fibrosis) or staining (benign pneumoconiosis) are associated with inhalation of metal oxides such as beryllium or aluminum (see page 151).

SYSTEMIC POISONING. Once a metal or a metal compound is absorbed into the body, a great number of organs may be affected. Each substance has its own unique behavior in the body (see Table 10).

LEAD TOXICITY — A SPECIAL PROBLEM

In recent years, research has increased our understanding of lead toxicity. It is now known that even the small amounts of lead we absorb from air pollution and contamination of food and water are causing health effects in us all and reduced mental acuity in our children.

Although lead has been used in art for hundreds of years, it is time we reconsider its use. For even if we manage to set up ventilation systems that will remove lead fumes and dust from our studios, it will contaminate the environment. The soil where your lead dust has settled will remain contaminated forever.

In addition, government regulations regarding the use and disposal of lead are incredibly strict and getting tougher. There are special standards in both the United States and Canada for workplaces where lead is used. Most studios and schools simply cannot afford to meet these standards.

As a result, schools and artists are often operating "outside" the law. Being caught could result in citations or lawsuits. The fines and damages could be especially severe because the violations are willful—that is we know that what we are doing is dangerous and illegal.

The answer is to begin immediately to seek alternatives to lead just as big business is finding substitutes for lead, for solvents which destroy the ozone layer, and for fuels which cause acid rain. Industry often resists making these changes because the substitutes will not be exactly like the old materials, will cost more, be less convenient, and so on.

Each of us must decide if we will use these same arguments to justify our use of lead.

TABLE 10	Hazards of Metals and Metal Compounds

Key

TOXICITY divided into LOCAL, and SYSTEMIC effects:

LOCAL effects are restricted to the chemical's potential for damaging the skin, eyes or respiratory system on contact through its toxic properties such as alkalinity, sensitization, or effects on surface tissues. Mechanical effects of the chemicals will not be included. IT IS ASSUMED THAT READERS KNOW THAT ALMOST ALL FINELY DIVIDED CHEMICAL POWDERS CAN CAUSE MECHANICAL DAMAGE TO LUNGS AND EYES AND CAN DRY AND ABRADE SKIN.

SYSTEMIC effects are restricted to the effects on various organ systems such as blood, kidneys, lungs, and brain. These effects are seen if elements are absorbed into the body after contacting the skin, respiratory system, or digestive tract. Only digestive tract absorption of very small amounts such as from swallowing of material cleared from the lungs or hand-to-mouth contact will be noted. EFFECTS OF MASSIVE INGESTION ARE EXCLUDED.

TVL-TWA: the American Conference of Governmental Industrial Hygienist's Threshold Limit Values which are Time Weighted Averages for the eight hour work day. They are expressed in milligrams per cubic meter (mg/m3). 10 mg/m3 is considered a nuisance dust level. TLV-TWAs lower than 10 indicate a greater toxicity. Occasionally a TLV-Ceiling will be included. This is a level which should not be exceeded even for an instant.

Table lay out:

NAME OF METAL (CHEMICAL SYMBOL)	TLV-TWA (mg/m³)
common sources: name, (formula), synonyms	fume
LOCAL toxic hazards	dust
SYSTEMIC toxic hazards	other

ALUMINUM (Al)
Alumina (Al_2O_3), alumina hydrate,
  aluminum oxide, corundum, emery;
Alumina hydrate ($Al[OH]_3$), alumina
  trihydrate; a chemically bound,
  nonhazardous constituent of clays and
  many minerals.

Al fume: 5
Al & oxide dust: 10
soluble salts: 2

LOCAL: Inhalation of fume is associated with lung scarring disease. Inhalation of oxides is associated with a form of pneumoconiosis (Shaver's Disease).

SYSTEMIC: Generally assumed to have no significant hazards, but some experts suspect it plays role in some chronic diseases like Alzheimer's disease.

ANTIMONY (Sb)
Antimony oxide (Sb_2O_3), antimony trioxide,
  stibium oxide, Pigment White 11;
Antimony sulfide (Sb_2S_3), antimony black,
  Color Index (C I.) 77050;
Lead antimoniate ($Pb_3[SbO_4]_2$), Naples Yellow,
  C. I. Pigment Yellow 41 (see also Lead);
Stibine gas (SbH_3), antimony hydride.

Sb & compounds: 0.5
stibine gas: 0.5

LOCAL: Fume and dust are potent irritants to skin, eyes, respiratory tract. Can cause ulcers of skin and upper respiratory tract.

SYSTEMIC: Absorption causes metallic taste, vomiting, diarrhea, irritability, fatigue, muscular pain, and may result in anemia, kidney and liver degeneration. Has adverse reproductive effects. Almost always contaminated with significant amounts of arsenic.

ARSENIC (As)
Arsenic oxide (As_2O_3), white oxide,
  arsenic trioxide, arsenous oxide;
Arsenic pentoxide (As_2O_5), arsenic acid;
Arsenic sulfide (AsS or As_2A_2), arsenic
  disulfide, ruby arsenic or red arsenic
  glass, realgar;
Arsenic trisulfide (As_2S_3), arsenious sulfide,
  orpiment, C. I. Pigment Yellow 39;
Copper acetoarsenite

fume, dust, compounds:0.2
arsine gas: 0.2

$([CuO]_3As_2O_3 \bullet Cu[Cu_2H_3O_2]_2)$,
C. I. Pigment Green 21, Paris Green;
Arsine gas (AsH_3).

LOCAL: Corrosive to the skin, eyes, and respiratory tract. Can cause skin cancer.

SYSTEMIC: Absorption can cause gastrointestinal distress, kidney damage, nerve damage, cancer, and reproductive effects.

BARIUM (Ba)
Barium carbonate $(BaCO_3)$, whitherite,   soluble compounds:0.5
C. I. Pigment White 10;   Ba sulfate: 10
Barium sulfate $(BaSO_4)$, barite, barytes,
blanc fixe, C.I. Pigment White 21,
Permanent White, Lithopone
(with zinc compounds);
Barium chromate $(BaCrO_4)$, C.I.Pigment Yellow 31.

LOCAL: The fume and the carbonate are slight irritants.

SYSTEMIC: Absorption can cause muscle spasms and contractions, bladder contractions, intestinal spasms, ringing of ears, irregular heart beat, heart rate may be slowed or stopped.

BERYLLIUM (Be)
Beryllium oxide (BeO), beryllia;   Be & compounds: .002
Beryl $(3BeO.Al_2O_3 \bullet 6SiO_2)$, glucinum oxide.

LOCAL: Irritates skin and can cause swelling and ulceration of nasal passages. Penetration of broken skin (e.g., cuts from beryllium-coated glass of old fluorescent lights) has produced skin tumors.

SYSTEMIC: Inhalation can cause severe, permanent lung disease, called beryllosis, which can be fatal. This disease is often misdiagnosed as sarcoidosis. Absorption can cause liver and spleen dysfunction, and cancer.

BISMUTH (Bi)
Bismuth trioxide (Bi_2O_3), bismuth oxide;   none

Bismuth nitrate (Bi$[NO_3]_3 \bullet 5H_2O]$);
Bismuth subnitrate.

LOCAL: No significant hazards.* (see footnote)

SYSTEMIC: Causes physiological response similar to lead, but much greater doses are required.

BORON (B)

Boric acid (H_3BO_3);
Borax ($Na_2B_4O_7 \bullet 10H_2O$);
Boron oxide (B_2O_3), boric oxide;
  component of borosilicate frits, Colmanite,
  Gerstley borate.

borates (tetra & sodium)
anhydrous (no H_2O): 1
decahydrate ($10H_2O$): 5
pentahydrate ($5H_2O$): 1
boron oxide: 10

LOCAL: Irritant to skin, eyes, and respiratory tract.

SYSTEMIC: Nausea, stomach pain, vomiting, diarrhea, kidney damage, death. Lethal amounts of boric acid have been skin-absorbed from old burn treatment medications.

CADMIUM (Cd)

Cadmium sulfide (CdS), greenockite, cadmium
  yellow, C. I. Pigment Yellow 37;
Cadmium oxide (CdO);
Cadmium selenide (CdSe), (see also selenium).

dusts & salts: 0.05
TLV-Ceiling, fume: 0.05

LOCAL: Irritant to skin, eyes, and respiratory tract. Chronic exposure can ulcerate nasal septum and yellow the teeth.

SYSTEMIC: Acute inhalation of fumes can cause fatal illness whose early symptoms are similar to metal fume fever (flu-like symptoms). Chronic exposure can cause lung and kidney damage, anemia, and cancer. Some cadmium compounds are insoluble, but many pigment and ceramic grade cadmium compounds contain enough soluble cadmium to be very hazardous. Has adverse reproductive effects.

CALCIUM (Ca)

Calcium carbonate ($CaCO_3$), calcite, whiting;
Calcium sulfate ($CaSO_4$ or $CaSO_4, 2H_2O$),

Ca carbonate: 10
Ca hydroxide: 5

plaster, gypsum, C.I Pigment White 25;
common element in many ceramic chemicals.

Ca oxide: 2

LOCAL: No significant hazards.*

SYSTEMIC: No significant hazards.*

CERIUM (Ce)
Cerium oxide (CeO_2), ceric oxide, cerium
dioxide, ceria; component of cerite,
monazite, orthite.

LOCAL: No significant hazards.*

SYSTEMIC: Inhalation of fume causes a lung disease called cer-pneumoconiosis.

CHROMIUM (Cr)
Chrome oxide (Cr_2O_3), chromium (III) oxide,
chromic oxide, chrome green,
C. I. Pigment Green 17;
Chromium trioxide (CrO_3), chromium (VI);
chromic acid;
Potassium dichromate ($K_2Cr_2O_7$), potassium
bichromate (chrome VI);
Iron chromate ($Fe_2[CrO_4]_3$), ferric chromate,
(chrome VI);
Lead chromate ($PbCrO_4$), chrome yellow,
C. I. Pigment Yellow 34
(chrome VI-see also Lead).

metal: 0.5
Cr (II) compounds: 0.5
Cr (III) compounds: 0.5
CR (VI) compounds: 0.05
strontium chromate,
C. I. Pigment Yellow
32 : .001

LOCAL: Irritating to skin, eyes, and respiratory system. Can cause severe skin allergies and slow-healing ulcers of skin and nasal passages.

SYSTEMIC: Moderately toxic. Cancer is associated with chrome (VI) compounds and chrome fume. Some experts think all chrome compounds can cause cancer.

COBALT (Co)
Cobalt oxides: cobaltous oxide (CoO), black
cobaltic oxide;

metal dust and fume: 0.05

(Co_2O_3), or cobalto-cobaltic oxide (Co_3O_4);
Cobalt carbonate (Co_2CO_3).

LOCAL: Mild skin, eye, and respiratory irritant. Can cause skin allergies.

SYSTEMIC: Inhalation causes asthma-like disease, pneumonia, and lung damage. Absorption causes vomiting, diarrhea, sense of hotness.

COPPER (Cu)

Copper oxides: black copper oxide (CuO); red copper oxide (Cu_2O); Copper carbonate ($CuCO_3$), green copper carbonate.	fume: 0.2 dusts & mists: 1

LOCAL: Irritates and discolors the skin. Respiratory tract irritant. Repeated inhalation of dust can cause sinus congestion and ulceration, and perforation of the nasal septum. Contact with eyes can cause conjunctivitis and discoloration and ulcers of the cornea.

SYSTEMIC: May cause allergies in some people. Inhalation of fumes can cause metal fume fever (flu-like symptoms). Absorption can cause nausea, stomach pains.

GOLD (Au)

Metallic gold and mercury/gold amalgams (in some lustres); Gold chloride ($AuCl_3$), gold trichloride.	none

LOCAL: Metallic gold has no significant hazards. Gold chloride and other gold salts may be irritating and cause allergies.

SYSTEMIC: Absorption of salts can cause anemia, liver damage, and nervous system damage.

IRON (Fe)

Iron oxides: magnetic iron oxide (FeO), ferrous oxide; ferric oxide (Fe_2O_3), hematite, Indian red, C. I. Pigment Red 101; ferrosoferric oxide (Fe_3O_4), black iron oxide, C. I. Pigment Black 11;	fume: 5 soluble salts: 1

Yellow ochre ($2Fe_2O_3 \cdot 3H_2O$), limonite;
Iron sulfate ($FeSO_4 \cdot 7H_2O$), crocus martis.

LOCAL: No significant hazards by skin or eye contact.* Inhalation can stain lung tissues causing a disease called Siderosis. This condition is considered benign, but it can fog lung X-rays.

SYSTEMIC: Inhalation of iron fume can cause metal fume fever (flu-like symptoms). Iron sulfate is irritating and toxic due to the sulfate radical.

LEAD (Pb)

Lead monoxide (PbO), litharge,	dust & fume: 0.15
C. I. Pigment Yellow 46;	lead chromate: 0.05
Lead tetroxide (Pb_3O_4), lead oxide,	OSHA Permissible
red lead, mennige, minium,	Exposure Limit for all
C. I. Pigment Red 105;	lead compounds: 0.05
Lead carbonate ($PbCO_3$), white lead, cerusite,	Canadian standard: 0.15
C. I. Pigment White 1;	
Lead sulfate ($PbSO_4$), white lead,	
C. I. Pigment White 2;	
Lead sulfide (PbS), galena, lead glance;	
Lead frits, e.g. lead monosilicate, lead	
bisilicate, C. I. Pigment White 16;	
Lead chromate (also see chromium);	
Naples yellow (also see antimony).	

LOCAL: No significant hazards.*

SYSTEMIC: Highly toxic. Acute exposure can cause colic, convulsions, coma and death. Chronic exposure can cause anemia, and brain, nervous system, and kidney damage. It accumulates in bones and tissues and may cause problems for prolonged periods of time. A hazard to the unborn fetus and to reproductive capabilities of both males and females. Children are even more seriously affected than adults and at lower doses.

LITHIUM (Li)

Lithium carbonate (Li_2CO_3);	none for compounds
Lithium-containing minerals: lepidolite,	used in art.
petalite, spodumene, and amblygonite.	

LOCAL: Irritating to skin, eyes, and respiratory system.

SYSTEMIC: Absorption can cause symptoms ranging from fatigue, dizziness, and gastrointestinal upset to more serious complications including tremors, kidney damage, muscular weakness, vision and hearing disturbances, coma, seizures, and death. Lithium carbonate is used medicinally to control manic depressive personality disorders which demonstrates that even milligram amounts can cause effects.

MAGNESIUM (Mg)

Magnesium carbonate ($MgCO_3$), magnesite
   (mineral form of magnesium carbonate);
Magnesium sulfate ($MgSO_4$), epsom salt
   (hydrated form);
Magnesium silicate ($MgO \bullet SiO_2$-ratio variable);

magnesite: 10

LOCAL: No significant hazards.*

SYSTEMIC: No significant hazards except inhalation of large amounts of fume could cause metal fume fever (flu-like symptoms). Large ingestions cause laxative effect.

MANGANESE (Mn)

Manganese dioxide (MnO_2), black oxide of manganese, pyrolusite, C. I. Pigment Black 14;
Manganese carbonate ($MnCO_3$).

fume: 1
dust &
compounds: 5

LOCAL: Mild irritant to skin and respiratory tract.

SYSTEMIC: Chronic inhalation can produce a degenerative nervous system disease similar to Parkinsonism. Early symptoms include languor, sleeplessness, weakness, muscle spasms, headaches, and irritability. Can also cause metal fume fever. Has adverse reproductive effects.

MERCURY (Hg)

Mercuric sulfide (HgS), cinnabar, vermillion,
   C. I. Pigment Red 106;
Metallic mercury and amalgams.

inorganic
compounds: 0.1
vapor: 0.05

LOCAL: Skin irritation and occasional skin allergies have been reported.

SYSTEMIC: Mercury and some of its compounds can be absorbed through the skin and can form vapors at fairly low temperatures which can be inhaled. Early symptoms of absorption are psychic and emotional disturbances. Symptoms can progress to tremors, kidney disease, and nerve degeneration. Has adverse reproductive effects.

MOLYBDENUM (Mo)

Molybdenum trioxide (MoO_3);
molybosilicates ($Mo[SiO_2]_x$);
Molybdate Orange (solution of lead molybdates, sulfates and chromates),
C. I. Pigment Red 104

soluble compounds: 5
insoluble compounds: 10

LOCAL: Not well studied. Slightly irritating to skin and respiratory system.

SYSTEMIC: Appears to be of low order of toxicity.

NICKEL (Ni)

Nickel oxides: nickel monoxide (NiO), green nickel oxide; dinickel trioxide (Ni_2O_3), nickelic oxide;
Nickel carbonate ($NiCO_3 \bullet 2Ni[OH]_2 \bullet 4H_2O$), green nickel carbonate;
Nickel chloride ($NiCl_2$).

metal: 1
insoluble compounds: 1
soluble compounds: 1

LOCAL: Can cause very severe skin allergies, commonly called "nickel itch," which can lead to ulceration and chronic eczema. Also irritating to eyes and mucous membranes.

SYSTEMIC: Inhalation of fume is associated with cancer. Ingestion of salts is associated with giddiness and nausea.

NIOBIUM (Nb)

Niobium metal (called "Columbium" by many metallurgists), often contaminated with tantalum;
Niobium chloride ($NbCl_5$).

LOCAL: Eye and skin irritant. Effects not well-studied.

SYSTEMIC: Known to cause kidney damage. Other effects not well-studied.

PLATINUM (Pt)

| Platinum chloride ($PtCl_4$), platinum tetra-chloride, chloroplatinic acid; Platinum black (finely powdered metal). | metal: 1 soluble salts: .002 |

LOCAL: Skin contact with salts can cause severe allergies. Inhalation can cause nasal allergies and "platinosis," a severe type of asthma.

SYSTEMIC: Some lung scarring may occur from chronic inhalation. Ingestion hazards are unknown.

POTASSIUM (K)

| Potassium carbonate (K_2CO_3), pearl ash, potash; Potassium hydroxide (KOH), caustic potash; A common constituent of many ceramic minerals, e.g., potash feldspars. | K hydroxide: 2 |

LOCAL: No significant hazards.* The hydroxide and carbonate compounds are eye, skin, and respiratory irritants.

SYSTEMIC: No significant hazards.*

PRASEODYMIUM (Pr)

| Praseodymium oxide (Pr_2O_3). | none |

LOCAL: No hazards known.

SYSTEMIC: When absorbed may depress coagulation of the blood. Not much known about toxicity.

RHODIUM (Rh)

| Rhodium chloride ($RhCl_3$), rhodium trichloride. | metal: 1 insoluble compounds: 1 soluble compounds: 0.01 |

LOCAL: Related to platinum, but apparently not a skin sensitizer.

SYSTEMIC: Not well studied. Slightly carcinogenic in animals. $RhCl_3$ is a potent mutagen.

SELENIUM (Se)

Cadmium selenide (CdSe),
  C. I. Pigment Red 108;
  and Yellow 35 (see also Cadmium);
Selenium photographic toners.

compounds: 0.2

LOCAL: Irritant to eyes, skin, and respiratory tract. When compounds come in contact with moisture or acid, they may release hydrogen selenide gas which is a vastly more potent irritant.

SYSTEMIC: Its toxicity is similar to that of arsenic. Symptoms of over exposure include a tell-tale garlic breath odor. Most damaging to liver, kidneys, spleen, bone marrow, and thyroid. A suspect carcinogen. Has adverse reproductive effects.

SILVER (Ag)

Metallic silver;
Silver chloride (AgCl);
Silver nitrate ($AgNO_3$);
Silver sulfide (Ag_2S), niello;
Silver/mercury amalgams (see also Mercury).

metal: 0.1
soluble compounds: 0.01

LOCAL: Silver salts can stain skin, and irritate mucous membranes. Silver nitrate is very caustic and burns skin and has caused blindness when splashed in the eyes. Silver fume can deposit in lungs to cause a benign pneumoconioses which can fog X-rays.

SYSTEMIC: Black silver deposits can migrate in the body to permanently stain the whites of the eye and the skin in a benign condition called "argyria."

SODIUM (Na)

Sodium carbonate (Na_2CO_3), soda ash,
  washing soda;
Sodium bicarbonate ($NaHCO_3$), baking soda;
Sodium bisulfite ($NaHSO_3$), sodium acid sulfite;
Sodium metabisulfite ($Na_2S_2O_5$);
Component of many ceramic chemicals and minerals.

Na bisulfite: 5
Na metabisulfite: 5

LOCAL: No significant hazards.* Sodium carbonate is an irritant to skin, eyes, and respiratory tract.

SYSTEMIC: No significant hazards.*

STRONTIUM (Sr)

Strontium carbonate ($SrCO_3$) strontianite;
Strontium chromate ($SrCrO_4$),
C. I. Pigment Yellow 32;
Strontium sulfate ($SrSO_4$), celestine.

Sr chromate: .001
(see chromium)
none for the other
Sr compounds

LOCAL: No significant hazards.*

SYSTEMIC: No significant hazards.*

TANTALUM (Ta)

Tantalum chloride ($TaCl_5$);
Tantalum oxide (Ta_2O_5).

metal & oxide dust: 5

LOCAL: Industrial skin injuries have been reported. Not well-studied.

SYSTEMIC: Systemic poisoning has not been demonstrated. Not well-studied.

TIN (Sn)

Tin oxides: stannous oxide (SnO); stannic
oxide (SnO_2), cassiterite,
white tin oxide;
Tin chloride ($SnCl_2$), stannous chloride, tin
dichloride.

metal: 2
oxide & compounds: 2

LOCAL: No significant hazards* except the fume deposits in the lungs to produce a benign pneumoconioses which fogs X-rays. The chloride salt is a skin, eye, and respiratory irritant.

SYSTEMIC: No significant hazards* for most compounds used in art.

TITANIUM (Ti)

Titanium dioxide (TiO_2), titania,
C. I. Pigment White 6;
minerals containing titanium: rutile, illmenite,
ferrous titanite, perowskite;
Titanium tetrachloride ($TiCl_4$).

titanium dioxide: 10

LOCAL: No significant hazards.* The chloride is highly irritating especially in the fume form.

SYSTEMIC: Generally thought safe, but some experts think it may cause a type of pneumoconiosis.

TUNGSTEN (W)

Tungsten carbide (WC);
Tungsten trioxide (WO_3), tungstic oxide,
  tungstenic ochre, wolframic acid;
components of minerals: scheelite, wolframite;
component in some ceramic frits.

insoluble compounds: 5
soluble compounds: 1

LOCAL: No significant hazards* to skin and eyes. Slightly toxic to respiratory tract.

SYSTEMIC: No significant hazards to insoluble compounds.*

URANIUM (U)

Uranium oxides: uranous oxide, UO_2; uranyl
  oxide, UO3; triuranium octoxide, U_3O_8;
  component in uranite, pitchblende;
Uranium nitrate ($UO_2[NO_3]_2 \bullet 6H_2O$),
  uranyl nitrate;
"Depleted uranium," uranium isotopes except for U^{235}.

soluble & insoluble
compounds: 0.2

LOCAL: Radioactivity could effect skin to cause cancer. The nitrate is easily skin-absorbed. "Depleted uranium," is as radioactive as other uranium chemicals.

SYSTEMIC: Highly toxic, radioactive carcinogen. Absorption results in severe kidney damage.

VANADIUM (V)

Vanadium pentoxide (V_2O_5);
Many mason and ceramic stains.

dust and fume: 0.05

LOCAL: Highly irritating to skin, eyes respiratory tract. Heavy exposures have caused chemical pneumonia. Can cause allergies.

SYSTEMIC: Can cause anemia, kidney disfunction, gastrointestinal disorders, nervous system damage, and cough.

ZINC (Zn)

Zinc oxide (ZnO), chinese white,
C. I. Pigment White 4;
Zinc chloride (ZnCl$_2$), zinc dichloride;
Zinc chromate (ZnCrO$_4$•7H$_2$O).

fume: 5
Zn oxide dust: 10
Zn chloride fume: 1
Zn chromates: 0.01

LOCAL: No significant hazards.* The chloride is a potent irritant to skin, eyes, and respiratory tract.

SYSTEMIC: Inhalation of zinc fume can cause metal fume fever (flu-like symptoms).

ZIRCONIUM (Zr)

Zirconium oxide (ZrO$_2$), zirconium dioxide,
baddeleyite;
Zirconium silicate (ZrSiO$_4$), zircon.

Zr compounds: 5

LOCAL: No significant hazards.* Rare allergies to zirconium deodorant products have been reported.

SYSTEMIC: No significant hazards.*

*No significant hazards UNLESS COMBINED WITH RADICALS CONTAINING OTHER HAZARDOUS ELEMENTS. Radicals are elements or combinations of elements bound to the metal. For example, the toxicity of potassium hydroxide (KOH) is not caused by potassium (K-), but by the caustic hydroxide radical (-OH). See Table 11, hazards of Radicals.

TABLE 11	Toxic Effects of Common Radicals

A radical is an element or group of elements that combines with a metal to form a compound. Radicals may affect the toxicity, solubility, and other characteristics of metallic compounds.

CARBIDE radicals (-C, carbon) usually do not contribute to toxicity. Carbide radicals are found in some abrasives such as silicon carbide (SiC) and tungsten carbide (WC). Diamonds are also a form of carbon. Carbon dioxide or carbon monoxide may be given off if carbides or carbon-containing materials are heated or fired.

CARBONATE radicals (-CO_3) usually do not contribute to toxicity. Carbon dioxide and toxic carbon monoxide may be given off if compounds are heated or fired.

CHLORIDE radicals (-Cl) usually increase solubility, reactivity, and irritant qualities. Heating or firing may release highly irritating hydrochloric acid gas or chlorine.

CHROMATES (-CrO_4). See Chromium in Table 10, Hazards of Metals and Metal Compounds, page 137.

CYANIDE compounds (-CN) should be avoided because they are very soluble and toxic. When in contact with acids, heat, or gastric fluids, highly toxic hydrogen cyanide gas is formed. This gas stops the body's cells from receiving oxygen. The victim dies quickly of asphyxiation. Cyanides usually are not very irritating to the skin, but electroplaters who are repeated exposed to cyanide solutions often develop rashes and skin eruptions.

FLUORIDE radicals (-F) usually increase solubility, reactivity, and irritant qualities. Fluorides also may produce long-term toxic reactions. Chronic fluorine poisoning or "fluorosis" is seen among miners of cryolite and other fluorine-containing minerals. The disease consists of sclerosis of the bones, calcification of ligaments, mottling of the teeth, anemia, gastric, respiratory, and nervous system complaints and skin rashes.

HYDROXIDES (-OH) can vary from being very soluble to very insoluble. Soluble hydroxides are caustic and irritating to skin, eyes, digestive tract, and respiratory system.

NITRATES (-NO_3) are most often very soluble which usually makes the metals in nitrate compounds more available to the body. They are often highly toxic by ingestion. All nitrates are powerful oxidizing agents and some can explode when exposed to heat or flame. Potassium, barium, and other nitrates are used in fireworks. May emit highly toxic nitrogen oxide gases during firing or glass-making.

NITRITES (-NO_2) are usually very toxic and strong oxidizers. Avoid.

OXIDE radicals (-0) usually do not contribute to toxicity.

PHOSPHATES (-PO_4) vary greatly in solubility and toxicity. Heating or firing phosphates may release highly toxic phosphorus oxides. Large doses of some phosphates can disturb the metabolism.

SILICATES (-SiO_2) usually are not very toxic. Unlike silica (free SiO_2), silicates do not cause silicosis although some silicates cause other less virulent pneumoconioses (lung diseases). Naturally occurring silicates are often contaminated with significant amounts of free silica.

SULFATE radicals (-SO_4) usually do not contribute to toxicity. They may emit highly irritating sulfur oxides during firing or glass making.

SULFIDES (-S) of metals are often insoluble. Many are irritating to the skin and eyes. Many sulfides are highly toxic by ingestion because they react with gastric acid to produce hydrogen sulfide gas. They emit sulfur oxides on heating or firing. If water vapor is present, hydrogen sulfide may also be released.

SULFITES (-SO_3) and *BISULFITES* (-HSO_3) usually are moderately toxic. They may emit sulfur oxides as they degrade with age, or when heated.

CHAPTER

12 | *MINERALS*

Minerals are used in almost all arts and crafts. Examples include all sculpture stones, gemstones, all clays and most ceramic chemicals, most abrasives, many paint, ink, and pastel extenders, some pigments, refractory and insulating materials for high temperature equipment, and more.

NATURAL MINERALS

It took Mother Nature ages to make our minerals. And since Mother Nature was not concerned with "quality control," she allowed inclusion of impurities in most minerals. Organic materials such as coal or asphalt contaminate some fire clay minerals. Sedimentary clays often contain a variety of organic matter deposited by ancient lakes and rivers with the clay.

Inorganic materials also may contain minerals. Trace metal impurities in gemstones, for instance, often are responsible for unique colors. Mineral talc (talcum) deposits usually contain significant amounts of other minerals such as silica and/or asbestos. Mineral impurities often must be considered when assessing the hazards of naturally occurring minerals.

SYNTHETIC MINERALS

Mother Nature is not the only mineral-maker. For thousands of years, potters have converted minerals from one form to another in their fires and kilns. Now more sophisticated equipment is used to make minerals such as synthetic gemstones and mineral fiber insulation.

Synthetic minerals can be tailored to fit our needs. Some types of synthetic gemstones can be made to possess exactly the same chemical and physical properties as pure natural gemstones. Synthetic mineral fibers can be tailored to have the same insulating properties as natural asbestos.

It should not be surprising then, that many synthetic minerals have health effects similar to those of natural minerals.

CHEMICAL VS. MINERAL HAZARDS

Like all matter, minerals are made of chemicals. In most minerals, these chemicals are arranged in a crystal structure with a definite chemical composition. Artists need information on both chemical composition (chemical analysis) and crystal structure (mineral analysis) of these materials, because both may affect health.

Some minerals contain very toxic chemicals. These toxic chemicals can affect the body if they are soluble—that is are released from the mineral into body fluids.

The mineral's crystal structure also may affect health. For example, asbestos minerals are made of harmless chemicals such as magnesium and calcium silicates. Asbestos is not soluble (inert) and does not release these chemicals in the body. But the asbestos minerals have long needle-like crystals which can penetrate tissues and cause cancer.

SOLUBILITY OF MINERALS. To find out if toxic chemicals in a particular mineral are soluble in body fluids, solubility tests are done. These tests place the mineral in contact with acid and water. Such tests do not precisely relate to body fluid solubility because body fluids contain not only acids and water, but bases, enzymes, and other materials. And solubility may differ in various body fluids such as digestive juices and lung fluids. For these reasons, the actual solubility of most minerals in various body fluids is not known precisely.

Artists also should consider that many of the minerals to which they are exposed are fine powders or dust from abrasive processes. These fine particles present a very large surface area to body fluids from which toxic metals may be released. If these small particles are inhaled, they may be retained in the lungs for a lifetime, giving the body years to dissolve or incorporate them. In addition, natural minerals often contain some soluble impurities.

For all these reasons, minerals containing highly toxic metals such as lithium, barium, and beryllium should be treated with caution regardless of laboratory solubility data. They may be considered as metal-containing compounds and their potential hazards can be looked up in Table 10, Hazards of Metal and Metal Compounds, page 133.

INSOLUBLE OR INERT MINERALS. Certain minerals have been actually observed after years of exposure to body fluids and are known to be insoluble and inert. For example, once inhaled, asbestos fibers and silica crystals are known to remain essentially unaltered in the lungs for a lifetime. Inert minerals are often associated with specific types of illnesses.

TOXICOLOGY OF INERT MINERALS

Inert minerals usually are not very hazardous to ingest and when inhaled, they all seem to dry and irritate the lungs to some degree. Their major effects, however, usually involve chronic lung diseases.

These diseases occur precisely because the minerals do not dissolve or break down in the lungs. Instead, they begin to accumulate in the lungs. The diseases they cause fall into certain categories.

PNEUMOCONIOSES, (meaning "dusty lungs" in greek) are diseases caused by inhalation of inert materials. Each type of pneumoconiosis is identified by the name of the dust which caused it. For example, talcosis is caused by talc inhalation.

Different mineral dusts cause diseases of varying severity. There are two major categories of pneumoconiosis: fibrogenic and benign.

FIBROGENIC PNEUMOCONIOSIS. This is a disease in which the lungs are scarred by mineral dusts. Minerals such as asbestos and silica cause severe forms of the disease. It is untreatable at all phases, can progress even after exposure has ceased, and its severity can range from shortness of breath to disability or death. Typically, the disease results from small exposures to dust over many years. However, even short exposures may be hazardous. Only a few weeks of heavy exposure to silica flour (400 mesh) has caused workers to die of silicosis a couple of years later. This form of the disease is called "progressive massive fibrosis."

Dusts which cause less severe fibrotic diseases and require inhalation of greater amounts of dust include: kaolin (clay uncontaminated with silica), alumina, and talc (uncontaminated with asbestos minerals). The diseases these cause are called respectively kaolinosis, aluminosis, and talcosis.

BENIGN PNEUMOCONIOSES do not result in lung scarring. However, some will alter the appearance of diagnostic lung X-rays causing doctors to do unnecessary medical tests if the cause of the X-ray change is not known. It also may obliterate X-ray evidence of other lung diseases causing other conditions to go untreated.

Examples of minerals which can cause benign pneumoconiosis include a barium sulfate mineral, barytes (causes baritosis), and ochres and other iron oxides such as rouge and rust (causes siderosis).

LUNG CANCER AND MESOTHELIOMA (cancer of the lining of the chest, abdomen or heart) are caused by inert, microscopic, needle-shaped partices such as those of asbestos and synthetic mineral fiber insulation.

HAZARDS OF COMMON MINERALS

The type of damage a particular mineral causes depends on its unique characteristics. To complicate matters, some minerals exist in more than one crystal form. It is important to know about these forms to assess health risks and to comply with governmental exposure regulations. The minerals with which artists should be familiar include asbestos, silica, feldspars, and clays. For other minerals, See Table 13, Hazards of Common Minerals, page 157.

ASBESTOS causes asbestosis and is associated with a number of cancers including mesothelioma and lung cancer. Even ingestion of asbestos may be hazardous causing intestinal and kidney cancer as some needle-like fibers migrate through the body.

Asbestos comes in a number of mineral forms:

CHRYSOTILE—serpentine groups of mineral, white asbestos
AMOSITE—cummingtonite-grunerite minerals, brown asbestos
CROCIDOLITE—blue asbestos

AMPHIBOLE ASBESTOS—can be found in three mineral forms:
TREMOLITE
ANTHOPHYLLITE
ACTINOLITE

Each of the amphibole minerals comes in two forms: fibrous and non-fibrous. The hazards of the fibrous forms are comparable with other forms of asbestos, but the hazards of the nonfibrous forms is being debated. Some people believe that these forms are not truly asbestos and their dusts are far less toxic than asbestos. Others believe that nonfibrous amphiboles mill into sharp thin cleavage fragments which cause illnesses like those caused by asbestos.

The United States Occupational Safety and Health Administration has reviewed studies of nonfibrous tremolitic talc miners and believes that this talc can be associated with increased risk of cancer. The risk appears to be less than for asbestos workers, but they have indicated that they will continue collecting data on this finding to see if regulation is needed.

Exposure to all fibrous forms of asbestos already is regulated in both Canada and the United States. The United States Permissible Exposure Limit (PEL) is .2 fibers per cubic centimeter of air (f/cc).* Canadian standards vary, with the laxest regulations being in the asbestos-mining province of Quebec. Their standard is 5 fibers per cubic centimeter of air (f/cc).

Clearly artists are not equipped to do air sampling and regulate their asbestos exposures. Until all the evidence is in, artists probably should avoid exposure to all types of asbestos, both fibrous and nonfibrous. Children certainly should never use any asbestos-contaminated materials.

SILICA, or silicon dioxide (SiO_2), is one of the earth's most common minerals. When silica is bound in compounds or minerals, it is not usually hazardous. However, inhaling unbound or "free" silica can cause a serious untreatable lung-scarring disease called "silicosis." Recently, an elevated risk of lung cancer has also been documented in people with silicosis.

---

* A typical male doing light work will inhale about a cubic meter of air per hour. This would mean at 0.2 f/cc a worker would inhale 1,600,000 fibers during an eight hour period. Heavy work can triple these figures because more air is inhaled. Many experts feel this standard does not provide sufficient protection for workers.

Free silica occurs in various crystalline and amorphous forms:

CRYSTALLINE SILICA—all forms have the same chemical formula (SiO_2) but the crystal structures differ.

QUARTZ, common constituent of sand, flint, and other rocks.

CRISTOBALITE can be formed from heat conversion of quartz geologically or when fired. About twice as toxic as quartz.

TRIDYMITE has roughly the same origins and hazards as crystobalite above.

AMORPHOUS SILICA or NON-CRYSTALLINE SILICA—the arrangement of silicon dioxide molecules is random and unorganized, whether natural or synthetic in origin. The synthetic silicas are manufactured and promoted as "safe" silica. There is considerable debate about their safety and many experts recommend handling them with the same precautions used for free silica. A separate Threshold Limit Value is expected to be set by the ACGIH in the near future. (See pages 32-33 for definitions of Threshold Limit Values.)

TABLE 12	Current ACGIH Standards for Silica	
TYPE OF SILICA	**TLV-TWA (mg/m³)***	
AMORPHOUS		
diatomaceous earth (unfired)	10.	total dust
precipitated silica**	10.	total dust
silica gel (sodium silicate)**	10.	total dust
silica fume (from manufacturing processes such as silicon chip making)	0.2	respirable dust***
fumed silica (e.g.Aerosol, Cabosil)**	——	to be proposed
CRYSTALLINE		
cristobalite	0.05	respirable dust***
quartz	0.1	respirable dust***
silica fused**	0.1	respirable dust***
tridymite	0.05	respirable dust***

*TLV-TWA in milligrams per cubic meter (see pp 32-33). **A synthetic product.
***Just that portion of the dust which can be inhaled deeply into the lungs—as opposed to total dust.

FELDSPARS are a group of minerals which combine silica (SiO_2) and alumina (Al_2O_3) with metal (alkali) oxides. The most common of these are sodium (in soda spars), potassium (in potash spars) and calcium (in lime spars). These metals are usually relatively insoluble and are not very toxic except for the caustic, irritating quality they may impart to the spar. Many other metals (such as magnesium [Mg], titanium [Ti], iron [Fe], barium [Ba], lithium [Li], and more) also may be present in the spar and these may be soluble to varying degrees. Analyses of spars should be obtained to estimate its health hazards and to understand its behavior in glazes or glass.

The major hazard associated with spars is the common presence of free silica contaminants.

KAOLIN AND OTHER CLAYS. "Kaolin" is a term usually used to describe white clays containing the clay mineral, kaolinite. However, the term "clay" refers to any of a number of minerals that dry to a hard form, which can be treated with heat to form a hard, waterproof material. The ones most commonly used in ceramics are minerals of various crystal structure arrangements of alumina, silica, and water. Other metals can be present in the structure of some clays.

The metal elements in clays are too well bonded to be soluble and their hazards come from their crystal structures. It is suspected that many clays can cause lung-scarring diseases after years of heavy exposure, but the disease best documented is "kaolinosis" which is seen in kaolin miners.

Since they are mined from the earth, clays usually contain many impurities. The major hazard associated with clay is the common presence of significant amounts of free silica contamination.

SYNTHETIC MINERAL FIBERS

Synthetic mineral fibers include ceramic fiber, and glass, slag, and rock wool. Research is beginning to show that microscopic needle-like inert materials whether of asbestos, glass, or ceramic origin may cause lung diseases and cancer. In June, 1987, the International Agency for Research on Cancer (IARC) recategorized glasswool, rockwool, slagwool, and ceramic fibers as being "possibly carcinogenic to humans" after evaluating data from laboratory experiments and from studies of workers in fiber-producing plants.

Ceramic fibers also have been shown to partially convert to christobalite (see Silica above) when they are heated to 870 °C (1600 °F) or above.

This means that ceramic fibers used as insulation in kilns and furnaces will convert as the equipment is used. Other man-made fibers may make similar conversions.

In spite of these hazards, most experts and the United States Environmental Protection Agency feel that the substitutes are less carcinogenic and toxic than asbestos. In addition, improvements in the manufacture of the fibers (increasing their diameter) will result in even better products in the future.

FRITS

Frits can be thought of as amorphous or as "less structured minerals." Ground glass, glass paints, metal enamels, and commercial ceramic glazes often are made of, or contain, frits. Frits were originally developed for the British pottery industry to reduce workers' deaths from poisoning by highly soluble raw lead compounds such as litharge and white lead.

Frits are made by melting various minerals and compounds together to form a glass-like material, sintering the glass by pouring it when molten onto cold metal or into cold water, then grinding it up into a powder.

SOLUBILITY OF FRITS. Lead frits are often inaccurately touted as being nontoxic and insoluble. Frit solubility is also measured by an acid test. In preparation for the test, the finest particles are washed out of the frit. Then the washed frit is mixed with a standard amount of acid for a couple hours, and the acid solution is then tested to see how much lead it contains.

This test has shown that although some frits are acid insoluble, frit solubility varies greatly. There are even some frits which are more soluble than raw lead compounds. Acid tests also have confirmed that a frits solubility is dependent on its chemical composition, how well it is manufactured, and its particle size.

Common acid solubility tests in which fine particles are removed prior to testing also may be misleading to glaze mixers and metal enamelists, since they may work with unwashed materials whose fine dust is more soluble.

In addition, recent studies have shown that some acid-insoluble lead frits are as soluble as raw lead compounds when ingested or inhaled by animals, or are placed in human body fluids such as lung and digestive fluids.

There is little or no data on the solubility of nonlead frits, yet these may contain barium, lithium or other toxic metals. Prudence dictates that all frits be treated with care.

GLASS

Glass can be manufactured in an infinite variety of compositions. Natural glasses, like obsidian and pumice also can vary in composition. Technically, fired ceramic glazes are also types of glass.

When powdered or ground fine, the hazards of these materials, like frits, will depend on the solubility of any toxic metals in the glass and on their ability to mechanically irritate eyes, skin and the respiratory system. Dust from grinding lead glass, for example, can be both irritating and toxic.

TABLE 13	**Hazard of Common Minerals** **Used in Ceramics, Sculpture, Lapidary, and Abrasives**

General information about common minerals is summarized in this table. Inhalation hazards are stressed since artists are most often exposed to airborne dust from these materials. Silica, asbestos, feldspars, and clays are often found in these minerals. The hazards of these materials are found in the body of the chapter. When toxic metals are present, refer to Table 10 in metals chapter.

AFRICAN WONDERSTONE (pyrophyllite, aluminum silicate) hazards are unstudied.

AGATE (chalcedony, flint, silica) see hazards of silica, pages 153-154.

ALABASTER (Calcium Sulfate) may cause eye and respiratory irritation. One of the least toxic stones. A nuisance dust.*

ALUMINUM OXIDE (see corundum).

AMBER (an organic fossil resin) no significant hazards.

AMETHYST (quartz) see silica, see pages 153-154.

AZURITE (see malachite).

CALCITE (calcium carbonate, chalk) A nuisance dust.*

CARBORUNDUM (silicon carbide) inhalation of large amounts may cause a type of pneumoconiosis. A nuisance dust.*

CERIUM OXIDE no significant hazards in dust form (fume can cause cer-pneumoconiosis).

CHALCEDONY (see agate)

CORNWALL STONE a rock (feldspathoid) which contains feldspar (see page 155), quartz, kaolinite (see kaolin, page 155), mica, and a small amount of fluorspar.

CORUNDUM (aluminum oxide) inhalation of large amounts is associated with a type of lung scarring called "Shaver's disease." A nuisance dust.*

CRYOLITE natural or synthetic sodium aluminum fluoride. Highly toxic due to the fluorine present. Used also as a pesticide.

DIABASE an igneous rock which contains various minerals. The term refers to different rocks in different countries. May contain feldspars and other minerals which are contaminated with silica.

DIAMOND (carbon) no significant hazards.

DOLOMITE (calcium magnesium carbonate) may contain some free silica.

ERIONITE a fibrous mineral unrelated to asbestos which has clearly been shown to cause the same diseases as asbestos in humans.

FLINT (quartz) see silica, pages 153-154.

FLUORSPAR (fluorite, calcium fluoride) is a skin, eye, and lung irritant. Highly toxic due to the fluorine present. Chronic inhalation can cause loss of appetite, weight, anemia, and bone and tooth defects.

GARNET (any of five different silicate minerals) may contain free silica. See silica, pages 153-154.

GLASS BEADS (various types of glass) do not cause silicosis. The dust is mechanically irritating to eyes and respiratory tract. If the glass contains toxic metals such as lead, poisoning can result from exposure to the dust.

GRANITE an igneous rock composed chiefly of feldspar and quartz with one more minerals such as mica included. Contains free silica.

GREENLAND SPAR see cryolite.

GREENSTONE a basaltic rock having green color from presence of chlorite, epidote, or other minerals. May contain free silica. Some stones sold as greenstone may contain asbestos minerals.

GYPSUM see alabaster.

ILMENITE a titanium-containing iron ore (see titanium and iron in Table 10, page 133).

JADE (jadeite or nephrite minerals) has no significant hazards.

JASPER (a black crystalline variety of quartz) see silica, pages 153-154.

LEPIDOLITE a lithium-containing mica. See mica, below, and lithium in Table 10, page 139.

LAPIS LAZULI is usually mixture of minerals with the principle mineral being lazurite which contains aluminum, silicon, sodium and sulfur. May cause skin and respiratory irritation. On ingestion, the sulfur in the mineral may be capable of forming highly toxic hydrogen sulfide gas with digestive acids.

LIMESTONE (calcium carbonate) may contain significant amounts of free silica.

MAGNESITE (magnesium carbonate) No significant hazards.

MALACHITE (hydrous copper carbonate, azurite) can irritate the eyes, nose, and throat. Known to cause nasal congestion and in severe exposure can cause ulceration and perforation of the nasal septum. Chronic exposure can cause anemia.

MARBLE (calcium carbonate) may contain some free silica. A nuisance dust if silica is not present.

MICA any of several silicates of varying chemical composition having a similar crystalline structure composed of thin sheets. Some natural micas contain free silica. Synthetic mica is also available.

NEPHELINE SYENITE a mixture of feldspars, free silica and other minerals.

OCHRES are clays containing iron oxides and occasionally manganese oxides. See kaolin, page 155, and iron and manganese in Table 10.

ONYX is a variety of quartz. See silica, pages 153-154.

OPAL (silica) is an amorphous silica which should be of low toxicity to the lungs, but large amounts may cause some lung scarring.

OPAX a frit of 92% zirconium dioxide, 6% lithium dioxide, and smaller amounts of titanium, iron, sodium, and aluminum. See zircon and lithium in Table 10, pages 139.

PEARL ASH see potash.

PERLITE a natural glass-like material which expands when heated. May contain significant amounts of free silica.

PETALITE a lithium feldspar. See feldspar, page 155, and lithium in Table 10.

PORPHYRY (conglomerate rock containing some feldspar) may contain significant amounts of free silica.

POTASH (potassium carbonate) is irritating and slightly caustic. A nuisance dust.*

PUMICE (a form of volcanic glass) may contain small amounts of free silica.

PUTTY (tin oxide) no significant hazards, inhalation of large amounts can cause benign pneumoconiosis (see page 152).

REALGAR (arsenic disulfide) is a highly toxic mineral causing skin irritation and ulceration. Inhalation can cause respiratory irritation, digestive disturbances, liver damage, peripheral nervous system damage, kidney, and blood damage.

SAND, SANDSTONE (quartz) see silica, pages 153-154.

SERPENTINE (magnesium silicate) usually is in the form of crysotile asbestos. See asbestos, pages 152-153.

SILICON CARBIDE see carborundum, above.

SLAG (glass-like material from smelting operations) may contain small but significant amounts of highly toxic metal impurities. May be contaminated with free silica.

SLATE (a rock formed from compression of clay, shale, etc.) may contain significant amounts of free silica.

SOAPSTONE see talc.

SODA ASH (sodium carbonate) slightly irritating. No significant hazards.

SODA SPAR are sodium-containing feldspars; see feldspars, page 155.

SODIUM SILICATE or water glass is sodium silicate. Some products contain free silica.

STEATITE see talc.

TALC a magnesium silicate platy mineral responsible for the slippery feel of soapstone and steatites. Talc causes a disease called "talcosis" when inhaled in large amounts. Many talcs, soapstones, and steatites are contaminated with many other minerals including amphibole asbestos and silica.

TRIPOLI (silica) is primarily an amorphous silica which should be of low toxicity to the lungs, but most varieties contain enough quartz to cause silicosis.

TRAVERTINE (calcium carbonate, a form of limestone, see limestone above)

TURQUOISE (mineral of copper aluminum and phosphate) may cause skin allergies and irritation of the eyes, nose and throat. May be contaminated with significant amounts of free silica.

VERMICULITE a plate-like, hydrated magnesium-iron-aluminum silicate mineral capable of being expanded (puffed up) with heat. Often found contaminated with tremolite or crysotile asbestos.

WHITING (calcium carbonate). Some natural sources contain free silica. When silica is not present, it is a nuisance dust.*

WOLLASTONITE a fibrous mineral unrelated to asbestos which may have some potential to cause cancer. Not well studied.

ZIRCON OXIDES or zirconia, see zircon in Table 10, page 146.

ZIRCONIUM SILICATE or zircon, see zircon in Table 10, page 146.

ZONOLITE see vermiculite.

---

*nuisance dust = 10 mg/m³, see page 130.

CHAPTER

13 *PLASTICS*

P lastics have revolutionized art. Artists now use plastics as vehicles in paints and inks, as casting materials, adhesives, structural elements, textiles, and much more.

WHAT IS PLASTIC?

A plastic or "polymer" is created when a chemical called a "monomer" reacts with itself to form large molecules, often in long chains. This reaction is called polymerization. For example, when a monomer called methyl methacrylate is polymerized, it becomes *poly*methyl methacrylate, better known as Lucite or Plexiglas. Natural polymers such as rubber and hardened linseed oil also are created this way.

Some polymers are capable of a second reaction in which the long chains are linked together laterally (side by side). This reaction is called crosslinking. For example, liquid polyester resin becomes a solid material when it is reacted with a crosslinking agent like styrene.

These long-chain and crosslinked polymers possess different properties when exposed to heat. Heat usually will deform or mold long-chain polymers into new shapes. These polymers are called thermoplastics. On the other hand, heat will not deform crosslinked polymers, and these are called thermoset plastics.

Chemicals which can cause monomers and resins to react have many trade names including activators, actuators, catalysts, curing agents, hardeners, or initiators. In this book the term "initiator" will be used in most cases.

GENERAL RULES FOR USING PLASTIC RESIN SYSTEMS

1. *Use the least toxic products.* Most monomers, initiators, and crosslinkers are very toxic. Obtain Material Safety Data Sheets (MSDS) on all plastic products and compare hazard information.

Reject plastics containing chemicals which are unduly toxic. For example, one chemical found in some polyurethane foam products, epoxy hardeners, foundry core binders, and other plastics, called methylenedianiline, is so toxic that the United States Occupational Safety and Health Administration (OSHA) is planning to set a permissible exposure limit for it at 10 parts per *billion.* Replace products containing such chemicals with safer ones.

2. *Prepare precautions in advance.* Investigate the hazards of plastic resin systems before using them. Read Material Safety Data Sheet and product literature precautions and be sure your shop is equipped with necessary protective equipment and ventilation. Be prepared to deal with spills and disposal of the materials.

3. *Follow product directions precisely.* If directions are followed, the polymerization reaction should bind the hazardous chemicals into the solid plastic. Handling, machining and tooling well-made solid plastic is usually not very hazardous. Exceptions are when the reaction is not complete because mixing was not uniform, the proportions were not correct, or some other factor. In these cases, unused monomer or other chemicals may be left to off-gas or render the plastic's dust toxic.

POLYESTER RESIN CASTING SYSTEMS

Hazardous chemicals used in these systems include: the crosslinking agent which is usually styrene; ketone solvents such as acetone used to dilute the resin, or for cleanup; the initiator, which is an organic peroxide such as methyl ethyl ketone peroxide; and fiberglass used for reinforcement.

Styrene is a highly toxic aromatic hydrocarbon solvent which can cause narcosis, respiratory system irritation, liver and nerve damage, and is a suspect carcinogen. Acetone is a less toxic solvent, but is extremely flammable. (See Table 5, Common Solvents and Their Hazards, page 89.)

Methyl ethyl ketone peroxide has caused blindness when splashed in the eyes, can form an explosive mixture with acetone, and converts to a shock-sensitive explosive material after a time. (See Organic Peroxides below for more complete discussion of hazards.)

Fiberglass dust can cause skin and respiratory irritation. There are many other compounds in polyester resin systems which initiate, promote, or accelerate the reaction. The hazards of many of these chemicals are not well-studied.

PRECAUTIONS FOR USING POLYESTER RESINS

1.Work only in local exhaust areas.Additional protection may be obtained by wearing a respirator with cartridges for organic vapors. Add a dust filter to the respirator if you use fiberglass or if you sand the finished plastic.

2. Wear gloves and chemical splash goggles when handling and pouring materials. Protection from some plastic resin chemicals requires special types of gloves. Ask the glove manufacturer for advice.

3. Wear clothing that covers your arms and legs. Remove clothes immediately if they are splashed with resins or peroxides. Always remove clothing completely after work, then take a shower.

4. Cover exposed areas of your neck and face with a barrier cream as protection in case of splashes.

5. Handle peroxides correctly by following the advice in the section on Organic Peroxides. Be especially careful to avoid splashes in the eyes, and never mix peroxides with acetone.

6. Use acetone, not styrene, for clean up. Cover your work area with disposable paper or plastic sheeting to make cleaning easier.

7. Follow all precautions for using solvents, such as cleaning up spills immediately, disposing of rags in approved, self-closing waste cans, and the like (see Chapter 9, Solvents, page 87-89).

8. When mixing small amounts of resins, use disposable containers and agitators such as paper cups and wooden sticks. If you need reusable containers, use polyethylene or stainless steel containers.

PLASTIC MOLD MAKING MATERIALS

SILICONE. Two types of silicone resin systems commonly are used to make molds. The first is a single-component system which cures by absorbing atmospheric moisture. The second is a two-component system which cures by means of a peroxide (see section on Organic Peroxides). Both systems contain solvents such as acetone or methylene chloride.

Single-component systems may release acetic acid or methanol into the air. Acetic acid vapors are highly irritating to the eyes and respiratory tract. Methanol is a nervous system poison (see Table 5, Common Solvents and Their Hazards, page 89). Two-component systems often contain chemicals which can damage the skin. Some also contain methylene chloride which can cause narcosis and stress the heart (see Table 5, Common Solvents and Their Hazards, page 89).

RUBBER. Rubber can be considered to be a plastic resin manufactured by nature. Water-based natural rubber latex systems are commonly used to make molds. Some kinds of latex contain chemicals which can irritate the skin, but natural rubber is one of the safest molding systems to use.

Solvent-containing rubber products are also used. In addition, rubber cement and some contact cements are rubber dissolved in solvents. These products usually contain very toxic solvents such as hexane which is especially toxic to the nervous system (see Table 5, Common Solvents and Their Hazards, page 89). When possible select rubber products which replace hexane with less toxic heptane.

PRECAUTIONS FOR USING SILICONE AND NATURAL RUBBER

1. Use with sufficient ventilation to remove acetic acid, solvents, and other vapors.

2. Wear protective gloves. Consult the manufacturer of the resin or latex about the proper gloves to use.

3. If any components are liquid, wear goggles when pouring or handling them.

4. Follow all solvent precautions when using products containing solvents.

EPOXY RESIN SYSTEMS

Epoxies are used for paint and ink vehicles, casting, laminating, and molding. They also are common adhesives and putties. Most are two-component systems. After they are mixed, the resulting epoxy gives off heat which vaporizes any solvents in it. An excess of hardener can cause the epoxy to heat to the point of decomposition and ignition.

Epoxy resins can irritate the skin. They also may contain varying amounts of solvents. Common solvents in epoxy include the glycidyl ethers which have caused reproductive and blood diseases in animals including atrophy of testicles, damage to bone marrow, and birth defects.

Epoxy hardeners are toxic and highly sensitizing to the skin and respiratory system. Almost 50 percent of industrial workers regularly exposed to epoxy develop allergies to them.

PRECAUTIONS FOR USING EPOXY RESINS

1. Wear goggles and gloves when using large amounts of epoxy. Do not mold epoxy putties by hand without wearing gloves; barrier creams do not provide sufficient protection.

2. Use large amounts of epoxy, either with local exhaust (such as a spray booth) or in front of a window exhaust fan.

3. Use liquid epoxies (those containing special solvents) in local exhaust and take special precautions to avoid skin contact. Check with glove suppliers to find which glove material will resist penetration of the particular solvent.

URETHANE RESINS

Polyurethane resin systems (do not confuse these with single-component polyurethane varnishes and paints which are safer) usually consist of a polyol polymer resin (which might also contain metal salts or amine initiators) and isocyanate crosslinkers. Foam casting systems also contain blowing agents such as freon.

Many artists, especially theatrical scene and prop makers, have used foam polyurethane casting systems. However, artists should avoid these systems for several reasons.

First, the isocyanate crosslinkers (which are related to the chemical which caused 2,000 deaths in Bhopal, India) are so irritating and sensitizing that they can cause acute asthma-like respiratory distress and other symptoms at very low levels. For this reason, the Threshold Limit Values (see pages 32-33 for definitions of Threshold Limit Values) for the crosslinkers are so low that most studios and shops cannot manage to achieve them. (For example, the Threshold Limit Value for one common isocyanate—toluene diisocyanate—is 0.005 ppm.)

Second, expensive air-supplied respirators must be used with isocyanates because there are no air-purifying respirators which provide proper protection.

Lastly, the final plastic product is still hazardous. When heated or burned can give off hydrogen cyanide, carbon monoxide, acrolein, and other toxic gases. Even cutting, sanding, and finishing the final product has been associated with skin and respiratory problems.

PRECAUTIONS FOR USING URETHANE RESINS

1. Do not allow anyone who has a history of allergies, heart problems, or respiratory difficulties to be exposed to urethane resins.

2. Use them in a local exhaust system large enough to enclose the entire project. If you also need respiratory protection, use an *air-supplied* respirator with full face mask.

3. Wear protective clothing and gloves during foaming and casting.

4. Use ventilation when sanding and cutting finished plastic, and wear protective clothing and gloves. Wear a dust mask and goggles if static electricity causes dust to cling to face and eyes.

OTHER RESIN SYSTEMS

There are a number of other resin systems but they are not used often in art. However, systems employing methyl methacrylate (MMA) alone or in combination with other monomers are used occasionally. Some of these systems need special precautions because they involve elevated pressures and/or temperatures.

Investigate the hazards of plastic resin systems before using them. Obtain Material Safety Data Sheets and other product information and be sure your shop is equipped with necessary protective equipment, spill control, and ventilation.

ORGANIC PEROXIDES

Organic peroxides (do not confuse these with hydrogen peroxide which is not as hazardous) are used to initiate many polyester, acrylic, and even some silicone polymerizations.

HAZARDS OF ORGANIC PEROXIDES. In general, organic peroxides burn vigorously and are both reactive and unstable. When heated, some are shock-sensitive and can explode. Some can burn without air because they release their own oxygen. This makes it dangerous to mix them with flammable or combustible materials. For example, if peroxides ignite after being spilled on clothing, the fire cannot be extinguished and must burn until spent.

Because of organic peroxides' fire and explosion hazard, they usually are sold mixed with inhibitors. Even so, these mixtures have been known to burn quietly until all the inhibitor is burned off; then the fire intensifies.

The toxic hazards of organic peroxides are largely unknown. In general, their vapors may cause eye and respiratory irritation, and many are sensitizers.

Organic peroxides react with oxygen in the air to form shock sensitive, explosive chemicals. Control peroxide inventories to dispose of old materials regularly.

PRECAUTIONS FOR USING PEROXIDES

1. Obtain Material Safety Data Sheets and product information on peroxides. Pay special attention to information about reactivity, fire hazards, and spill procedures.

2. Keep date of purchase and date of opening on the container label. Dispose of peroxides after six months if unopened or after three months once opened. Never purchase peroxides if containers are damaged or irregular.

3. Store peroxides separately from each other and from other combustibles. Always keep peroxides in their original containers.

4. Do not store large amounts of peroxides without consulting fire laws and OSHA standards.

5. Do not heat peroxides or store them in warm areas or sunlight.

6. Never dilute peroxides with other materials or add them to accelerators or solvents.

7. Wear protective goggles when containers are open or when pouring peroxides.

8. When mixing small amounts of resins and peroxides, use disposable containers. Soak all tools and containers in water before disposing of them.

9. Clean up spills immediately in accordance with Material Safety Data Sheet directions. Inert materials such as unmilled fire clay usually are recommended to soak them up. Clean up peroxide-soaked material with nonsparking, nonmetallic tools; do not sweep them because fires have started from the friction of sweeping itself.

10. If peroxide spills on your clothing, remove your clothes immediately and launder them separately and well before wearing them again.

11. When discarding unused peroxide or fire clay/peroxide mixtures, first react them with a 10 percent sodium hydroxide solution to prevent fires. Otherwise, unused peroxide can be reacted with resin and the solid plastic discarded safely.

FINISHED PLASTICS

Rather than working with resin systems, it is easier and safer to work with sheets, films, beads, or blocks of finished plastic. Even so, when plastics are cut or heated, decomposition products are released and these products can be hazardous. Processes during which this can occur include sawing, sanding, hot knife or wire cutting, press molding, drilling, grinding, heat shrinking, vacuum forming, plastic burnout casting, torching, and melting. In general, the gases and smoke produced from the finished plastics during high-heat processes are usually more dangerous than those produced at lower temperatures.

Some plastics are especially hazardous to cut or heat. Among these are polyvinyl chloride (which produces hydrochloric acid gas) and all nitrogen-containing plastics such as polyurethane, melamine resins, urea formaldehyde, and nylon (which produce hydrogen cyanide gas).

In addition, the dusts of some plastics are very sensitizing, and this dust will contain many potentially hazardous additives such as plasticizers (used to achieve the desired softness), stabilizers, colorants (dyes and pigments), fillers, fire retardants, inhibitors, accelerators, and more. Some of the common plasticizers (some of the phthalate esters) are known to cause cancer in animals. However, the vast majority of these additives' hazards are unknown.

Some plastics adhesives also contain toxic solvents which require precautions (see Table 5, Common Solvents and Their Hazards, page 89).

PRECAUTIONS FOR WORKING WITH FINISHED PLASTICS

1. Use good dilution ventilation or local exhaust ventilation. Use water-cooled or air-cooled tools, if possible, to keep decomposition to a minimum. When heat forming plastics, use the lowest possible temperature.

2. Add vacuum attachments to sanders, saws, and other electric tools to collect dust.

3. Wear dust goggles and a dust mask if static electricity causes particles to cling to face and eyes. Remember that the dust mask provides protection only against particles. No mask will protect you from all the emissions from plastics. Organic vapor respirators will trap some decomposition gases and vapors. Acid gas cartridge respirators will collect hydrochloric acid gas from decomposing polyvinyl chloride plastics. However, there are no approved cartridges or filters for emissions such as hydrogen cyanide, isocyanates, and nitrogen oxides.

4. Clean up all dust carefully by wet mopping or specially filtered vacuums. Do not sweep.

5. Use precautions for solvents (page 87) when using plastics adhesives.

GLUES AND ADHESIVES

Most glues and adhesives are either synthetic or natural polymers. Most are less hazardous than casting plastics simply because smaller amounts are used. Some common ones are in Table 14.

TABLE 14	Hazards of Common Adhesives

AIRPLANE GLUE: plastic dissolved in solvent, usually acetone. No hazards except solvents.

CYANOACRYLATE, "SUPER GLUE," "KRAZY GLUE:" plastic monomer which cures on exposure to air. Potent eye irritant. Fast curing-time can cause unplanned adhesion of body parts.

"ELMER'S," WHITE GLUE, PVA: polyvinylacetate plastic in a water-based emulsion. One of the least hazardous glues unless poorly manufactured (these contain unreacted monomer).

EPOXIES: see above.

GLUE STICKS: plastic and/or mucilage materials. No known significant hazards.

RUBBER CEMENT: rubber dissolved in solvent, often n-hexane. No hazards except for solvents.

SILICONE ADHESIVES: see above.

UREA FORMALDEHYDE and PHENOL FORMALDEHYDE: Resin dissolved in solvents or water-based materials. Also a plywood and pressboard adhesive. These off-gas formaldehyde. Avoid if possible.

WALLPAPER PASTE: usually wheat or methyl cellulose and preservatives. May contain large amounts of pesticides and fungicides. Use wheat or methyl cellulose paste made for children. These have no significant hazards.

WHITE PASTE, LIBRARY PASTE: no significant hazards.

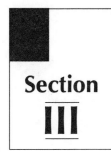

Section

III

Precautions for Individual Media

CHAPTER 14 | PAINTING AND DRAWING

The diseases caused by painting and pigment grinding have been observed since Ramazini wrote about them in 1713. Back then, painters did not know about the chemical hazards in their paints as we do now.

WHAT ARE PAINTS?

Today artists use a vast array of different paints; however, these products have many properties in common because almost all of them contain pigments suspended in vehicles or bases.

Vehicles usually contain a liquid such as an oil, a solvent, or water. Cleaners and thinners for most paints are these same liquids or liquids which are compatible with them. For example, turpentine will thin and clean up oil paints.

WHAT ARE DRAWING MATERIALS?

Drawing materials also are pigments suspended in vehicles. Some drawing material vehicles include wax (crayons), inert minerals (pastels, conte crayons, chalks), and liquids (solvent and water-based inks and marking pens). Pencils contain "leads" made of graphite and clay ("lead" pencils) or pigmented clay/binder mixtures (colored pencils).

The hazards of both painting and drawing materials arise from exposure to their pigments, vehicles, and solvents.

PIGMENT HAZARDS

There are only a few hundred pigments which are light-fast enough to be used in art. These pigments are used in oils, acrylics, alkyds, pastels, colored pencils, and all colored materials used in high-quality fine arts products. The hazards of these pigments are discussed in Chapter 10, Pigments and Dyes, page 98-99).

Paints with fugitive pigments (those which fade with time or exposure to light) can be used for work which is not expected to endure many years, such as theatrical scenery or props, commercial art, or children's art work. Artists who use untraditional paints such as consumer wall paints will also find that the pigments in these paints fade. Fugitive pigments are often complex organic chemicals whose long-term hazards are not well-studied.

Inhalation is the route by which exposure is most likely. Processes during which pigments could be inhaled include: working with raw powdered pigments; using dusty chalks or pastels; sanding or chipping paints; airbrushing or spraying paints; and heating or torching paints until pigments fume.

Skin contact with pigments is less hazardous. Pigments usually are not absorbed in significant amounts by skin contact. However, some contaminants in pigments such as PCB's (polychlorinated biphenyls) could be skin absorbed. And some pigments can cause dermatitis or skin irritation. Preventing skin contact through good hygiene can prevent these problems. Good hygiene also can prevent accidental ingestion of paint pigments.

VEHICLE HAZARDS

Common vehicles include oils, wax, water, egg yolk, casein, resins, and polymer emulsions and solvent solutions. Vehicles usually also contain additives such as stabilizers (to keep ingredients in suspension), preservatives, plasticizers, antioxidants, fillers, wetting agents, retarders, and more. These additives affect paint characteristics such as drying time and workability. The hazards of many of these additives have not been well researched. And manufacturers often are reluctant to divulge the identity of these additives.

Vehicle preservatives can be especially hazardous since their purpose is to kill microorganisms. Common paint preservatives include formaldehyde (sometimes in the form of paraformaldehyde or formalin), phenol, mercury compounds, bleach, and a host of commercial fungicides and pesticides.

Even though these additives are present in small amounts, they have caused illness in artists. For example, a mural artist developed mercury poisoning some years ago from soluble mercury preservatives used in her paints.

Vehicle ingredients can be divided into volatile (will evaporate into the air) and nonvolatile components. Since nonvolatile ingredients do not become airborne, they usually present no significant hazard to artists unless they are used in techniques that make them available to be inhaled, such as spray painting. Some resins and vehicle solids are associated with allergies.

Volatile vehicle ingredients, on the other hand, can be inhaled by artists while they work or while paints or inks are drying. Acrylic paints, for example, usually contain ingredients which release ammonia and formaldehyde gases while they dry. Permanent markers contain solvents which evaporate and can be inhaled.

SOLVENT HAZARDS

Solvents may be found in paints and inks or may be used to thin and clean up materials. Solvents are also found in products used with painting and drawing such as varnishes, shellacs, lacquers, and fixatives. These products include resins such as damar, mastic, copal, lac, shellac, acrylic, and other plastic resins dissolved in solvents. (Some of these resins have been known to cause allergies.)

Solvents commonly used in paints, thinners, varnishes, etc., include turpentine, paint thinner, mineral spirits, methyl alcohol, ethyl alcohol, acetone, toluene, xylene, ethyl and other acetates, and petroleum distillates. The hazards of these and other solvents are discussed in Chapter 9, Solvents, page 83.

GENERAL PRECAUTIONS FOR PAINTING AND DRAWING MEDIA

The hazards of each type of painting or drawing will depend on the toxicity of the ingredients of the materials and how much exposure oc-

178

curs during use. The most hazardous exposure to paints will occur if they are air-brushed, sprayed, or otherwise made airborne. These processes always require local exhaust ventilation.

When paint and ink are applied by brushing, rollering, dipping and other methods which do not cause pigments and vehicles to become airborne, precautions will vary depending on the hazards of each paint or ink. See Tables 15 for precautions for specific media.

TABLE 15	Ventilation and Precautions for Painting and Drawing Media

The following hazards and precautions apply only to paint and ink techniques such as brushing, rollering, and dipping which to not cause pigments and vehicles to become airborne:

ACRYLIC PAINTS (WATER-BASED EMULSIONS) are composed of synthetic acrylic resins and pigments with many additives usually including an ammonia-containing stabilizer and formaldehyde preservative. The small amounts of ammonia and formaldehyde released during drying can cause respiratory irritation and allergies. Formaldehyde has caused cancer in animals. A low rate of dilution ventilation such as that provided by a window exhaust fan should be sufficient.

ACRYLIC PAINTS (SOLVENT-BASED) are synthetic acrylic resins and pigments dissolved in solvents. The solvents should be identified and ventilation sufficient to keep the solvent's concentration at a safe level should be provided.

ALKYD PAINTS are alkyd resins and pigments dissolved in solvents. Provide dilution ventilation at a rate sufficient to keep solvent's concentrations at safe levels.

ARTIST'S OILS are pigments mulled into oils such as pre-polymerized linseed oil. There usually are no volatile ingredients, but oil paints are commonly thinned and cleaned up with solvents such as paint thinner. Dilution ventilation sufficient to keep solvent exposure low should be provided. Some people use oil paints without solvents and clean brushes and skin with baby oil followed by soap and water. This is a very safe way to work and requires no special ventilation.

CASEINS are made from dried milk, pigments, and preservatives. Some contain ammonium hydroxide which can be irritating to the skin and eyes and dust from the powdered paint should not be inhaled. There are usually very strong preservatives added because the casein is a good source of food for microorganisms. When painting with brushes or rollers, ordinary comfort ventilation should be sufficient.

CHARCOAL has no known significant hazards.

CONSUMER OIL PAINTS AND ENAMELS contain pigments, fillers, and a variety of solvents. A common solvent for these paints is paint thinner. Sufficient dilution ventilation should be provided.

CONSUMER LATEX PAINTS are primarily pigments and water emulsions of various plastic resins. Most also contain between 5 and 15 percent solvents. On occasion, these solvents are the highly toxic glycol ethers (see Table 5, Common Solvents and Their Hazards, page 89) which can be skin-absorbed and inhaled. Dilution ventilation and proper gloves should be provided. Men and women planning families and pregnant women should avoid exposure to paints containing the glycol ethers.

CRAYONS are pigments in wax. Most have no significant hazards because the pigments are contained. Techniques which involve melting crayons may produce irritating wax decomposition products which would require exhaust ventilation.

DRAWING INKS may contain hazardous dyes and solvents. Skin contact should be avoided. Ventilation is needed only if extraordinary amounts are used or if the solvents are especially toxic.

FRESCO consists of pigments ground in lime water (calcium hydroxide) which is corrosive to eyes, skin, and respiratory tract. Gloves and goggles should be worn.

ENCAUSTICS are dry pigments suspended in molten white refined wax such as beeswax along with drying oils, Venice turpentine, and natural resins. Working with dry pigments is very hazardous. Heating waxes can release highly irritating wax decomposition products such as acrolein and formaldehyde. Torching the wax surface also can cause pigments to fume. The solvents and wax and pigment fumes require local exhaust ventilation.

EPOXY PAINTS are two part epoxy resin systems and containing highly toxic and sensitizing organic chemicals (see Chapter 13, Plastics, page 167) and diluents (solvents). Some contain highly toxic glycidyl ether solvents. Wear gloves, goggles, and avoid inhalation with local exhaust ventilation or respiratory protection.

GOUACHE is an opaque water color which contains pigments, gums, water, preservatives, glycerin, opacifiers, and other ingredients. The opacifiers may be chalk, talc, and other substances. Formaldehyde may be used as a preservative. Ordinary comfort ventilation should be sufficient ventilation unless very large amounts are used.

MARKING PENS contain pigments or dyes in a liquid. The liquid may be water or a solvent. Water-based markers are safest. Of the solvent-based markers, those containing ethyl alcohol are the safest. Others may contain very toxic solvents. Solvent-based markers should be used with some ventilation.

PASTELS, CHALKS AND CONTE CRAYONS are pigments in binders and chalk (calcium carbonate), talc, barytes (barium sulfate mineral), or other powdered inert minerals. Oil pastels are much safer because they contain small amounts of oils and waxes which keep dust from getting airborne. "Dustless" chalks and conte crayons also are easy to use safely because they contain binders which prevent creation of respirable-sized dust particles (see page 32). Unfortunately, it is almost impossible to use dusty pastels and chalks without being exposed to pigment and vehicle dust. A dust mask and ventilation (such as working very near a window exhaust fan) may reduce exposure.

PENCIL AND GRAPHITE drawing usually exposes artists to such small amounts of dust that they are not hazardous. Very large amounts of graphite can cause black lung disease similar to that which afflicts coal miners.

TEMPERA PAINTS are pigments suspended in emulsions of substances such as oils, egg, gum casein, and wax. Preservatives are added to kill microorganisms which would feed on the vehicles. If no solvents are used in these paints, ordinary comfort ventilation should be sufficient for working with liquid paints.

WATERCOLORS (dry cakes) are composed of pigments, preservatives (often paraformaldehyde) and binders such as gum arabic or gum tragacanth. Liquid watercolors may also contain water, glycerine, glucose, and other materials. Both liquid and dry watercolors may give off small amounts of formaldehyde, but they generally need no exhaust ventilation.

RULES FOR PAINTING AND DRAWING

1. Choose studio locations with safety in mind. Floors, tables, and shelving should be made of materials which can be easily cleaned. Isolate the studio from living spaces unless you intend to use materials with no significant hazards such as watercolors and pencils. Never use toxic paints, solvents, or drawing materials in kitchens, bedrooms, living rooms, etc.

2. Obtain Material Safety Data Sheets (MSDSs) on all paints, inks, thinners, varnishes, and other products. If paint pigments are not identified by their Color Index names or numbers, ask your supplier for this information. Some suppliers' catalogs list the Color Index names of their paint pigments. These suppliers should be favored over less informative ones.

3. Use water-based products over solvent-containing ones whenever possible.

4. Buy premixed paints and avoid working with powdered pigments if possible. Pigments and paints are most hazardous and inhalable in a dry powdered state.

5. Choose brushing and dipping techniques over spray methods whenever possible.

6. Use Material Safety Data Sheets and product labels to identify the hazards of any toxic solvents, preservatives or other chemicals in paints and drawing materials. Look up the hazards of the pigments in Table 6.

7. Plan studio ventilation to control the hazards of the materials and processes you use. For example, if solvents are used, provide sufficient dilution ventilation to keep vapors below their Threshold Limit Values (see pages 32-33). If powdered paints or pigments are used, plan local exhaust ventilation (e.g., figure 6) or use a glove box (figure 14).

8. Avoid dusty procedures. Sanding dry paints, sprinkling dry pigments or dyes on wet paint or glue, and other techniques which raise dust should be discontinued or performed in a local exhaust environment or outdoors.

9. Spray or airbrush only under local exhaust conditions such as in a spray booth. A proper respirator may provide additional protection. Use a dust/ mist respirator for water-based paints. Use a paint, lacquer, and enamel mist (PLE) respirator for solvent-containing products.

10. Follow all solvent safety rules if you use solvent-containing products (see pages 87-89), and give extra attention to studio fire safety.

11. Avoid skin contact with paints and pigments by wearing gloves or using barrier creams. Use gloves with dyes. Wash off paint splashes with safe cleaners like a) baby oil followed by soap and water, b) nonirritating waterless hand cleaners, or c) plain soap and water. Never use solvents or bleaches to remove splashes from your skin.

12. Wear protective clothing, including a full-length smock or coveralls. Leave these garments in your studio to avoid bringing dusts home. Wash clothing frequently and separately from other clothing. Wear goggles if you use caustic paints or corrosive chemicals.

13. If respirators must be used, follow all rules regarding their use (see Chapter 8, Respiratory Protection, pages 71-79).

I4. Avoid ingestion of materials; eat, smoke, or drink outside your workplace. Never point brushes with your lips or hold brush handles in your teeth. Wash your hands before eating, smoking, applying make-up and other personal hygiene procedures.

I5. Keep containers of paint, powdered pigments, solvents, etc., closed except when you are using them.

I6. Work on easy-to-clean surfaces and wipe up spills immediately. Wet mop and sponge floors and surfaces. Do not sweep.

17. Follow Material Safety Data Sheet advice and purchase a supply of materials to control spills and for chemical disposal (e.g., kitty litter, solvent spill kits).

18. Dispose of waste solvents, paints, and other materials in accordance with health, safety, and environmental protection regulations.

19. Always be prepared to provide your doctor with precise information about the chemicals you use and your work practices. Arrange for regular blood tests for lead if you use lead-containing paints or pigments.

SPECIAL PRECAUTIONS FOR PAINT REMOVING

Occasionally artists must remove paints from objects or walls. Paint removers are either highly toxic solvent mixtures or strong caustic removers. Gloves, goggles, protective clothing, and ventilation are needed. Some new methods may be less hazardous. One involves applying a caustic material, covering the material with a special cloth, and later removing the cloth and adhered paint as one flexible sheet.

Other methods of removing paint include chipping, sanding, or heating with torches or heat guns. These methods are all hazardous, especially if the paint being removed contains toxic pigments such as lead.

Dust from chipping and sanding is toxic to inhale or ingest. If removal of lead paint from walls is being done, use precautions similar to those for asbestos removal. First, the area should be isolated with taped walls of plastic sheeting. Then an exhaust fan should be installed to draw air out of the isolated area to keep it under negative pressure (so air cannot escape back into unisolated areas). In addition, respiratory protection, protective clothing, and scrupulous hygiene should be practiced.

Torching or heat gunning paint is just as hazardous. These methods create toxic paint decomposition products. Torching or heat gunning lead paint also produces a fine lead fume which has been shown to cause lead poisoning in those removing the paint. Fine lead dust or fume also can cause health effects for years afterward if it contaminates living areas.

CHAPTER 15 *PRINTMAKING*

A ll printmaking techniques rely on the use of inks of various types. There are four basic printmaking techniques: screen printing, lithography, intaglio, and relief:

SCREEN PRINTING uses a fine-meshed framed screen on which areas have been stenciled or blocked with a resist. Ink is then drawn (squeegeed) across and through the screen to the paper or other material which is being printed.

LITHOGRAPHY involves acid-etching smooth limestone surfaces on which areas have been blocked with wax pencils or crayons. Oil-based ink is rollered onto the damp stone. It adheres to the waxy areas and is repelled by the wet stone. The print is then made by running the stone through the lithographic press.

INTAGLIO is done by engraving or etching an image onto a metal plate. Ink is then forced into the grooves and depressions, the unetched areas are wiped clean, and the plate and a sheet of dampened paper are run through an etching press.

RELIEF is done by carving away parts of a materials such as wood (see Chapter 28, Woodworking, page 281) or linoleum with knives and gouges. The remaining raised surface is inked and pressed onto paper.

WHAT ARE PRINTMAKING INKS?

Traditionally, printmaking inks are oil-based or water-based materials which dry or set by evaporation, by polymerization, or by penetrating the material on which they were printed. In recent years new inks have come into use which cure with heat, infrared, or ultraviolet light. In addition special inks have been developed which glow, puff up, or sparkle.

However, both traditional and modern printmaking inks are made up of two basic components: pigments and vehicles.

PIGMENTS

Pigments used in printmaking are essentially the same as those used in painting. Artists are sometimes not aware of this because the printmakers and painters may use different names for the same pigment. For example, bone black which is made from charred animal bones is called "Frankfourt black" by printers and "ivory black" by painters.

Printmakers who make their own inks are at the greatest risk from pigments. The hazards of pigments can be found in Table 6, Pigments Used in Paints and Inks, page 102.

TRADITIONAL VEHICLES

The most common vehicles are mixtures of oils, mixtures of solvents and oils, and polymer emulsions. The oil base of lithography and etching inks are linseed oil and burnt plate oil (boiled linseed oil and driers).

Vehicles also contain additives such as stabilizers (to keep ingredients in suspension), chemical driers, preservatives, plasticizers, antioxidants, antifoaming chemicals, fillers, and more. The hazards of many of these chemicals have not been well researched.

Printmaking vehicles are quite complex because they must have exactly the right physical properties for the particular printmaking technique. The properties that must be controlled include drying time, tack, flow, stiffness, and more. For this reason, printmakers often alter their vehicles by adding oils, solvents, chemical driers, retarders, and the like to change ink performance. Printmakers usually refer to these chemicals as "modifiers."

Ink modifiers include: nontoxic tack reducers and stiffeners such as Crisco, vaseline, cup grease, magnesium carbonate, and aluminum stearate; moderately toxic tack oils such as oil of cloves and oil of lavender; toxic solvents such as petroleum distillates; and highly toxic lead and manganese driers and aerosol anti-skinning agents.

SOLVENTS

Many solvents are used in printmaking as ink components, modifiers, and clean-up products.

Common printmaking solvents might include kerosene, benzine, mineral spirits, gum turpentine, denatured alcohol, and acetone (see Table 5, Common Solvents and Their Hazards, page 89). The water-based inks also may contain toxic solvents such as the glycol ethers.

Cleaning presses, rollers, plates, screens, and the like can cause hazardous amounts of solvents to become airborne. Screens in particular may need large amounts of solvents for cleaning. Often it is cheaper and safer to use inexpensive screens and discard them after use.

RESISTS AND BLOCKOUT STENCILS

Both water-based and solvent-containing materials can be used to resist inks in various printmaking methods. Water-based materials usually have no significant hazards. Included are water-soluble glues, liquid wax (wax emulsions), latex rubber, and water-based friskets.

Solvent-containing resists and block outs include tusche (contains a very small amount of solvent), lacquers, shellac, polyurethane varnishes, and caustic enamels. These products all create toxic solvent vapors during use.

Stencil films may be adhered to screens or plates or removed from them with water-based or solvent-containing adhering fluids and film removers. Solvents commonly found in these materials include acetates, alcohols, and acetone.

Printmaking techniques have expanded in recent years to include photographic processes that can be used to create resists for screen printing or etching. The hazards of many of the chemicals involved in these new inks and photo chemicals are not well known. Some of them will be covered in the chapter on photography.

ACIDS AND CAUSTICS

Acids and other corrosive chemicals are used in intaglio, lithography, and some photo processes. These are very corrosive to the eyes, skin and respiratory system. They are most toxic in their concentrated form.

Hydrochloric acid, nitric acid, and Dutch mordant (potassium chlorate/water/hydrochloric acid) used in etching and lithography can cause skin and eye burns and respiratory system damage. There is no effective air-purifying respirator for nitric acid so local exhaust ventilation must be used. Hydrochloric acid can be replaced with less hazardous ferric chloride solutions in many etching processes. Ferric chloride etching usually requires no special local exhaust ventilation. Good dilution ventilation should suffice.

Phosphoric acid used for cleaning stones is highly corrosive to the skin, eyes, and respiratory tract. Caustic soda (sodium hydroxide) sometimes is used for stone cleaning. It also is highly caustic to skin and eyes.

Phenol (carbolic acid) is highly toxic by both skin absorption and inhalation. Skin contact with concentrated phenol for even several minutes can be fatal. Dilute solutions can cause severe skin burns.

MISCELLANEOUS CHEMICALS

Rosin dust can cause severe allergies. When confined in aquatint boxes, a spark, flame, or static discharge can cause rosin dust to explode (similar to grain elevator explosions).

Some kinds of French chalk (talc) are contaminated with asbestos.

PRECAUTIONS FOR PRINTMAKING

1. Plan the studio with health and safety in mind. Floors, shelving, tables, and other surfaces should be made of materials that can be easily cleaned. Floors should be capable of supporting heavy presses. Isolate studio from eating, recreation, or living areas.

2. Install ventilation which is appropriate for the processes you will do. For example, use window exhaust fans for dilution of small amounts of solvent and kerosene vapors. Install chemical fume hoods or slot hoods for acid baths.

3. Obtain Material Safety Data Sheets (MSDSs) or ingredient information on all products used. If ink pigments are not identified by their Color Index names and numbers or by Chemical Abstracts Service numbers, ask your supplier for this information.

4. Use Material Safety Data Sheets and product labels to identify the hazards of any toxic solvents, acids, or other chemicals in products and choose the least toxic materials.

5. Reduce solvent use. Use water-based inks and other products whenever possible. Use disposable screens for screen printing rather than cleaning them with solvents. Use water-based film adhering fluids or film removers when possible.

6. Follow all solvent safety rules if you use solvent-containing products (see Chapter 9, Solvents page 87-89). Pay special attention to solvent fire safety rules in the studio.

7. If respirators are worn, follow all regulations regarding their use (see Chapter 8, Respiratory Protection, pages 71-79).

8. Protect against acids, caustics, or other irritating chemicals by wearing chemical splash goggles, gloves, aprons, and other protective clothing as needed. Use these chemicals with local exhaust systems. Install an eye wash fountain (and emergency shower if large amounts are used). Have first aid equipment on hand for chemical burns and have emergency procedures posted.

9. Keep containers of inks, pigments, solvents, acids, and other materials closed except when you are using them.

10. Avoid working with powdered materials. Buy premixed inks and other products. If toxic powders must be handled, weighed, or mixed, perform these processes where local exhaust ventilation is available or use a glove box (see figure 14).

11. Avoid dusty procedures. French chalk, wood, or rosin should be used in ways that raise as little dust as possible. If dust cannot be avoided, wear a toxic dust respirator.

12. Use aquatint processes which do not raise dust when possible. One such method uses nonaerosol, pump-sprayed rosin solution. Otherwise, construct rosin boxes with nonsparking parts to avoid dust explosions. Do not use flame or heat sources near the box.

13. Avoid aerosol spray products whenever possible. If they must be used, provide local exhaust conditions such as a spray booth and/or a proper respirator (e.g. a dust/mist respirator for water-based sprays; a paint, lacquer, and enamel mist (PLE) respirator for solvent-containing products).

14. Provide local exhaust such as slot hoods or recessed canopy hoods for heating or burning processes such as heating plate oil, wood burning tools, etc. Have first aid burn treatments handy.

15. Keep all tools sharp and all machinery in good working order. Use presses with stops to keep the beds in place. Provide local exhaust ventilation systems, guards and lockouts for table saws and other machinery. Have first aid equipment for trauma on hand. Post and practice emergency procedures.

16. Avoid ingestion of materials by eating, smoking, or drinking outside the studio. Wash your hands before eating, smoking, applying make-up, or other personal hygiene tasks.

17. Avoid skin contact with inks by wearing gloves or using barrier creams. Avoid hand wiping plates. Wash off ink splashes with safe cleaners like, 1) baby oil followed by soap and water, 2) nonirritating waterless hand cleaners, or 3) plain soap and water. Never use solvents or bleaches on your skin.

18. Wear protective clothing, including a full-length smock or coveralls. Leave these garments in your studio to avoid bringing dusts home.

19. Clean up spills immediately. Follow Material Safety Data Sheet advice and have handy proper materials for controlling spills and for chemical disposal, especially for acids and solvents.

20. Wet mop and sponge floors and surfaces. Do not sweep.

21. Dispose of all inks, pigments, spent acids, and other chemicals in accordance with health, safety, and environmental protection laws.

22. Always be prepared to provide your doctor with precise information about the chemicals you use and your work practices. Arrange for regular blood tests for lead if you use lead-containing paints or pigments.

CHAPTER

16 *TEXTILE ARTS*

Batik dyers, costume makers, scene painters, weavers, and other artists who work with dyes, and textiles, are at risk of exposure to dye chemicals and fiber dusts.

DYE HAZARDS

Although there are thousands of commercial dyes, only a few hundred have been studied for long term effects. Of those tested many were found to cause cancer, birth defects and other toxic effects. The chemistry and hazards of dyes are discussed In Chapter 10, pages 99-100.

Many dyes also must be used with hazardous dye-assisting or mordanting chemicals. These chemicals are added to dye baths to help dyes react with fabrics properly. A list of common dye assisting chemicals and their hazards can be found in Table 16, Hazards of Mordant and Dye Assisting Chemicals, pages 199-200.

Modern textile artists also color fabrics with paints and silk screen inks. The hazards of these materials are discussed in Chapter 14 and 15.

EXPOSURE TO DYE PRODUCTS

Dyes are most hazardous in the powdered state. Skin contact and inhalation of even very small amounts of dyes in this concentrated form should be avoided.

Dyes sold in liquid form are safer to handle. Liquid dyes still can be hazardous because they have strong preservatives and inhibitors in them to keep the dye from degrading. Some also contain solvents including acetone, toluene, xylene, carbitol (diethylene glycol ether) and other solvents.

Dyes applied in hot baths release steam which may contain small amounts of toxic chemicals from dye impurities and decomposition products. Local exhaust ventilation should be installed above hot dye baths.

DYE TECHNIQUES

Dyes are used by artists in batik, tie-dyeing, discharge dyeing and a number of other techniques.

BATIK dyeing traditionally employs fiber reactive dyes (see Table 7, The Hazards of Dyes by Class, page 122-124) on silk. However, batik techniques are now used with a number of different dye classes on many fabrics, on paper, and other materials.

The batik process uses wax (beeswax, paraffin, etc.,) as a dye resist. The wax is heated to melting and applied to the fabric. After the resisted fabric is dyed, the wax is removed by ironing the fabric between sheets of newsprint, or by applying solvents such as dry cleaning fluids, mineral spirits, etc.

Heated wax is a fire hazard. Hot wax or the vapors rising from wax pots can explode into flame easily, so open flames, gas burners, and the like should not be used to heat wax. Instead, equipment such as crock pots and electric frying pans may be used if their controls can be set accurately at the lowest temperature at which the wax remains liquid.

Heated wax also emits highly irritating chemicals, including acrolein and aldehydes such as formaldehyde. Wax emissions require exhaust ventilation because there are no suitable air-purifying respirators for acrolein. Some artists avoid using heated wax by applying cold wax emulsions which are suitable for some purposes.

Irons for pressing wax out of fabrics also should be set at the lowest temperature required for wax removal. Exhaust ventilation such as table-level window exhaust fans should be provided. If solvents are used for wax removal, all the rules for solvent use should be followed (see Chapter 9, Solvents, pages 87-89). Some artists boil fabrics to remove most of the wax and then send them to professional dry-cleaners for complete removal.

For some purposes, much safer vegetable matter batik resists which can be washed out with strong soap and water now are being developed and sold.

TIE DYEING is done by applying dyes to fabrics which have been tied tightly. Concentrated dye solutions are usually used making exposure to these solutions more hazardous by skin or eye contact.

DISCHARGE DYEING, DYE STRIPPING, AND BLEACHING involves applying chlorine bleaches or other harsh chemicals to dyed fabrics. These chemicals remove dyes by destroying their chemical bonds. In the process, dyes may be broken down into even more hazardous chemicals. For example, benzidine dyes may be broken down to free benzidine; aniline (azine) dyes may release highly toxic aniline.

Using bleach to remove dye stains from your skin would have the same effect. Bleach also irritates and damages the skin. Skin contact with dyes should be avoided, but in case of accidental contact, it is best to let stains wear off.

Some of the highly toxic break-down products of dyes are volatile and can be made airborne especially if dyeing is done in hot baths. Some of these chemicals are likely to be absorbed through the skin. Gloves and ventilation must be provided when dye stripping or discharge dyeing.

PRECAUTIONS FOR DYERS

1. Plan the dye room with health and safety in mind. Floors and surfaces should be made of materials which are easily sponged clean and which will not stain. General ventilation rates should not be so high that dusts are stirred up.

2. Install ventilation systems appropriate for the work done. For example, provide local exhaust such as slot hoods or recessed canopy hoods for heating dye pots, reverse dyeing, wax heating and removal, and all other processes which release toxic air borne substances. Vent dryers and similar equipment.

3. Obtain Material Safety Data Sheets (MSDSs) on all dyes and textile paints. If dyes and pigments are not identified by their Color Index names and numbers or by their Chemical Abstracts Service numbers (see page 43), ask your supplier for this information. Try not to use dyes without at least knowing their classes. Look up hazards of each dye class in Table 7, page 122-124.

4. Use Material Safety Data Sheets and product labels to identify the hazards of any toxic solvents, acids, or other chemicals in dyes, paints, inks, mordants, or other materials. If solvents are used in dyes or for removal of wax, follow all precautions for solvents (see pages 87-89), and pay special attention to fire safety.

5. Choose water-based products over solvent-containing ones whenever possible.

6. Buy premixed dyes if possible. Dyes packaged in packets which dissolve when dropped unopened into hot water also can be handled safely. Dyes and pigments are most hazardous and inhalable in a dry powdered state.

7. Weigh or mix dye powders or other toxic powders where local exhaust ventilation is available or use a glove box (see fig.14, page 101).

8. Keep containers of powdered dyes and pigments, solvents, etc., closed except when you are using them.

9. Avoid procedures which raise dusts or mists. Sprinkling dry dyes or pigments on wet cloth, airbrushing, and other techniques which raise dusts or mists should be discontinued or performed in a local exhaust environment such as a spray booth.

10. Avoid skin contact with dyes by wearing gloves. If skin staining does occur, wash skin with mild cleaners and allow remainder to wear off. Never use solvents or bleaches to remove dye splashes from your skin.

11. Melt and remove wax at the lowest possible temperatures. Do not heat wax with open flames such as on gas stoves. Use devices like electric stoves or fry pans with good heat control mechanisms. Use wax emulsion products when possible. Irons used to remove wax should be set as low as possible. Sending fabrics to professional dry-cleaners is a viable, but expensive alterative. Investigate nonwax resists as substitutes.

12. Wear protective clothing, including a full-length smock or coveralls. Leave these garments in your studio to avoid bringing dusts home. Wash clothing frequently and separately from other clothes.

13. Protect eyes by wearing chemical splash goggles if you use caustic dyes or corrosive chemicals. Install an eye wash fountain (and emergency shower if large amounts are used).

14. Clean up spills immediately. Follow Material Safety Data Sheet advice and have handy proper materials to handle spills and disposal. Wet-mop and sponge floors and surfaces. Do not sweep.

15. Avoid ingestion of materials by eating, smoking, or drinking outside your workplace. Never point brushes with your lips or hold brush handles in your teeth. Never use cooking utensils for dyeing. A pot which seems clean can be porous enough to hold hazardous amounts of residual dye. Wash your hands before eating, smoking, applying make-up, or other personal hygiene procedures.

16. Dispose of dyes, mordants, and other chemicals in accordance with health, safety, and environmental protection laws.

17. Always be prepared to provide your doctor with precise information about the chemicals you use and your work habits. Arrange for regular blood tests for lead if you use lead-containing textile paints or pigments.

FIBER HAZARDS

For centuries, occupational diseases such as dermatitis, skin and pulmonary anthrax, and weaver's cough (brown lung) have been associated with exposure to some vegetable and animal textile fibers. Now new man-made fibers and chemical treatments of textiles have added some occupational hazards to the list.

VEGETABLE FIBER HAZARDS. Fiber from plants such as flax, hemp, sisal, and cotton have been associated with a debilitating disease commonly called "brown lung" or byssinosis. It is usually only seen among heavily exposed textile factory workers. Its early symptoms, including chest tightness, shortness of breath, and increased sputum flow, commonly appear when the worker returns to work after being away a few days. The condition is reversible if exposure ceases, but after ten or twenty years of exposure, the disease can progress without further exposure and may be fatal.

Long years of exposure to hemp, sisal, jute, and flax dusts is associated with chronic bronchitis, emphysema, and various allergic conditions. Some of these illnesses may be caused by mildew, fungus spores, dyes, and fiber treatments like permanent press or sizing rather than by the fiber itself. Artists noticing recurring symptoms when working with fibers should investigate the possible causes of such reactions and see their doctors.

SYNTHETIC FIBER HAZARDS. Very little is known about the hazards of synthetic fibers such as rayon, acetate, nylon, acrylics, and so on. Their dusts have been reported to cause irritation when inhaled. Fiberglass textiles, of course, will cause considerable irritation to the skin and respiratory tract. Whether more serious diseases result from exposure to synthetic fibers will not be known until years of data from industrial experience has been gathered. In the meantime, prudence dictates minimizing exposure to them.

ANIMAL FIBER HAZARDS. Fibers used by artists may include wool, silk, hair from goats, horses, rabbit, dogs, and other animals. Allergies to such fibers or animal dander are well-known and can affect fiber artists. But many reactions to animal fibers are from mold, mildew, spores, and the like which can contaminate fibers.

There are other contaminants as well. For example, greasy wool can contain sheep dip. Uncarded or dirty wool or hair can contain little twigs and grass seeds which can cause injury to weavers and spinners.

ZOONOSES—diseases which can be transmitted from animals to man— also may afflict users of animal fibers. For example, inhalation of invisible anthrax spores from wool or hair harvested from diseased animals can cause a virulent, often fatal infectious disease.

Artists also should encourage stricter government enforcement of import regulations and testing of all animal products to prevent contaminated products from entering their countries. Failure to detect a shipment of anthrax-contaminated Pakistani wool in the United States resulted in the death of an artist-weaver in 1976.

Other diseases which affect those working with animal products include Q fever, mange, lice, and more. Even working with dog hair can be hazardous since dog tapeworm larva can cause hyatids (cysts) to form in the liver, skin, and other areas of the body.

Cleaning animal fibers will remove some of these hazards, but not all. It is safer to buy pre-washed, disinfected fibers. Artists using suspect materials may wish to be immunized for anthrax, although the shots also cause side effects which must be considered.

FIBER TREATMENT HAZARDS. Many fiber treatments such as formaldehyde-emitting permanent press treatments, sizing, fire retardants, stain-guarding chemicals, mothproofing, and the like, have been shown to cause allergies and other effects. Many of these chemicals have not been well-studied. The complex organic chemical fire retardant called "tris" was not found to be a carcinogen until years after it was in common use in children's sleepwear.

Artist's who have unusual reactions to working with particular materials should also consider fiber and fabric treatment as a possible source of the difficulty. When applying fiber treatments themselves, artists should obtain as much information about the chemicals as possible.

MOTHRPOOFING chemicals are usually pesticides and require care when they are used. Two chemicals commonly used for mothproofing and mothballs are paradichlorobenzene (PDB) and naphthalene. Threshold Limit Values for PDB and Naphthalene are 75 and 10 parts per million respectively. This confirms that both are very toxic but that PDB should be the preferred treatment chemical.

PDB is moderately toxic and has been shown to be an animal carcinogen in United States National Toxicology Program tests. Naphthalene is currently being tested for its cancer-causing ability. It is moderately toxic causing anemia, liver, and kidney damage. To certain people of Black, Mediterranean, and Semitic origins with genetic glucose-6-phosphate dehydrogenase deficiencies, naphthalene is highly toxic causing severe anemia.

WEAVING, SEWING, AND OTHER FABRICATION TECHNIQUES

Weaving, spinning, sewing, knitting, macrame, embroidery, tapestry, and similar processes involve sitting or remaining still, and using the hands in repetitive actions for long periods of time. Such tasks require careful positioning of the body. For example, looms must be properly tuned, chair heights and sewing machine foot pedals must be adjusted to fit the individual artist.

Frequent breaks should be taken and posture should be varied as often as possible. Many weavers find exercising to relieve strain is helpful.

Eyes also can be strained if lighting is not of the proper intensity and direction. Ergonomic problems, eye strain, and other health effects from exposure to Video Display Terminals may result if weavers use computers to generate patterns.

PRECAUTIONS FOR FIBER ARTISTS

1. Fibers and textiles should be purchased from reliable suppliers who will provide information about the origin of the materials, the dyes or fiber treatments which have been applied, and so on.

2. Purchase cleaned or washed fibers or textiles when possible. If raw, uncleaned materials are used, get advice on best methods for cleaning and disinfecting fibers.

3. Do not use mildewed or musty materials. Store fibers in clean dry places to avoid growth of microorganisms.

4. Avoid dust. For example, use proper-sized needles in loom shuttles. Damp mop or sponge up dusts rather than sweeping or vacuuming. Shake out fabrics away from the workplace.

5. Obtain information on moth-proofing, sizing, permanent press, and other treatments which have been applied to your materials. When applying treatment chemicals yourself, obtain Material Safety Data Sheets and/or ingredient information and follow precautionary instructions.

6. Adjust looms, chair heights, etc., for ergonomic comfort. Take breaks (perhaps five minutes each half hour), stretch and exercise to relieve strain.

7. Provide proper lighting for weaving and other work (see page 38).

8. Follow precautions for VDT use if computers are used (see page 38).

9. Artists exposed to fiber dusts should have pulmonary function tests periodically. Weavers using raw animal fibers should keep up with their tetanus shots and consult with experts about other immunizations appropriate for the raw materials used. Always be prepared to provide your doctor with precise information about the materials you use and your work practices.

TABLE 16	Hazards of Mordants and Dye Assisting Chemicals

ALUM (potassium aluminum sulfate) Some people may be allergic to it, but no special precautions are needed when using it.

AMMONIA (ammonium hydroxide)* Avoid concentrated solutions. Household strength ammonia is diluted and less hazardous. Inhalation of its vapors can cause respiratory and eye irritation. Wear gloves and avoid inhalation.

AMMONIUM ALUM (ammonium aluminum sulfate) Hazards are the same as those of alum (see above).

CAUSTIC SODA (lye, sodium hydroxide)* Very corrosive to the skin, eyes, and respiratory tract. Wear gloves and goggles.

CLOROX (household bleach, 5 percent sodium hypochlorite)* Corrosive to the skin, eyes, throat, and mucous membranes. Wear gloves and goggles. Mixing with ammonia results in the release of highly poisonous gases (nitrogen trichloride, nitrogen oxides, chlorine, etc.). Mixing with acids releases highly irritating chlorine gas.

COPPER SULFATE (blue vitriol)* May cause allergies and irritation of the skin, eyes, and upper respiratory tract. Chronic exposure to copper sulfate dust can cause ulceration of the nasal septum.

CREAM OF TARTAR (potassium acid tartrate) No significant hazards.

FERROUS SULFATE (copperas)* Slightly irritating to skin, eyes, nose, and throat. No special precautions necessary.

FORMIC ACID (methanoic acid)* Highly corrosive to eyes and mucous membranes. May cause mouth, throat, and nasal ulcerations. Wear gloves and goggles.

GLAUBER'S SALT (sodium sulfate) Slightly irritating to skin, eyes, nose, and throat.

OXALIC ACID* Skin and eye contact may cause severe corrosion and ulceration. Inhalation can cause severe respiratory irritation and damage. Wear gloves and goggles.

POTASSIUM DICHROMATE (potassium bichromate, chrome)* Skin contact may cause allergies, irritation, and ulceration. Chronic exposure can cause respiratory allergies. A suspect carcinogen. Wear gloves and goggles.

SALT (sodium chloride)* Some all-purpose dyes contain enough to be toxic to children by ingestion. No other significant hazards.

SODIUM CARBONATE * Corrosive to the skin, eyes, and respiratory tract.

SODIUM HYDROSULFITE (sodium dithionite)* Irritating to the skin and respiratory tract. Stored solutions decompose to give irritating and sensitizing sulfur dioxide gas. Mixtures with acids will release large amounts of sulfur dioxide gas. Wear gloves.

SULFURIC ACID (oleum)* Highly corrosive to the skin and eyes. Vapors can damage respiratory system. Heating generates irritating and sensitizing sulfur dioxide gas. Wear gloves and goggles.

TANNIN (tannic acid)* Slight skin irritant. Causes cancer in animals. Handle with care.

TIN CHLORIDE (tin, stannous chloride)* Irritating to the skin, eyes, and respiratory tract. Wear gloves and goggles.

UREA No significant hazards.

VINEGAR (dilute acetic acid) Glacial (pure) acetic acid is highly corrosive and the vapors are irritating. Vinegar (about 5 percent acetic acid) is safer. Mildly irritating to the skin and eyes.

---

* Can be poisonous if ingested. Keep out of reach of children.
credit: M. Rossol, "Fiber Arts Hazards and Precautions," Center for Occupational Hazards, New York, 1985

17 LEATHER AND OTHER ANIMAL PRODUCTS

For centuries, occupational diseases including zoonoses and allergies have been associated with the use of animal products such as leather, horn, bone, ivory, and shell. In recent years, statistical studies of leather workers have shown high rates of bladder and nasal sinus cancer.

HARVESTING AND TANNING

Workers harvesting leather from animals and birds are exposed to a host of zoonoses—diseases which can be transmitted from animals to man. Many of these diseases are discussed in Chapter 16, Textile Arts, pages 195-197. In the United States and Canada, rabies is also known to be transmittable during harvesting.

Once harvested, leather is preserved with tanning chemicals. Extracts from certain plants which are natural sources of tannic acid are still used for "vegetable tanning" of sole and heavy duty leathers.

Many other leathers are tanned with minerals such as the sulfates of chromium, aluminum, or zirconium. Many synthetic chemicals are now used to tan leather. Some of these are sulfonated phenol or naphthols condensed with formaldehyde. A few special leathers and skins for taxidermy and natural history specimens also may be treated with arsenic and powerful pesticides.

HAZARDS OF TANNING CHEMICALS

Tannin is a suspect carcinogen. Chrome sulfates and some other chrome compounds are sensitizers and suspect carcinogens. Synthetic tanning chemicals such as sulfonated phenols are very toxic. The use of these toxic and sensitizing tanning chemicals may explain in part why workers exposed to leather dusts have high rates of cancer and other occupational illnesses.

Tanners should also remember that human skin can be tanned. Tanning chemicals should be kept off the skin.

LEATHER WORKING

Tools such as knives, awls, punches, and a host of specialized tools are used in each type of leather work. Care should be taken to keep these tools in good repair and sharp, and to use them safely.

Sanding of leather can be done by hand or with electric sanders. This sanding dust contains leather, tanning chemicals, dyes, and glues. Dust exposure should be prevented with local exhaust ventilation and/or respiratory protection. Goggles should be worn to prevent eye injury.

DYEING

Leather dyes, like textile dyes, tend to be hazardous chemicals (see Chapter 10, Pigments and Dyes, pages 99-100). Traditional leather dye products contain solvents from very toxic classes such as chlorinated hydrocarbons, glycol ethers, and aromatic hydrocarbons (see Table 5, Common Solvents and Their Hazards, page 89). Some leather dyes are dissolved in ethyl alcohol. These are safer to use.

Safer still are the new water-based acrylic leather dyes. Although there may be small quantities of water-miscible solvents in these products, it is assumed that these dye products are the least toxic.

CEMENTING

There are a number of leather glues on the market. Barge cement and rubber cements are the most common. Barge cement contains toluene and petroleum distillates (see Table 5, Common Solvents and Their Hazards, page 89). Rubber cements often contain normal hexane (n-hexane) which is a potent nerve toxin (see Chapter 9, Solvents, page 84.)

Inhalation and skin contact with all solvent-containing glues should be avoided.

Some new water-emulsion glues for leather have been developed. Choose these when ever possible.

CLEANING AND FINISHING

Cleaning can be done with oxalic acid or saddle soaps. Saddle soap has no significant hazards unless it is preserved with strong pesticides. Oxalic acid is corrosive to skin, eyes, digestive, and respiratory tracts. Once absorbed, oxalic acid is damaging to the kidneys.

Finishes for leather may consist of oils such as neatsfoot oil and waxes, most of which have no significant hazards. Other types of leather finish are lacquers and resins dissolved in solvents. Skin contact and inhalation of these is hazardous.

OTHER ANIMAL PRODUCTS

BONE, ANTLER, IVORY, and HORN are used in many crafts. Toxic solvents are used to dissolve fats and oils from these materials when they are freshly harvested. Harvesting and tooling these materials also has been associated with zoonoses. There are known cases of anthrax resulting from harvesting and working with these materials, including a fatal case of anthrax contracted while tooling ivory into piano keys.

The most common diseases associated with these materials is irritation and allergic response to their dusts. Dusts from abrasives used to sand these materials may also be hazardous (see Table 13, Hazards of Common Minerals used in Ceramics, Sculpture, Lapidary, and Abrasives.

SHELLS including mother-of-pearl, abalone, and coral are commonly ground and sanded. Dust from these processes causes respiratory allergies, especially if the shell is not properly washed and contains organic matter.

Inhalation of mother-of-pearl dust can cause fevers, respiratory infections, and asthmatic reactions. Years ago, repeated inhalation of mother-of-pearl dust by adolescents working in the pearl button industry caused defects and lesions of the long bones of their arms and legs.

FEATHERS for crafts and for pillow stuffing can cause "feather-pickers disease" which is characterized by chills, fever, coughing, nausea, and headaches. These symptoms usually abate when the individual develops a tolerance for feathers. Tolerance may take weeks or even years to develop. Some people become permanently allergic to feathers.

Mothproofing chemicals such as paradichlorobenzene or naphthalene are commonly applied to feathers (see Chapter 16, Textile Arts, page 197). Allow mothball odors to dissipate before working with feathers.

PRECAUTIONS FOR WORKING LEATHER AND OTHER ANIMAL PRODUCTS

1. Obtain Material Safety Data Sheets on all chemicals and choose the safest products when possible.

2. Work on easy to clean surfaces and wipe up spills and dust immediately. Follow Material Safety Data Sheet advice and have handy proper materials for controlling spills and for chemical disposal. Wet-mop and sponge floors and surfaces. Do not sweep.

3. Practice scrupulous personal hygiene. Do not eat, smoke, or drink in the workplace. Wash hands and change out of work clothing before leaving the studio. Wash work clothes frequently and separately from other clothes.

4. Avoid skin contact or inhalation of tanning chemicals by using exhaust ventilation and/or respiratory protection and gloves. Use chemical splash goggles when using corrosive chemicals. Purchase pretanned leather when possible.

5. Keep tools sharp and all machines in good repair. Prepare for accidents by having first aid materials for trauma and post emergency procedures. Keep tetanus immunization up-to-date.

6. Clean leather with saddle soaps or other detergent and soap cleaners when possible. Avoid oxalic acid cleaners.

7. Clean shell, bone, horn, antler, and other animal products well before working with them. Buy precleaned materials when possible.

8. Control sanding dusts of all leather and animal products with local exhaust ventilation and/or respiratory protection (with a dust filter or cartridge).

9. If dyes are used, follow all precautions for dyers (see Chapter 16, Textile Arts, pages 193-194). Choose acrylic water-based leather dyes or dyes dissolved in ethyl alcohol when possible.

10. Follow all rules for solvent use when working with solvent-containing dyes, glues, and finishes (see Chapter 9, Solvents, pages 87-89).

11. Always be prepared to provide your doctor with precise information about the materials you use and your work practices.

CHAPTER

18 | *CERAMICS*

O ccupational illnesses, such as lung disease (silicosis) and lead poisoning, have been associated with pottery-making for hundreds of years. Unfortunately, these illnesses and others are still seen in ceramic artists and hobbyists and their families today. Ceramic hazards occur during three basic processes: working with clay, glazing, and firing.

CLAY HAZARDS

Most art and craft potters use one of two methods when making clay objects: manipulating wet clay by methods such as hand building or wheel throwing; and slurrying the clay into a liquid slip and casting it with molds.

HAZARDOUS INGREDIENTS. Whether hand-formed or slip cast, the term "clay" has come to mean any mineral material which can be used to make ceramic or porcelain objects. Most of these "clays" are composed of a number of mineral ingredients mixed together to produce a body which will fire at a particular temperature and have particular qualities.

Some ingredients in.these "clays" include true clays (such as fire clay, china clay, and red clays), sources of silica (such as powdered flint, quartz, or sand), and many other minerals including feldspar, talc, and wollastonite. Most clays will also have small amounts of additives such as: barium compounds to control scumming; bentonite to increase plasticity; grog (ground fire brick), vermiculite, or perlite to give texture; metal oxides to impart color; and the like. Slip clays additives may include stabilizers such as gum arabic to keep the mixture in suspension, and biocides to control mold and fungus.

Those clays and minerals which are mined from the earth usually contain many impurities. The actual composition of a particular ingredient may vary greatly from place to place in the mine or deposit. Researching the hazards of these ingredients usually means getting their chemical and mineral analyses. This information should be readily available from your suppliers because they need it for their right-to-know programs for their workers.

Once you have identified all the ingredients of your products, the hazards can be looked up. Almost all clays and clay mixtures contain significant amounts of silica (see pages 153-154). Hazards of other minerals, such as talc and wollastonite, can be found in Table 13, Hazards of Common Minerals used in Ceramics, Sculpture, Lapidary, and Abrasives, page 157. Metal compounds such as barium sulfate can be looked up in Table 10, Hazards of Metals and Metal Compounds, page 133.

PHYSICAL HAZARDS. In addition to toxic chemicals, there are physical hazards from the heavy work, from noise, and other hazards.

OVERUSE AND STRAIN INJURIES. There are also many overuse injuries which can occur while wedging, throwing, or hand building with clay. Many potters have acquired injuries such as carpal tunnel syndrome, a condition involving compression of the median nerve at the wrist. Often, wedging and/or throwing are the cause.

Hand, back, and wrist muscle injuries can also occur from sitting at the potters wheel for too long, especially if posture is incorrect. Injuries from lifting sacks of clay, molds, and the like are common among both potters and ceramicists (see Chapter 4, Physical Hazards and Their Control, Over-Use Injuries, page 39).

NOISE loud enough to damage hearing may be created by machinery such as pug mills and badly installed kiln ventilation. Wearing hearing protection such as ear plugs should prevent hearing loss (see Chapter 4, Physical Hazards and Their Control, pages 35-37).

OTHER PROBLEMS which are noted among clay workers include chapping and drying of the skin, and bacterial and fungal infections of the skin and nail beds.

Since wet clay commonly harbors bacteria and molds, some people may develop allergies to clay dust, and people with preexisting asthma and allergies may find their conditions worsen with exposure to clay. Avoiding dusty procedures is always advisable to prevent development of allergies. People with severe allergies would be wise to choose a different craft.

Wet clay is also a good medium of exchange for disease-causing bacteria and viruses. It is not recommended for hospital and institutional art or therapy programs if patients are carriers of infectious diseases such as hepatitis B.

GLAZE HAZARDS

Common glazes are a mixture of minerals (see Table 13, Hazards of Common Minerals Used in Ceramics, Sculpture, Lapidary, and Abrasives, page 157), metallic compounds (see Table 10, Hazards of Metals and Metal Compounds, page 133), and water. Commercial glazes usually contain frits and additives such as gum stabilizers and preservatives. Preservatives in commercial glazes are usually small amounts of toxic pesticides or bacteriocides. Gum stabilizers usually are not very toxic.

HAZARDOUS INGREDIENTS. In general, metallic elements function in glazes as fluxes (causing the glaze to melt properly) and colorants. Their toxicity varies greatly. Some very safe ones are iron, calcium, sodium, and potassium. Some low fire glazes contain very toxic fluxes and colorants including lead, cadmium, antimony, and arsenic. Middle range and high fire glazes may have large amounts of highly toxic fluxes such as barium and lithium. Toxic colorants which can be in both high- and low-fired glazes include uranium, chromium, cobalt, manganese, nickel, and vanadium. Some lustre glazes also contain highly toxic mercury and arsenic.

Lustre glazes usually contain metallic alloys and compounds, highly toxic solvents such as chloroform and other chlorinated or aromatic hydrocarbons (see Table 5, Common Solvents and Their Hazards, page 89), and tack oils such as oil of lavender. Tack oils are hazardous primarily when they decompose during firing (see Carbon Monoxide and Other Organic Decomposition Products below.)

Glazes are often used in conjunction with colorant materials such as metallic oxides, stains (e.g., Mason stains), underglazes, engobes, ceramic decals, and the like. These materials rely primarily on metallic compounds for coloring (see Table 10 Hazards of Metals and Metal Compounds, page 133).

There are also new ceramic paints on the market which look like fired ceramic glazes when dry. These usually contain plastic resins and solvents. The hazardous ingredients in these glaze paints are solvents and resins (see Chapters 9 and 10, Solvents and Pigments).

LEAD GLAZES. Those choosing to use lead glazes, should consider the health effects of lead (see pages 132-133), the solubility of lead frits (see page 156), and the leaching characteristics of lead glazes (see Finished Ware Hazards below). They also need consider the expense of compliance with (or being caught in violation of) Canadian or United States occupational and environmental lead laws. Ideally, lead glazes should be phased out of use for art and craft work.

WORKING WITH GLAZES. Glazes are potentially hazardous at all stages of use including during glaze making, application, firing, and when glazed pottery is used as food utensils.

GLAZE MAKING is one of the most hazardous tasks potters perform because it involves weighing and mixing the powdered ingredients. Methods of controlling the dust should be employed (see Chapter 7, Ventilation).

APPLICATION of glazes can be done by brushing, dipping, spraying, air brushing, and occasionally by dusting dry ingredients onto wet ware. Brushing and dipping methods are preferred because they produce less dust. Spraying, air brushing, and dusting should only be done in a spray booth or outdoors.

Many other glazing processes are potentially hazardous and should be evaluated for safety. For example, melting paraffin to use as a glaze resist can be a fire hazard and result in exposure to toxic wax decomposition products. Local exhaust ventilation should be provided for this process, direct flame should not be used to heat the wax (e.g., use an electric fry pan), and the temperature of the paraffin should be kept as low as possible. Water/wax emulsions which are applied without heat are safer.

FIRING

VENTILATION. When clays and glazes are fired, they release various gases, vapors, and fumes. Some common emissions from kilns include carbon monoxide, formaldehyde and other aldehydes, sulfur dioxide, chlorine, fluorine, metal fumes, nitrogen oxides and ozone (see Table 17, Sources of Toxic Kiln Emissions, page 216).

For this reason, all firing processes require ventilation. Different types of firing need different types of ventilation. Some types can only be done safely outdoors. All indoor kilns, whether electric or fuel-fired, need exhaust ventilation. Table 18 describes proper ventilation for various types of kilns.

FIRE/ELECTRICAL SAFETY. Fire hazards should be considered when planning pottery or ceramic studios. Consult local fire officials or other experts to be sure your studio meets all local fire regulations and electrical codes.

Large kilns should be located in areas in which there are no combustible or flammable materials. Even small electric kilns should be at least three feet from combustible materials such as paper, plastic, or wood. Electric kilns also should be raised at least a foot above the floor to allow air to circulate underneath. Wooden floors under small electric kilns can be protected by asbestos-substitute fiber boards, or refractory brick.

To prevent fires and damage to ware, electric kilns should be equipped with two automatic shut-offs in case one fails. (Three types to choose from are pyrometric shut-offs, cone operated shut-offs, and timers.)

KILN BUILDING. Many potters choose to build their own kilns. This process may expose potters to many hazards including asbestos-substitutes (some are suspect carcinogens), fire brick dust (usually contains silica), heavy lifting, and noise (if hard bricks are wheel cut).

If dust-producing tasks cannot be done in local exhaust or outdoors, respiratory protection approved for toxic dusts should be used. Hearing protection should be used if brick cutting or other noisy processes are done (see Chapter 4, Physical Hazards and Their Control, section on Noise, pages 35-37).

Connecting kilns to gas or electric lines should be done or approved by licensed electricians and/or gas company employees.

FINISHED WARE HAZARDS

Potters and ceramicists often are not aware that they may be liable if the ware they sell harms someone. Potters, like commercial chinaware makers, could be held responsible for injuries or damages incurred if their ovenware shatters from heat, or if lead or other toxic metals from their glazes contaminates food.

LEACHING. The problem of glaze solubility (leaching) is particularly complex. Leaching glazes solubilize, slowly releasing all their ingredients into food (albeit sometimes at varying rates). Most glazes leach faster in acid solutions such as orange juice. Standard laboratory leaching tests are done in acid solutions. But there is reason to believe that some may solubilize faster in contact with alkaline foods such as beans or some green vegetables.

Many factors influence glaze solubility including composition of the glaze, small amounts of certain impurities, heating and cooling cycles during firing, fumes from other glazes fired in the kiln, and more. Commercial producers have found that testing programs are the only way to guarantee glaze performance. Potters should consider doing the same.

Some ceramicists have relied on premixed glazes which are sold as "lead safe," meaning that they are not expected to leach lead or cadmium into food if the firing and application of the glazes are done properly. However, over- or under-firing, application over an unsuitable underglaze (such as one containing copper), the contamination of a glaze from using an unclean brush, and many other factors can render a "lead safe" glaze dangerous.

Potters often mistakenly think that only low fire lead glazes are hazardous with food. Now it is known that some high fire glazes can leach dangerous amounts of barium, lithium, and other metals. It is true that the Canadian and the United States consumer protection laws currently only regulate lead and cadmium release from ceramics. However, in 1989, the United States Food and Drug Administration (FDA) called for data on leaching of other metals from lead-free glazes to investigate their safety. And whether regulated or not, potters are still liable for harm toxic glazes cause consumers.

Potters should consider either having reliable laboratories periodically test their ware, or to use glazes which contain no toxic metal-containing ingredients. These safer glazes would rely on glaze chemicals containing sodium, potassium, calcium, and magnesium fluxes.

Glazed ware which will not pass leaching tests should have a hole drilled in it to render it unusable or it should be labeled with a permanent fired decal. In the United States, the decal must state: FOR DECORATIVE USE ONLY—NOT FOR USE WITH FOOD. (New wording proposed by the FDA is: NOT FOR FOOD USE—MAY POISON FOOD.)

GLAZE TESTING. Glazes can be tested by sending pieces to certified laboratories. Usually cups are easiest to ship and test. The cost may run from as little as $50.00 to as high as $ 400.00 for testing six cups for two metals. Good laboratories can test for many different metals at your request.

There is also a company which markets two home lead ceramic tests— one a twenty-minute screening test and the other a more accurate twenty-four hour test. These do not replace proper laboratory tests, but will identify a possible problem with lead (and in some cases other metals) leaching.

The tests can be purchased for around $30.00 each and they contain enough materials to do 100 tests. They are available from Frandon Enterprizes, 511 North 48th Street, Seattle, WA 98103, (206) 633-2341.

RULES FOR WORKING WITH CLAY AND GLAZES

1. Plan studios with clean up procedures in mind. Floors should be sealed and waterproof. Tables, shelving, and equipment should be made of materials which can be easily sponged clean. Enough space should be left between tables and equipment to make cleaning easy.

2. Construct kilns from refractory brick and castables when possible. Avoid asbestos and synthetic fiber insulation. Wall off existing fiber insulation with brick or metal barriers. Repair or dispose of fiber insulation with precautions similar to those required for asbestos abatement. Follow all occupational and environmental regulations when disturbing, repairing, or disposing of asbestos-containing materials.

3. Install proper ventilation for the types of kilns you use (see Table 18).

4. Keep all tools, machinery, and potter's wheels in good condition. Be especially vigilant about electrical condition since water is always present.

5. Plan fire protection carefully. Locate kilns in areas free of combustible materials. Equip electric kilns with two automatic shut-offs in case one fails. Consult fire officials or other experts for advice on proper fire-fighting systems and/or extinguishers. Do not locate water sprinkler heads above kilns or other hot and/or high voltage equipment. Hold regular fire drills.

6. Prepare for emergencies. Have a first aid kit handy. Post and practice emergency procedures.

7. Use proper personal protective equipment. Wear infrared-blocking goggles when looking into glowing kilns (see figures 4 & 5, pages 58-60), asbestos-substitute gloves when handling hot objects, impact goggles when grinding or chipping, dust masks if needed, and so on.

8. Obtain Material Safety Data Sheets on all materials used in the studio such as clays, glazes, and grind wheels. In addition, obtain mineral and chemical analyses of clays, glazes, and other minerals from suppliers. Avoid materials containing highly toxic ingredients such as lead and asbestos, and treat materials containing over one percent free silica as toxic, providing ventilation and/or respiratory protection.

9. If lead is used on the job, employers must be prepared to meet complex OSHA Lead Standard regulations in the United States or the OHSA Regulations respecting Lead in Canada.

10. Practice good hygiene. Wash hands carefully and use a nail brush after glazing. Work on surfaces that are easily cleaned with a damp sponge and wipe up spills immediately.

11. Avoid skin problems. Keep broken skin from contact with clay and glazes. Wash hands and apply a good emollient hand cream after work. People with skin problems can wear surgical or plastic gloves while working.

12. Wear protective clothing such as smocks, tightly woven coveralls, and hair covering. Avoid flammable synthetic fabrics. Change clothing when leaving the pottery rather than carrying dusts home. Wash clothing frequently and separately from other clothes.

13. Avoid repetitive strain injuries. Make repetitive and/or forceful movements of the hands and arms in short bursts and take frequent rests. Never work to the point of exhaustion or pain. Change positions frequently. When wedging, keep the wrist in a neutral or mid-joint position, and use the weight of the body rather than just the muscles of the upper limb. In general, good posture, avoidance of extreme overweight, and exercise to keep muscles strong are all useful in preventing overuse injuries.

14. Avoid lifting injuries. Store heavy bags of clay and other materials at heights (on benches or shelves) where lifting can be done without bending the back. Storage on trolleys may even avoid the need to lift. When lifting is necessary, it should be done with the legs, keeping the back straight to avoid injury.

15. Avoid dusty processes when possible. Examine all dust-producing procedures such as mixing clay and glazes, sanding greenware, and reprocessing clay. Identify procedures which can be replaced. For example, premixed clay can be purchased instead of mixing it. Buying premixed clay is usually economical if the cost of providing proper ventilation for mixing is considered.

16. Install local exhaust areas for processes that create toxic airborne materials such as glaze spraying, mixing powdered chemicals, for grind wheels, and the like. Spray booths are suitable for glaze spraying and many other processes. Some dusty tasks can be done in front of a strong window exhaust fan or outdoors. (see Chapter 7, Ventilation).

17. If respirators must be used, they should be approved for the process (see Table 4, Respiration Filters and Cartridges, page 76) and follow all rules regarding respirator use (see Chapter 8, Respiratory Protection).

18. Clean floors without creating dust. Do not sweep. Use wet mopping and hosing methods. Ordinary household, industrial, shop, and water-filled types of vacuums will collect only large dusts while releasing the invisible respirable dusts back into the air. Proper vacuums include those which pick up wet material from the floor, or those with high efficiency (HEPA) filters.

19. Dispose of all old clays and glazes, grinding dusts, and other waste materials in accordance with occupational and environmental protection regulations.

20. Always be prepared to provide your doctor with precise information about the chemicals you use and your work practices. Have lung function tests included in your regular physical examinations. Arrange for regular blood lead tests if you use lead-containing frits, glazes or other materials.

21. Provide customers with food-safe ware (see Finished Ware Hazards above).

TABLE 17	Sources of Toxic Kiln Emissions

CARBON MONOXIDE is formed when carbon-containing compounds are burned in limited oxygen atmospheres such as in electric kilns. Carbon sources include organic matter found in most clays and many glaze materials, from wax resists, stabilizers in slip clays, tack oils in lustres, and other organic additives in clays and glazes. Amounts of carbon monoxide over the Threshold Limit Value have been measured near electric kilns.

OTHER ORGANIC DECOMPOSITION PRODUCTS. When organic materials burn, large numbers of compounds in addition to carbon monoxide are created. Many of these also are toxic. Formaldehyde is one such emission which has been measured in significant amounts near electric kilns.

SULFUR OXIDES. Many clays and glaze ingredients contain significant amounts of sulfur-containing compounds. When these are fired they give off sulfur oxides which form sulfurous and sulfuric acids when they combine with water. These acids etch the metal kiln parts above ports and doors and also are highly damaging to the respiratory system.

CHLORINE AND FLUORINE. These gases are released when fluorine- and chlorine-containing clay and glaze chemicals such as fluorspar, iron chloride, and cryolite are fired. Both gases are very irritating to the respiratory tract. Fluorine also is associated with bone and tooth defects.

METAL FUMES. Fumes are formed when some metals and metal-containing compounds are fired. Complex reactions which occur during glaze firing make it difficult to predict precisely at what temperature metals will volatilize and oxidize to form a fume. Some toxic metals which commonly fume include lead, cadmium, antimony, selenium, copper, chrome, and nickel. The fumes may be inhaled or they may settle on surfaces in the studio. Some fumes can contaminate the kiln and deposit on ware in future firings.

NITROGEN OXIDES AND OZONE. These gases may be produced by decomposition of nitrogen-containing compounds or by the effect of heat and/or electricity on air in the kiln. They are strong lung irritants.

OTHER EMISSIONS. One of the strongest arguments for venting all kilns is the unpredictability of emissions. Pottery magazines and textbooks often suggest projects which result in the firing of nails, paper, plastic, wood, wire, and many other items. One magazine even suggested throwing mothballs into hot electric kilns to create reduction atmospheres. This practice would release highly toxic emissions including cancer-causing benzene. Projects such as these combined with the unpredictability of clay and glaze composition make ventilation necessary.

TABLE 18	Types of Kiln Ventilation

ELECTRIC KILNS either should be equipped with canopy hoods, negative pressure ventilation systems, or isolated in a separate room which is provided with very rapid dilution ventilation.

FUEL-FIRED KILNS create large amounts of toxic emissions from the burning of the gas, oil, wood, or other heat sources. Most of these emissions will be drawn through the stack or chimney. The stack should be tall enough to keep emissions from drifting into areas where they are unwanted. Unless they are located outdoors, fuel-fired kilns also need a canopy hood to collect emissions which escape the stack's draw and gases generated during firing techniques such as reduction (when more fuel is introduced than the kiln can burn).

SALT FIRING probably can be done safely only outdoors. Salt firing produces gases such as highly corrosive hydrochloric acid gas. The process can be made safer if salt is replaced with other sodium-containing compounds such as sodium bicarbonate. Kiln stacks should be placed where emissions cannot affect people. If back-up respiratory protection is needed, respirators should be full-face types with acid gas and fume cartridges. (See Chapter 8, Respiratory Protection.)

RAKU FIRING also is best done outside. Theoretically, the firing could be done indoors in almost any type of kiln, but the very smoky reduction phase of the process requires an outdoor location. Even outdoor firing will not provide sufficient ventilation if materials used for reduction release highly toxic chemicals. This can happen if sawdust from chemically treated wood or if leaf and plant materials sprayed with pesticides are accidentally used.

OTHER FIRING TECHNIQUES such as pit firing, sawdust firing, and waste-oil firing are touted in magazines and texts. The materials and methods used in these processes should be investigated and evaluated, and precautions should be planned before attempting them.

CHAPTER

19 *GLASS*

S tudies have shown that a large percentage of glassblowers develop lung problems and significantly decreased lung capacities. The cause or causes of these changes are unknown.

Glass workers also develop other physical problems for which the causes have been associated with hazardous materials or processes. These hazards are encountered during four basic stages in glassblowing: 1) making glass, 2) working (blowing) the glass, 3) annealing, and 4) finishing. The hazards of lampworking and slumping will also be discussed.

MAKING GLASS

Because glass is a "supercooled liquid" rather than a compound or mineral, there is no limit to the varieties and mixtures of glass ingredients possible. Adding a pinch or two of another ingredient to a mixture will produce a "different" glass.

However, there are several basic divisions or classifications of glass. These are usually referred to by the names of their primary fluxes (components which cause the glass to melt). For example, glasses called "borosilicates" employ boron compounds as their major fluxes.

The most common types of clear glass are lead/potash, borosilicates, and soda/lime. White or opal glasses usually come in two varieties, calcium phosphate/silica and alumina/silica/ fluorine glass. Other chemicals are also added to glass melts to alter their properties.

The common glass forming chemicals are the same ingredients used in ceramics. For example, silica, feldspars, lead compounds and frits, boron, and zinc compounds are used. The hazards of these minerals and metal-containing compounds can be looked up in Table 10, Hazards of Metals and Metal Compounds, page 133, and Table 13, Hazards of Common Minerals Used in Ceramics, Sculpture, Lapidary, and Abrasives, page 157.

Glass colorants are often added to the melt. These also are generally the same chemicals used to color ceramic glazes and enamels. They may include compounds of cadmium, chrome, cobalt, copper, gold, iron, manganese, silver, and uranium. The hazards of these metals can be looked up in the Table 10, Hazards of Metals and Metal Compounds, page 133.

These glass-making and coloring compounds are weighed and put in the glass furnace to melt. The powdered chemicals can be inhaled while weighing and charging the furnace. The melting of the glass causes toxic gases and fumes to be given off. Gas furnaces also may give off carbon monoxide gas. Excellent dust control and exhaust ventilation for the furnace are needed.

A safer way to obtain glass is to purchase premixed glass or glass cullet (scrap glass) from glass factories. Some glass blowers recycle scrap glass bottles. Using glass from these sources eliminates handling toxic powders and reduces formation of toxic gases and fumes in the furnace.

Furnaces also must be vented to reduce heat in the work area. Fatigue, rashes, and stroke from heat are common problems among glassblowers. Hot glowing furnace brick and molten glass give off infrared radiation. Protective infrared goggles should be worn to prevent infrared cataract which historically has been called "glassblower's cataract."

WORKING THE GLASS

Glassblowing is heavy physical work in a hot, hazardous environment. The glass is worked while molten and glowing. Sharp glass splinters and shards are created when pieces are discarded, transferred to the pontil, or knocked off the pontil into the annealing oven. Avoiding cuts, burns, and accidents takes constant vigilance and glass workers should be prepared to treat burns and cuts. Some old-time glassblowers keep ice cubes on hand to treat small burns.

Wet wooden tools are often used to form glass and smoke from over-heating these can be inhaled while working. Some practices such as marvering (rolling the hot glass on a cold surface such as metal) colorant chemicals onto the glass, will cause hot toxic gases and fumes to be created.

Work surfaces and benches often have been insulated with asbestos board. Dust raised when these surfaces are abraded has been associated with asbestos-related disease in glassblowers.

ANNEALING

Annealing is done at lower temperatures than melting. Annealing ovens add heat to the workspace, but the amount of heat should be easily dissipated by the shop's general ventilation system. However, if fuming (putting metal chlorides into the oven to create iridescent surfaces) is done in the annealing oven, the irritating fumes created require local exhaust such as a movable canopy hood.

Fiber insulation, such as asbestos or ceramic fiber (see pages 152-156), used in annealing ovens is likely to become disturbed and made airborne as glass is continually put in and removed. Refractory brick contains some free silica, but is much safer.

Annealing is done to relieve stresses in the glass. Improperly annealed glass may crack or shatter, often without warning. There are polarized lights and other instruments which can detect unrelieved stress. Having glass shatter while polishing it can be dangerous. Having it shatter in a show room is not only dangerous, it is embarrassing.

FINISHING GLASS

Dry grinding and polishing of glass can create abrasive dust. Some of the least toxic abrasives and polishing compounds are alumina, tin oxide, silicon carbide, diamond, and cerium dioxide (see Table 13, Hazards of Common Minerals Used in Ceramics, Sculpture, Lapidary, and Abrasives, page 157).

Dry grinding also produces glass dust. This dust is a mechanical irritant to the eyes and respiratory system. It also may be toxic depending on the type of glass being ground. For example, lead/potash glass dust, like a lead frit, can be a source of lead poisoning. Glass colored or opacified with highly toxic chemicals such as arsenic or antimony also can produce hazardous dust.

Wet grinding and polishing methods should be used when possible to reduce exposure to grinding dusts. Some dust will be suspended in the water mist which rises from these tools. Breathing this mist should be avoided.

Mist from these tools also may contain disease-causing microbes. Hazardous microorganisms such as those causing Legionnaires Disease have been isolated from wet grinding water reservoirs. Frequent cleaning keeps these organisms from establishing themselves in the reservoir.

Both wet and dry grinding and polishing dusts containing highly toxic components may be costly to dispose of properly. Consult local environmental protection authorities for further information.

DECORATING GLASS

Glass can also be decorated by etching, sand blasting, painting, and other techniques. These processes are discussed in Chapter 22, Ceramic, Glass, and Enamel Surface Treatments, page 241.

BUILDING/REPAIRING OVENS, FURNACES, ETC.

Furnaces, glory holes, annealing ovens, and other studio equipment are often constructed of hazardous materials. The safest materials are refractory brick and castables. A wide variety of these are on the market. High alumina refractories are extremely resistant to glass. Soft insulating brick is not, but can be protected from direct contact with a layer of hard brick or alumina refractory.

Other construction and insulation materials include asbestos, ceramic and other synthetic fiber products (see pages 152-156). Repair or disposal of equipment constructed with these fiber products can release large amounts of highly hazardous dusts. Repair and disposal of asbestos containing-materials must be done in accordance with occupational and environmental protection regulations. Complying with these regulations is usually costly, but being caught violating them can be even more costly.

LAMPWORKING

Lampworkers use small torches (usually propane, butane, methane, or natural gas and oxygen) to heat glass rods and tubes to form or "blow" into objects and figures. Lampworking hazards include thermal burns, cuts, infrared radiation, fire hazards, and toxic chemicals in some colorants and surface treatments. The hazards of surface treatments can be found in the Chapter 22. Lampworkers can follow those Precautions for Glassworking (below) which are applicable.

SLUMPING AND FUSING

Glass slumping is the process of changing the shape of glass by heating it to temperatures exceeding 530 degrees Centigrade (1000 degrees Farenheit) so it will soften and bend under its own weight. Fusing is the process of heating pieces of glass together until they adhere.

These processes are usually done in electric kilns. Follow all precautions for using ceramic kilns including ventilation (see page 211).

Slumping hazards include burns and cuts, the use of colorants and surface treatments (see Chapter 22, Ceramic, Glass, and Enamel Surface Treatments), thermal shock shattering of improperly annealed glass or from fusing of incompatible glasses, and exposure to mold release powders, fiber paper, kiln washes and the like. Artists doing glass slumping may follow those Precautions for Glassworking (below) which are applicable.

The materials used for molds or to protect forms are of several types. Included are shelf primers, kiln washes, and ceramic fiber mats and papers. Most kiln washes and primers contain sources of free silica such as flint. Firing may convert the silica to more toxic cristobalite (see page 153). Obtain ingredient information and use suitable precautions. Avoid inhalation of dust from these materials and practice good dust control.

Avoid ceramic fiber mats and papers. These may be associated with asbestos-like illnesses, and after repeated firing they partially convert to crystobalite (see pages 155-156). Thin layers of refractory materials or insulating brick can be substituted in some cases.

PRECAUTIONS FOR GLASSWORKING

1. Plan studios with health and safety in mind. Floors should be cement or other noncombustible material. Walls should be fire resistant. Ceilings should be high enough to accommodate swinging blow pipes. Construct adjacent bathroom facilities and a walled-off recreation area. Artists should be able to clean up and retire to a clean room to drink fluids to replace those lost through perspiration, to rest, and the like.

2. Construct furnaces and other equipment from refractory brick and castables when possible. Avoid asbestos and synthetic fiber insulation. Wall off existing fiber insulation with brick or metal barriers. Repair or dispose of fiber-insulated equipment with precautions like those required for asbestos abatement. Follow all occupational and environmental regulations when disturbing, repairing, or disposing of asbestos-containing materials.

3. Plan fire protection carefully. Eliminate all combustibles from the area and provide a source of water on the premises. Do not install water sprinkler heads above furnaces, electric annealing ovens, and similar hot and/or high voltage equipment. Consult fire marshalls or other experts for advice on proper fire-fighting systems and/or extinguishers which meet local and federal safety codes. Post fire procedures and hold drills.

4. Provide excellent local exhaust for the furnace to remove heat and toxic gases. Gas furnaces will need both stack and canopy exhausts. Vent electric annealing ovens if fuming or lustre glazing is done in them.

5. Provide good general ventilation for the workspace to reduce heat. Follow rules to avoid heat stress and repetitive strain injuries (see page 39-40).

6. Provide local exhaust for any processes which create toxic emissions such as hot marvering of colorants, etching, or fuming (see Chapter 22, Ceramic, Glass, and Enamel Surface Treatments, page 244, for precautions for glass surface treatments).

7. Use cullet or second melt glass if possible to avoid the hazards of making glass. Handle shards of broken glass cullet with great care or purchase special "chain mail" types of safety gloves which protect glass handlers from cuts.

8. Obtain Material Safety Data Sheets, formulas and analyses of your glass-making and/or colorant ingredients. Look up their hazards and use the safest materials possible. Especially try to avoid highly toxic ingredients such as arsenic, antimony, cadmium, and uranium colorants, cyanide reducers, and fluorine compounds.

9. Avoid exposure to powdered glass ingredients or colorants. Weigh them in local exhaust areas, outdoors, or use respiratory protection. Transfer them carefully to avoid creating dust. Clean up spills immediately. Prepare for spill control and chemical disposal.

10. Protect eyes by wearing infrared-blocking goggles, which are also impact resistant, whenever looking at glowing hot materials, working with materials which might shatter, or whenever eyes are at risk. (See figures 4 and 5 pages 58-60.)

11. Wear protective clothing similar to welders'. For example, do not wear polyester or other synthetic fibers which will melt to the skin at high heat. Avoid pockets, trouser cuffs, and socks which can catch hot chips. Remove jewelry and tie back hair or wear a hair covering. Wear shoes with soles not easily penetrated by broken glass. Leave clothing in the studio to avoid tracking dusts home. Wash clothing frequently and separately from other clothes.

12. Take frequent work breaks when doing hot work and drink plenty of water (with one teaspoon of salt added per gallon if replacing water lost by perspiration). People with heart or kidney disease, who are very overweight, or who have impaired reflexes, dexterity or strength should not engage in glassblowing.

13. Avoid ingestion of materials by eating, smoking, and drinking in the separate facility outside the work area. Wash hands before eating, applying make-up, and other hygiene tasks.

14. Keep containers of cool water and/or ice handy for cooling tools and treating small burns. Have a first aid kit equipped with treatments for burns and cuts. Post and practice emergency procedures.

15. Practice constant good housekeeping to prevent cuts caused by stepping on broken glass. Never allow trip hazards in the work area.

16. Clean the studio with methods that do not raise dust such as wet mopping or hosing down.

17. Use polarized light sources or other equipment to check finished glass for stress and adjust annealing temperatures and time accordingly.

18. Dry grinding and polishing wheels also should be equipped with local exhaust. All wet and dry grinding and polishing wheels should have machine guards and face guards. Wear impact resistant goggles when grinding.

19. Use wet grinding equipment rather than dry when ever possible. Wet grinding equipment should be cleaned while wet to avoid dust exposure. Water tanks should be cleaned often to keep microorganisms from establishing themselves.

20. Obtain Material Safety Data Sheets on grind wheels and abrasives. Avoid those containing silica and other toxic substances when possible.

21. Dispose of all grinding and polishing dusts, used chemicals, waste glass, and other materials in accordance with good hygiene and waste disposal regulations.

22. Always be prepared to provide your doctor with precise information about the chemicals you use and your work practices. Have lung function tests included in your regular physical examinations. If lead materials are used, arrange for regular blood tests for lead.

CHAPTER 20

STAINED GLASS

L ead poisoning is the major hazard in stained glass work. Lead is used in traditional stained glass to bind pieces of glass together in frames of lead came (channeled lead strips) or in lead-soldered seams coated with copper foil.

NEW MATERIALS

Traditional lead solder methods are likely be replaced in the near future. This is due to the increasing enforcement of lead laws and regulations in the United States and Canada. In the United States, the OSHA Lead Standard requires any workplace where lead is used more than thirty days per year to do air sampling. If lead found in these tests is above a certain amount (.03 milligrams per cubic meter), then regular air monitoring, medical surveillance, special ventilation, and many other costly provisions must be met.

Many glass studios could not afford to meet these standards. Fortunately, new lead-free solders developed for plumbing water pipes will work for stained glass purposes. They are not as easy to use, but more and more stained glass craftspeople are turning to them. In addition, it is likely that lead-free solders will be modified and improved in the near future.

Solders appropriate for stained glass work are made of silver, tin, copper, and zinc. Some lead-free solders contain antimony and these are too toxic. Lead- and antimony-free solders cost about twice what lead solders cost, but they are cheaper than the cost of meeting the lead laws.

Some craftspeople are also changing from lead came to channels of zinc and other metals. With these lead-free materials and certain other precautions, it even may be possible to do stained glass in schools and home workshops safely.

TRADITIONAL LEAD CAME AND SOLDER HAZARDS

Until better lead substitutes are available, traditional stained glass artists and production studio workers must consider the hazards of lead.

LEAD. Cases of lead poisoning among stained glass workers and hobbyists in the medical literature confirm the major hazard of this craft. In some cases, family members and children of stained glass hobbyists who did not work with lead were also poisoned. This phenomena is similar to that observed among the children and wives of industrial lead workers who were affected by small amounts of lead dust and fumes carried home on workclothes and shoes.

There are a number of ways stained glass workers and their families may be exposed to lead. For example, handling lead came will transfer small but significant amounts of lead oxides to the hands. This contamination can be transferred to clothing, food eaten while working, or to other people who are touched. Cutting the came and cleaning or polishing it with whiting creates tiny lead flakes and dust which can be blown or tracked into other areas.

Soldering can also result in contaminating the whole home or studio with lead. Iron soldering or torching solder seams (e.g., copper foil method) creates invisible lead fume which can remain airborne for hours and later may settle on surfaces at a considerable distance from the operation.

OTHER HAZARDOUS METALS. Traditional lead/tin solders may also be a source of other hazardous metals. A lot of these solders also contain significant amounts of highly toxic arsenic and antimony. These metals contaminate lead ore and still are present many in inexpensive solders.

Not only are the fumes of arsenic and antimony highly hazardous to inhale during soldering, but in contact with acids—such as the acid fluxes or patina chemicals—they form extremely toxic arsine and stibine gas. Though the amounts of the metals and their gases may be small, their extreme toxicity can make exposure to them significant.

FLUXES. The solder fluxes themselves, such as zinc chloride and other acid fluxes, are skin, eye, and respiratory irritants. Rosin fluxes are not much used in stained glass work, but they can cause allergies and asthma. Fluoride fluxes are especially toxic and should be avoided if possible. For more detailed information, see Chapter 24, Metal Surface Treatments, Fluxes, page 254-255.

INSULATION. Asbestos board table tops, gloves and other insulated materials may also be a hazard. These should be replaced with asbestos substitutes.

SURFACE TREATING CAME AND SOLDER

METAL COATINGS. Lead came and solder seams are often coated with other metals for the visual effect or to prepare them for treatment with patinas. Copper may be electroplated onto soldered seams from highly toxic chemical baths which may even employ cyanide (see Chapter 24, Metal Surface Treatments, Electroplating, pages 255-257). Or areas may be "tinned" to give them a coating of solder. Tinning solder fluxes usually contain fluorides and can be very hazardous to use.

Lead surfaces must be scrupulously cleaned in order to be coated with metal or patina. Some of these metal cleaners contain strong caustics, strong acids, chemicals which release hydrofluoric acid, or solvents including the glycol ethers (see Table 5, Common Solvents and Their Hazards, page 89).

PATINAS. Once the surface is prepared the patina can be applied. Patinas are generally of two types:1) those which react with the metal surface to form metal compounds such as sulfides or oxides, and 2) those which dissolve metal from the metal surface and replace it with a different metal deposited from the patina chemicals. Both types are composed of chemicals of varying toxicity and they usually produce toxic gases or vapors during application.

Common patina chemicals include copper sulfate and acid solutions which give off sulfur dioxide during use, selenium-containing patinas which may give of highly toxic hydrogen selenide gas, patinas containing highly toxic antimony sulfide. (For further information, see Chapter 24, Metal Surface Treatments, Patinas, page 254 and Table 10, Hazards of Metals and Metal Compounds, page 133.)

WORKING WITH GLASS

Scoring and breaking glass is obviously a safety hazard. Hands and eyes are most at risk from injury. Other glass-shaping methods involve mechanical cutting and grinding for purposes such as beveling and precision cutting. Dry grinding methods produce dust which can be hazardous to inhale. Glass dust, like enamels and frits, may cause mechanical injury to tissues and may release their toxic elements in body fluids. For example, lead glass dust could be a source of lead poisoning.

Wet grinding, polishing, and cutting tools are safer. See page 241. Slumping and fusing glass also are covered in Chapter 19, Glass.

DECORATING GLASS

All glass, whether free blown, lampworked, slumped, fused, or cut for stained glass, can be decorated. There are many glass decorating methods including abrasive blasting (sand blasting), fuming, painting, hydrofluoric acid etching or frosting, and electroplating. The hazards of these procedures are described in Chapter 22.

PRECAUTIONS FOR STAINED GLASS WORK

1. Plan studios and shops with health and safety in mind. If lead will be used, the studio must be completely isolated and separate from living areas. Never allow children into areas where lead or other toxic chemicals are used. Floors and surfaces should be made of materials which are easily sponged and mopped clean.

2. Install ventilation systems appropriate for the work to be done. For example, provide local exhaust, such as slot vents or (if local codes permit) a window exhaust fan at work table level, for soldering, tinning, dry cleaning (with whiting), or polishing, applying patinas or any other operation which produces toxic emissions or dust.

3. Plan for fire safety. Install proper fire extinguishers and post and practice fire evacuation procedures.

4. Have electroplating done professionally, if possible. Otherwise have safety experts help plan and design studio equipment, ventilation, and emergency facilities.

5. If slumping and fusing are done, see Chapter 19, Glass, page 223. If glass painting is done, see Chapter 22.

6. Obtain Material Safety Data Sheets on all solders, abrasive grits and wheels, patinas and other products. Avoid solders and other products containing significant amounts of arsenic, antimony, or other highly toxic metals.

7. Substitute lead-free solders and cames whenever possible. If lead is used on the job, employers must be prepared to meet complex OSHA Lead Standard regulations in the United States or the OHSA Regulations respecting Lead in Canada.

8. Provide local exhaust ventilation for dry grinding and polishing equipment. Equip grind wheels with face guards. Remember, dust from grinding lead glass also can be a source of exposure to lead.

9. Use wet grinding, polishing and cutting methods whenever possible. Equipment should have face guards. Wet grinding equipment should be cleaned when wet to avoid dust exposure. Water reservoirs should be cleaned often to remove scum or other microbe growth.

10. Wear impact/dust goggles (see figures 4 and 5, pages 58-60) when cutting, grinding, or polishing glass.

11. Have first aid treatment handy for cuts and accidents. Post emergency procedures. Special "chain mail" types of safety gloves can be used for especially hazardous procedures.

12. Do not eat, smoke, or drink in the studio. Wash hands before eating, applying make-up, and other hygiene tasks.

13. Wear protective clothing such as a smock or coveralls, shoes and hair covering. Leave work clothing, hair covering, and shoes in the studio to avoid taking dusts home. Wash clothing frequently and separately from other clothes.

14. Clean the studio with methods which do not raise dust such as wet mopping. Clean floors and sponge surfaces frequently. Clean up shards and scraps often.

15. Replace or encapsulate all asbestos materials and insulation. Follow all health, safety, and environmental protection regulations whenever disturbing, repairing or disposing of asbestos or asbestos-containing materials.

16. Read product literature, Material Safety Data Sheets, and other information on metal cleaners and patinas carefully. Many will require special gloves, goggles, ventilation, and respiratory protection. Follow Material Safety Data Sheet advice and have materials on hand for spill control and chemical disposal.

17. Dispose of all grinding and polishing dusts, spent or neutralized acids and other chemicals, waste glass and other materials in accordance with health, safety, and environmental protection regulations.

18. Always be prepared to provide your doctor with precise information about the chemicals you use and your work practices. If lead is used, arrange for regular blood tests for lead. Keep your tetanus immunization up-to-date.

CHAPTER

21 *ENAMELING*

E namelers are exposed to several hazards including infrared radiation, acids, powdered glass enamels. Enameling is usually done on copper, silver, or gold. However, there are enamels for other surfaces including steel, aluminum, ceramic, and glass.

WHAT ARE ENAMELS?

Enamels are essentially powdered colored glass frits (see frits, pages 156-157). The glass-making frit ingredients may include silica, borax, lead compounds, lithium compounds, and other fluxes. The enamel colorants and opacifiers may include many different metal salts.

It is possible for artists to manufacture their own enamels from these materials. However, grinding and mixing these raw chemicals is hazardous. Commercially manufactured enamels are safer and easier to obtain and use.

The composition of the enamel will determine the material to which it can be fused (depending on its coefficients of expansion with heat). Most art and craft enamels are designed to remelt at low temperatures (730 degrees Centigrade, 1350 degrees Farenheit) and to adhere copper or silver.

LEAD-BEARING AND LEAD-FREE are the two major types of enamels. Lead-bearing types are the most common and can cause lead poisoning. Lead-free enamels are often borosilicate glass and usually only their colorants are hazardous. However, neither type is suitable for use with children since they are both ground glass and most contain some toxic metals.

COLORANTS AND OPACIFIERS are metal compounds which usually are fused into frits during manufacture. Enamel manufacturers' rarely divulge the identity of these chemicals.

Common colorants include cadmium, cobalt, copper, manganese, antimony, selenium, chrome, and nickel. Most opaque lead enamels are opacified with arsenic. In the past, manufacturers used radioactive colorants such as uranium and thorium. Examples include Thompson's Forsythia and Burnt Orange enamels, which have been discontinued. Sale of radioactive enamels now is banned in the United States. Old stocks of such enamels should be discarded.

ENAMEL SOLUBILITY

Some enamels are so soluble in water that they dissolve (degrade) even in humid air. These enamels are easily recognized as those which must be washed before use or else they will produce cloudy or otherwise inferior results. These are the most soluble types, but all enamels are soluble in varying degrees (see Frit Solubility, pages 156-157). For this reason, all enamels that contain toxic metals should be treated as very toxic materials.

Finer particles of enamel dust present more surface area and, hence, are more soluble and toxic. Although most enamels are sieved to 40 or 80 mesh (too large to be airborne), much finer particles are also present in the enamel. These can be seen as a dust which floats up when enamels are transferred from one container to another.

Once fired, enamels usually are too soluble to be used for eating utensils. Lead, cadmium, barium, and other toxic metals can leach into food or drink. Have enameled utensils tested as you would ceramics if you wish to use or sell them (see pages 212-213).

ENAMELING HAZARDS

Enameling is potentially hazardous during 1) application of enamels, 2) kiln firing, 3) preparation of metal to receive enamels, 4) soldering, and 5) during many specialty processes such as hydrofluoric acid etching of fired enamels, and electroplating.

These processes are used with many different enameling techniques. Some of these include cloisonne (soldered wires separate colors), champleve (enamels fired in acid-etched depressions), basse-taille (etched, engraved, chased, or stamped metal covered with layers of transparent enamels), pallion (fusing gold or silver foil into enamel), grissalle, limoges, plique-a-jour, repouse, and sgraffito.

APPLICATION. The degree of hazard during enamel application is related to the degree to which the enamel can be inhaled or contaminate hands, hair, or clothing. Least hazardous are methods that do not raise dust such as wet charging damp enamel with spatulas, or dipping and painting enamels that are mixed with resin and solvents (here the hazards are primarily the solvent vapors). Far more hazardous methods include dusting the powder onto the metal by hand or through a screen, and spraying or air brushing enamels.

The hazards of various enamel adhesives and fixatives are related to their composition and the degree to which the user is exposed to these ingredients. Spray products containing solvents are the most hazardous and should be used with local exhaust ventilation. Obtain ingredient information and use accordingly.

Grinding and polishing of fired enamel surfaces is often done with carborundum or other abrasives under water. Such methods do not raise dust, but waste enamel material should be discarded carefully.

KILN FIRING. Toxic metal fumes from enamel ingredients may emanate from kilns, especially if enamels are over-fired or if bits of enamels flake onto kiln furniture or elements. During the firing process heat can cause burns, and long term exposure to infrared radiation can cause cataracts.

METAL PREPARATION. The metal surface that is to be enameled must be prepared to receive enamel. Metal preparation techniques include cleaning, pickling, etching, engraving, chasing, grinding, filing, and more.

CLEANING is done to prepare metal for enamels and to remove fire scale. Mechanical methods of cleaning metal can be done with pumice, steel wool, wire brushes, or buffers. These methods are the safest.

PICKLING hot metals in acid solutions is a more hazardous way of cleaning metal. Acid vapors constantly rise from acid baths. During pickling, still greater amount of vapors and mists are created.

Pickling solutions are usually dilute sulfuric acid, nitric acids, or solutions of sodium bisulfate. Some commercial jewelry cleaning methods employ cyanide solutions. Cyanide solutions should never be used. Sodium bisulfate (often sold as Sparex) is the least hazardous, but it, too, releases irritating vapors.

ACID ETCHING for techniques such as champleve' is especially hazardous. Nitric acid is commonly used to etch copper. This method liberates highly dangerous nitrogen dioxide gas, which, when inhaled, can cause serious lung damage, including chemical pneumonia. Hydrochloric acid also etches copper, but can be replaced with ferric chloride solutions. Ferric chloride etching is slower, but considerably safer.

OTHER PROCESSES such as engraving, chasing, grinding, buffing, and cutting may be done. Machine tools can be purchased that have guards and exhaust ventilation connections. Cutting, engraving, and similar processes can result in cuts, eye injuries, and the like.

Further information on the hazards of these and other metal working processes may be found in the Chapter 24, Metal Surface Treatments.

SOLDERING creates metal fumes and emissions from fluxes. Lead, gold, and silver solders are commonly used in enameling. Lead fume is very hazardous (see page 228). Silver and gold solders often contain cadmium, which is released as cadmium fume when heated. Cadmium in this form is associated with lung and kidney damage and lung cancer. Cadmium-free silver solders usually contain antimony, which is somewhat less toxic but still can cause serious health effects (see Table 10, Hazards of Metals and Metal Compounds, page 133).

Fluxes for soldering may be zinc chloride and other chlorides, fluoride compounds, or organic resins such as rosin. Of these, fluoride fluxes are most acutely toxic and cause long term hazards such as bone and tooth defects. Zinc and other chloride fluxes release respiratory irritants. Rosin is known to cause allergies.

OTHER TECHNIQUES such as creating matte or etched enamel surfaces with hydrofluoric (HF) acid is a occasionally done. Paste forms of HF are safer than liquid acid solutions. Follow all HF precautions (see page 244).

Electroplating of metal enamel pieces with gold, copper, and other metals is also done. Cyanide plating baths are too toxic for use by most artists. The hazards of other bath chemicals should be researched carefully before embarking on plating.

PRECAUTIONS FOR ENAMELING

I. Choose a studio location that is compatible with all necessary fire protective equipment and ventilation needed for the type of enameling you will do. Never locate studios in or near living or eating areas. Floors and surfaces should be made of materials that are fire resistant and easily mopped and sponged clean.

2. Provide all kilns with ventilation such as recessed canopy hoods, or place them near a window exhaust fan.

3. Keep areas around kilns and other hot processes free of flammable and combustible materials. Sufficient work space should be provided around kilns. Fire extinguishers or other approved fire control equipment should be installed. Post and practice emergency fire procedures.

4. Replace or encapsulate all asbestos pads, gloves, kiln insulation, and other materials. Follow all health, safety, and environmental protection regulations whenever disturbing, repairing, or disposing of asbestos or asbestos-containing materials.

5. Provide sufficient space around kilns for user to work safely and comfortably.

6. Protect against burns by wearing asbestos-substitute or leather gloves. Avoid wearing synthetic clothing, loose sleeves, or other items which could melt, burn, or catch fire from radiated heat. First aid kits should be stocked with appropriate thermal burn treatments. Post emergency burn treatment procedures.

7. Wear protective clothing such as a smock or coveralls and work shoes. Leave shoes and work clothing in the studio to avoid taking dusts home. Wash work clothes frequently and separately from other clothes.

8. Protect eyes during firing with infrared-blocking goggles. Welding goggles of shades 2-6 will work but they may be too dark to see enamel fuse. Use lightly colored goggles designed specifically to block infrared. (see Figures 4 and 5, pages 58-60).

9. Do not eat, smoke, or drink in the studio. Wash hands before eating, applying make-up, and other hygiene tasks.

10. Investigate the composition of your enamels, fixatives, and all other products you plan to use by obtaining Material Safety Data Sheets and other product information from suppliers.

11. Choose the safest enamels. Lead-free should be chosen over lead-based. Reject enamels colored with radioactive metal salts. Avoid, or handle with extra care, enamels colored with highly toxic metals such as arsenic and cadmium.

12. Examine methods of applying enamels and choose those which control dust best and employ the least toxic adhesives, fixatives, etc. Wash enamels if possible. Dusting, spraying, or air brushing methods should be avoided or only done in local exhaust.

13. Clean up enamel spills immediately. Use wet cleaning methods to avoid raising dust. Do not allow dust to remain on floors to be tracked into other areas.

14. Select metal cleaning and pickling, methods which can be done safely in your studio. Mechanical hand-rubbing with steel wool or pumice is the safest method. Never use cyanide cleaning methods. Sodium bisulfate (Sparex) is one of the least hazardous pickles. If acids or Sparex are used, follow precautions for acids (see next rule).

15. Use of acids requires installation of eye wash fountains. Emergency showers must be installed if large amounts of strong acids (more than a quart) are stored or used. Acid baths for cleaning, pickling, or etching require local exhaust (such as chemical fume hoods or placing baths in front of a window exhaust fans). Respirators equipped with acid-gas cartridges may be worn as back-up to ventilation for most acids except nitric acid. Other personal protective equipment includes chemical splash goggles, aprons, and gloves.

16. Stock first aid kit with appropriate acid burn treatments. Post first aid and emergency procedures.

17. Prepare for spills of acids and other chemicals in advance with supplies of neutralizing chemicals, absorbants, etc. Spills of some kinds of acid and other chemicals must be reported to local environmental authorities. Check federal and local (state, provincial, municipal) regulations.

18. Have especially hazardous work such as electroplating done professionally off-site when possible. Otherwise, have safety experts help plan and design studio equipment, ventilation, and emergency facilities for hazardous processes.

19. If soldering is done, provide local exhaust ventilation—work close to a window exhaust fan or on a slot vented table. Obtain reliable ingredient information on solders and choose the safest ones. Avoid solders containing cadmium, arsenic, and antimony. Avoid fluorine fluxes when possible.

20. All dry buffing and grinding wheels require machine guards, face guards, and local exhaust ventilation. Heavy equipment also needs lockout mechanisms. Impact resistant goggles should be worn when working.

21. Obtain Material Safety Data Sheets on abrasive grits and wheels. Choose those free of silica and other toxic minerals when possible.

22. When sawing, cutting, and doing other mechanical metal work, keep tools sharp and employ safe techniques. Stock first aid kit with supplies to treat cuts and abrasions.

23. Dispose of all spent or neutralized acids, waste enamels, and grinding, polishing dusts, and the like in accordance with health, safety, and environmental protection regulations.

24. Do not make enameled items for use with food or drink unless the piece has passed laboratory tests for release of toxic metals. Other pieces should have the warning "not for use with food, for decorative use only" fired permanently on the bottom.

25. If lead is present in solders, enamels, or any enameling materials, arrange for regular blood tests for lead. Always be prepared to provide your doctor with information about the chemicals you use and your work practices.

CHAPTER

22

CERAMIC, GLASS, AND ENAMEL SURFACE TREATMENTS

T he surfaces of ceramics, glass, and enamels can be treated in many ways to produce artistic effects. Some of these treatments are hazardous.

CUTTING AND GRINDING

These methods can be used for purposes such as beveling, cut glass techniques, and incising. Dry grinding and cutting wheels and tools produce dust which can be hazardous to inhale. Dust from glass, enamels, and glazes may cause mechanical injury to tissues and may release their toxic elements in body fluids. For example, dust from grinding lead glass or glazes can be a source of lead poisoning. Dust from grinding fired ceramics contains silica (cristobalite-see pages 153-154).

Wet grinding, polishing, and cutting tools are safer. But some produce dust-containing water mists which are hazardous to inhale. Water reservoirs also may become contaminated with disease-causing microorganisms that can be inhaled with the mist. Running water lubrication systems are more sanitary.

ABRASIVE BLASTING

This method is currently a popular decorating technique. Hand-held blasting guns and enclosed cabinet blasting are two methods in use. Both direct a blast of abrasive material against a surface to etch it or clean it. Common abrasives include sand, metal, slag, garnet, aluminum oxide, silicon carbide, glass bead, and organic substances such as walnut shells, sawdust, apricot pits, plastic, and the like. See Table 13, Hazards of Common Minerals Used in Ceramics, Sculpture, Lapidary, and Abrasives, for the hazards of common abrasives.

Sand or other sources of free silica should not be used for abrasive blasting because it is such a serious health hazard. Abrasive blasting with sand produces large amounts of very fine silica dust that has been shown to cause a type of rapidly developing silicosis (progressive massive fibrosis), which can be contracted in as little as a few weeks of exposure and is usually fatal within a year or two. For this reason, sand blasting is outlawed in some countries (not in the United States and Canada).

Regardless of the toxicity of the abrasive, all inert dusts are hazardous in quantity. Protective measures must be devised. One method is to use blasting cabinets, which are sealed and kept under negative pressure. In this case the user needs no additional protective gear except when dust is released during processes such as changing the abrasive. However, the cabinet will only provide protection as long as it is well-maintained. Unfortunately, it is common to see blasting cabinets in schools and studios in poor repair and leaking toxic dusts.

Hand-held blasting equipment usually requires the user to wear protective gear and work in an isolated or outdoor environment. Protective gear for large work may include air-supplied respiratory protection, eye protection, gauntlet gloves, and protective clothing and shoes.

FUMING

Fuming metallic salts (usually chlorides) onto surfaces to create an iridescent look is a technique popularized by Tiffany. It is the process of depositing a thin layer (only a molecule or two) of metal on the glass surface which give an "oil on water" appearance. Different metals will produce different colors. Metals that have been used in fuming include tin, iron, titanium, vanadium, cadmium, and uranium.

Fuming can be done by introducing the metal compounds into an annealing oven or by spraying a water solution of the chlorides and acids onto surfaces when hot. Both methods cause the metal compounds to fume and to dissociate. The resulting emissions are highly irritating to the respiratory system and eyes. Cadmium and uranium are too toxic for use in this manner by studio artists. Vanadium is also very toxic and probably should not be used. Superb ventilation is needed for these processes.

PAINTING

Painting on glass and ceramic surfaces can be done with a number of materials. Some "glass paints" are really enamels fired onto glass. These paints are usually lead frits and metal colorants whose dust can be hazardous. Some are premixed in solvents and tack oils. See Chapter 21, Enameling, page 237, for precautions.

Lustres or metallic paints, which are similar to lustre glazes, contain metal alloys and compounds. Some may even contain amalgams of mercury. Often these are mixed with solvents and oils. See Chapter 18, Ceramics, page 209.

Glass stains are usually silver nitrate, gamboge, water and gum arabic. Mirroring is done with solutions containing ammonia, silver compounds, and reducing compounds such as rochelle salts.

Vapors given off during painting of solvent-containing paints and lustres are toxic. Silver nitrate can cause skin burns and can damage the eyes. The emissions during firing of paints and enamels include metal fumes and decomposition products of organic chemicals such as tack oil, gum arabic, etc.

There are also new glass and ceramic paints which do not need firing. These are polymer materials which dry to look like glazes or enamels. Most contain toxic solvents which can be inhaled during painting.

Sometimes paints and lustres are silkscreened onto surfaces. The resists can be photo etched. Many of the solvents, emulsions, and cleanup materials for these processes are toxic. See Chapter 29, Photography and Photoprinting, for the hazards of photo chemicals.

ETCHING

Etching or frosting with hydrofluoric acid (HF) is one of the most hazardous processes in surface decorating. HF is insidious because it does not cause pain on contact. Later, often hours later, severe pain onsets, indicating that the acid has penetrated the skin and is destroying tissues deep beneath the point of entry. Surgery and amputation are sometimes needed.

In addition, the absorbed fluorine from the acid can cause systemic poisoning. As little as a half cup of this acid spilled on a person has resulted in death.

Etching creams which release HF on contact with the glass are less hazardous but also can cause burns. Material Safety Data Sheets for some of these products are deceptive because they list the two major ingredients without making it clear that the combined chemicals release HF.

Vapors rising from an HF acid bath can seriously damage lungs, causing chemical pneumonia. Long term exposure is associated with kidney, liver, bone, and tooth damage.

Etching surfaces of glazes, enamels, or glass that contains arsenic and/or antimony can result in the formation of extremely toxic arsine and stibine gases. Though the amounts of the metals and their gases may be small, their extreme toxicity can make exposure to them significant.

Special precautions for HF acid etching include the use of gloves resistant to HF, goggles, a face shield and protective clothing and shoes. Some glassworkers use two pair of gloves as extra protection against leaks. An eye wash fountain and emergency shower should be installed near the operation. HF burn treatment should be handy and personnel taught how to use it. Emergency procedures should be understood by all personnel. Local exhaust is needed to remove the gases and vapors created during etching.

Artists wishing to use HF should obtain and follow additional safety procedures outlined in special data sheets on HF, such as the one published by the National Safety Council in Chicago.

ELECTROPLATING

Although this technique is usually done on metals, it can also be applied to ceramics, enamels and glass under certain circumstances (see Chapter 24, Metal Surface Treatments, pages 255-257 for details).

SPECIAL PRECAUTIONS FOR SURFACE TREATMENT PROCEDURES

1. Obtain Material Safety Data Sheets and other reliable ingredient information on surface treatment chemicals. Material Safety Data Sheets often will recommend the use of special gloves, goggles, ventilation, and respiratory protection. Follow Material Safety Data Sheet advice and have handy materials for spill control and chemical disposal.

2. Use Material Safety Data Sheet information to try to avoid products containing lead, hydrofluoric acid, and other highly toxic ingredients whenever possible.

3. Also obtain detailed information about the surface to be treated. Avoid treating or acid etching surfaces of glazes, enamels, or glass containing significant amounts of arsenic, antimony, or other highly toxic metals. These metals may volatilize from the surface during some treatments. Blasting such surfaces creates highly toxic fine dust.

4. Provide excellent ventilation, such as slot vents or a window exhaust fan at work table level, for dry cleaning (with whiting), or polishing, applying acids, or any other operation that produces toxic emissions. Dry grinding and polishing equipment should have built-in local exhaust systems.

5. Use wet grinding, polishing, and cutting methods whenever possible. Wet grinding equipment should be cleaned when wet to avoid dust exposure. Water reservoirs should be cleaned often to remove scum or other microbe growth.

6. Have highly hazardous processes such as HF acid etching or electroplating done professionally, if possible. Otherwise have safety experts help plan and design studio equipment, ventilation, and emergency facilities.

7. Dispose of all neutralized acids, grinding dusts, spent abrasives and other waste materials in accordance with health, safety, and environmental protection regulations. Some wastes containing only relatively small amounts of highly toxic chemicals such as fluorides and arsenic can be very expensive to dispose of properly.

CHAPTER 23 | *SCULPTURE, LAPIDARY, AND MODELING MATERIALS*

Stone, cement, plaster, self-hardening clays, plasticine, wax, and papier mache are commonly used to sculpt and model. Most of these traditional materials can be used safely when appropriate precautions are taken.

STONES

Many stones used in sculpture and lapidary are the same minerals that are used in ceramics, glass, and as abrasives. For example, flint, steatite, dolomite, and fluorspar stones can be used for sculpture. When these same stones are ground to a powder, they can be used to make ceramic glazes and glass. For another example, garnet may is used as both a gem and a sand paper abrasive.

Artists are exposed to dust and flying chips when stones are shaped for sculpture or lapidary work by chipping, carving, grinding, and polishing. These operations can be done by hand or with electric tools. Electric tools produce large amounts of dust. Hand operations are the least hazardous, but flying chips still can damage eyes.

In addition, hand tools can slip and large stones can fall to cause injuries. Lifting heavy stones and tools can lead to strain injuries.

Electric tools also are associated with vibration syndrome or "white fingers" disease. It is a progressive circulatory system disease which constricts flow of blood to the hands (sometimes also to the feet) causing pain and numbness (see page 37). Noise from percussive hammering, electric tools, and other equipment also can damage hearing (see page 35).

The toxicity of dust from sculpture stones varies. Some stones contain significant amounts of asbestos. These are too hazardous to use under the conditions found in craft and sculpture studios. Other stones may contain hazardous ingredients, including free silica, talc, or caustic metallic compounds.

In order to choose stones whose dust will be the least toxic, artists need both chemical and mineral analyses of the stones, including the amounts of impurities in them. Abrasives used in grinding and polishing stone may also produce hazardous dusts. The hazards of many common minerals used in sculpture, lapidary, and abrasives are listed in Table 13.

CEMENT

Cement is a mixture of fine ground lime, alumina, and silica which will set to a hard product when mixed with water. Other chemicals commonly found in cement include various iron compounds, traces of chrome, magnesia, sodium, potassium, and sulfur compounds.

In addition to these naturally occurring contaminants, there are many substances added to cement to improve adhesion, strength, flexibility, curing time, and water evaporation. Usually these are plaster, various plastic resins, and latex solids.

The primary hazards of cement are skin and respiratory irritation from the alkaline compounds. Skin burns are a common problem among cement workers and severe ulcers can develop from contact with wet cement.

Allergies to cement dust are also commonly seen in cement workers. A major cause is reaction to small amounts of chrome compounds in some cements. Some researchers also feel that the statistically significant number of cases of lung cancer seen among some workers is caused by chrome (hexavalent type) in cement.

PLASTER

Plaster or plaster of paris is calcium sulfate. It occurs in nature as gypsum and as alabaster. Plaster dust is irritating to the eyes and slightly irritating to the respiratory system. Plaster may also contain additives such as lime which make the dust more irritating. Ventilation or respiratory protection should be used to avoid exposure to excessive amounts of dust.

Heat is produced during the setting reaction. Severe burns have resulted when children and adults cast their hands in plaster.

RULES FOR WORKING WITH STONE, CEMENT, AND PLASTER

1. Wear impact/dust goggles when shaping or chipping materials. See figures 4 and 5, pages 58-60.

2. Wear steel-tipped shoes with heavy materials or equipment.

3. Move all heavy stones and other objects in accordance with correct lifting and carrying procedures.

4. Obtain mineral and chemical analyses of sculpture stones. Good Material Safety Data Sheets will include this data. Use the least toxic varieties which meet your artistic needs. Avoid stones containing asbestos or radioactive elements.

5. Purchase electric grinding and polishing tools that are equipped with local exhaust connections for removing dust from the studio. To control other sources of dust, practice good hygiene and clean up.

6. If respiratory protection is needed, match the respirator filters to the type of dust produced. Do not expect air-purifying respirators to contend with heavy amounts of dust (over 10 times the Threshold Limit Value). For high dust level, air-supplied respirators may be needed.

7. Avoid skin contact or wear gloves when working with wet cement.

8. Purchase electric tools with low vibrations amplitude and comfortable hand grips. Do not grip tools too tightly, take frequent work breaks, and do not work in cold environments to reduce risk from vibration syndrome.

9. Purchase quiet tools and exhaust fans, or wear hearing protection (see pages 35-37).

10. Do not cast body parts in plaster unless provisions are made for dissipation of heat. There should also be a barrier of vaseline or similar material between the skin and any casting material.

MODELING MATERIALS

Modeling can be done with many products including nonhardening clays such as plasticine, air-setting and oven-setting clays, papier mache, and wax. (The hazards of sculpture clays such as terra cotta are the same as those of ceramic clays—see Chapter 18, Ceramics.)

SELF-HARDENING CLAY. The hazards of self-hardening and oven-setting clays are very complex. Most manufacturers of these products will not reveal all of their contents. However it is known that most are clay mixed with plastic resin materials that contain hardening agents and plasticizers. Some of these plastics and their additives are known to cause dermatitis and allergies. Some are suspect carcinogens. Oven-curing products can cause some plasticizers to volatilize or fume. These plasticizers then may contaminate ovens, kitchens, and studios. (See Chapter 13, Plastics.)

To work safely with self-hardening clays, protect your hands with gloves. If severe reactions occur, stop using the product. Try to obtain reliable ingredient information on these products. Provide ventilation or respiratory protection if sanding or mixing of the product raises dust. Do not use kitchen ovens or other equipment or utensils that will be used subsequently for food. For children, a modeling material made from flour and salt is a more suitable alternative.

NONHARDENING CLAYS, such as plasticine, are usually made of clays mixed with oils and petrolatum. Other ingredients may include sulfur dioxide and other preservatives, vegetable oils, aluminum silicate, and very small amounts of turpentine. The colored clays contain pigments or dyes.

A few reports of skin allergies and respiratory symptoms have been reported among users of plasticine due to the presence of turpentine or when too much sulfur dioxide preservative has been added. In general, however, these are usually very safe materials. Discontinue use if skin or respiratory reactions occur.

WAX used in sculpture and jewelry making is relatively safe to use unless it is heated to the point where it smokes or dissociates. Processes which can produce sufficient heat to dissociate wax include lost wax casting, sculpting wax with hot tools, ironing out batik wax, and over heating wax for ceramic glaze resists.

When wax breaks down with heat many toxic and irritating compounds are formed including acrolein and formaldehyde. Acrolein is an exceedingly potent lung irritant for which there is no suitable air-purifying respirator cartridge. Provide proper ventilation.

PAPIER MACHE that is formed of plain paper pieces and white glue has no significant hazards. It would only be hazardous if paper with toxic inks or an unsafe glue were used.

Powdered or instant papier maches, however, may contain very hazardous ingredients. Many paper mache powders, even those for children, used to be asbestos/glue mixtures. Some products still may be made with asbestos-contaminated talcs.

Now some papier mache powders are ground up magazines mixed with glue and fillers. The problem with these products is that slick magazine paper contains talc and other fillers, and the inks may contain lead, cadmium and a host of organic pigments of varying toxicity. Although the amounts of the toxic chemicals are fairly small the materials are usually ground so fine that considerable amounts can be inhaled.

To use papier mache safely, obtain reliable ingredient information and choose the safest product. There are good papier mache products that employ ground clean (uninked) cellulose. Avoid inhaling dust by providing ventilation for any mixing or sanding operations.

CHAPTER 24
METAL SURFACE TREATMENTS

Metals can be treated by many processes that also are used for nonmetal surfaces (see Chapter 22, Ceramic, Glass, and Enamel Surface Treatments). For example, metals can be etched and photo-etched, abraded and sandblasted, or painted. This chapter will consider procedures which are used primarily on metal surfaces including cleaning and degreasing, applying patinas, using fluxes, electroplating and annodizing, gilding, and niello work.

CLEANING AND DEGREASING

Metals must be very clean if solders are to adhere, if patinas are to take, and so on. Metals must be cleaned again after soldering, brazing, forging and similar processes, to remove flux residues, fire scale, and the like. For these purposes, many different metal cleaners are used.

Most metal cleaners and degreasers are solvents, hydroxides, ammonia, acids, or combinations of these. Other cleaners for metals include hand-rubbed abrasives such as putty and whiting, or Sparex and other acidic solutions for cleaning fire scale off hot metals. Cyanide cleaners also are used for cleaning cast metal. The hazards of these types of cleaners are listed in Table 19.

PATINAS AND METAL COLORANTS

Patinas and metal colorants usually employ very toxic chemicals. Toxic gases and vapors may be emitted during the reaction with the metal as well.

One of the most common colorants is liver of sulfur (potassium sulfide). When applied to metals this compound will darken the metal and release highly toxic hydrogen sulfide gas. This gas can be identified by its "rotten egg" odor. Many of the patinas and colorants rely on sulfides and similar reactions may occur.

When planning to use patinas, research the hazards of both the patina and the byproducts of its reaction with metals. Be aware that some patina Material Safety Data Sheets do not list the hazardous byproducts created during use of the product. The hazards of some common patinas and metal colorants are found in Table 20.

FLUXES

Many fluxes today are very complex mixtures of chemicals. Many types of chlorides, fluorides, and borates may be found in fluxes. Organic fluxes may contain a variety of organic chemicals including stearic acid, glutamic acid, oleic acid, other fatty acids, and organic amines and organic sulfates. Rosin fluxes may be "activated" with bromides and hydrochlorides. There also are other compounds which are used in vehicles such as petroleum gel, polyethylene glycol, alcohols, and water.

Some of these compounds are toxic in and of themselves. And all of them release irritating or toxic emissions when they are used. The plume of smoke rising from soldering or brazing should be considered toxic.

Fluxes can be categorized by their main ingredients into the following groups:

ACID fluxes (and acid core solders) usually are chlorides of zinc, ammonium or other matals.
BORAX fluxes containing boron compounds.
FLUORIDE fluxes containing fluoride compounds.
ORGANIC fluxes containing fatty acids.
ROSIN fluxes (and rosin core solders) contain pine rosin (colophony).

A number of the chemicals in these fluxes and their hazards are listed in Table 20. In general, acid fluxes are the safest to use for most art processes and fluoride fluxes are among the more hazardous.

RULES FOR USING DEGREASERS, PATINAS, AND FLUXES

1. Protect skin and eyes by wearing gloves, aprons and chemical splash goggles when handling acids, caustics, solvents, and other irritating chemicals. Install eye wash fountains near where they are used. If large amounts of caustics or acids are used, install emergency showers.

2. Provide local exhaust ventilation by working in front of a window exhaust fan, a slot hood, or a similar system. (Most degreasers, patinas, and fluxes give off toxic gases and vapors.)

3. Choose the safest materials by comparing Material Safety Data Sheet information. In general, acid fluxes are the least toxic. Avoid fluoride fluxes if possible. Try to avoid patinas containing sulfides (which release hydrogen sulfide gas). Avoid cleaners containing cyanides.

4. Follow directions for use carefully.

5. Never mix different types of fluxes. Some mixtures can produce especially toxic emissions and most will not perform properly. Never mix different cleaners or patinas unless you understand fully the chemical reactions which may occur.

6. Remove all residue from degreasing before soldering or heating metal (some will release highly toxic gases such as phosgene on heating).

ELECTROPLATING AND ANODIZING

Electroplating relies on depositing a metal out of an electrolyte solution by running a current from a metal anode to the object to be plated which acts as a cathode. Even materials which do not conduct electricity can be made to plate by sealing them with wax or lacquer and then coating them with a conductive material like graphite or metal paint.

Anodizing is an electrolytic process in which certain metals (aluminum, magnesium, and several others) that naturally produce a film of metal oxide on their surfaces can be made to accept even thicker and more stable metal oxide coatings. A number of different metals can be employed to produce the coating including titanium and niobium. These metallic oxides also will accept dyes and pigments making it possible to obtain finishes in many colors including black. The lustre of the underlying metal gives the coating a metallic sheen.

Many different electrolytic solutions are used in plating and anodizing. Copper can be plated from a solution of copper sulfate and sulfuric acid. Many other types of plating such as gold and silver employ cyanide solutions. Anodizing electrolytes are usually sulfuric, oxalic and chromic acids.

Sulfuric, oxalic, and chromic acid baths are highly irritating to skin, eyes, and respiratory system. Cyanide baths are moderately toxic by skin contact and highly toxic by inhalation or ingestion. Acid, heat, even carbon dioxide from the air will cause the formation of deadly hydrogen cyanide gas from cyanide solutions. Acute inhalation of either cyanide salts or hydrogen cyanide gas can be fatal.

Before being treated, metals must be scrupulously cleaned. Skin and eye damaging cleaners are used such as caustic soda and other hydroxides (see Table 19, Metal Cleaners and Degreasers). Once in the bath, large electrical currents are applied which can cause electric shocks. If lacquers or metal paints are used, these may contain toxic solvents.

PRECAUTIONS FOR ELECTROPLATING AND ANODIZING

1. Protect skin and eyes by wearing gloves, aprons and chemical splash goggles when handling acids, caustic soda, and solvents. Install eye wash fountains. If large amounts of caustics or acids are used, install emergency showers.

2. Try to avoid using cyanide salts. If they must be used, consult safety experts when designing and installing equipment and local exhaust ventilation for the baths. Train all personnel about the hazards and emergency procedures. Keep a cyanide antidote kit available (if someone on staff is qualified to use it) or notify the local hospital to be prepared for cyanide poisoning. If local hospitals are not prepared, a cyanide kit should be taken with a victim to the hospital.

3. Avoid spraying lacquers or solvent-containing paints. If they must be sprayed, use a spray booth or wear a proper respirator.

4. Instruct all personnel about electrical hazards. Install ground fault interrupters and other electrical safety features.

5. Look up the hazards of the metals and metal compounds used (see Table 10, Hazards of Metals and Metal Compounds, page 133), especially some of the rare metals employed in some anodizing procedures.

GILDING

Metal gilding (as opposed to goldleaf gilding of wood and plaster) may be done with gold and silver amalgams. The amalgams are made by mixing or heating mercury and gold or silver together. The amalgams are applied to the metal and heated until the mercury vaporizes, leaving the gold or silver on the surface.

This gilding method is not recommended for studio work. Mercury is highly toxic and can be absorbed by the skin and the vapor inhaled (see Table 10, Hazards of Metals and Metal Compounds, page 133). If the method is used, first investigate and comply with all applicable toxic substance regulations. Avoid skin contact with mercury and heat mercury amalgams only under excellent local exhaust ventilation.

Work on a tray or on a surface designed to contain spilled mercury. Since mercury vaporizes at room temperature, it must be stored in sealed containers. When in use, constant ventilation must be provided. Mercury spills must be scrupulously cleaned up. Small amounts of spilled mercury left in sink traps or floor cracks can produce significant amounts of mercury vapor.

Mercury spill kits containing ferric chloride or other chemicals which will react with mercury should be available. Do not vacuum (except with vacuums specially developed for mercury spills).

NIELLO

In this process, silver, copper, and lead are melted and poured into a crucible with sulfur. The mixture is remelted, sintered, and ground finely. Then it is mixed with ammonium chloride into a paste, applied to the metal, and heated.

Lead poisoning can result from inhaling lead fumes during heating or lead sulfide dust during grinding of the mixture. All procedures should be done in local exhaust. A proper dust mask should be worn when dealing with the powder and excellent hygiene should be practiced.

| TABLE 19 | Metal Cleaners and Degreasers |

ACIDS such as hydrochloric, sulfuric and nitric acid are used in some metal cleaners. These are highly irritating, can damage eyes, skin, and respiratory system, and should not be mixed with other cleaners unless it is known they will not react.

AMMONIA is a respiratory irritant and may be found in both solvent and hydroxide cleaners. Ammonia can react with bleach and inorganic acids such as hydrochloric acid to release highly toxic gases. Care should be taken not to mix ammonia-containing products with acid cleaners, fluxes and acid-containing patinas, or with scouring powders that contain dry bleach.

CYANIDE cleaning mixtures are in common use in the jewelry industry for cleaning cast metal. Cleaning with a mixture of cyanide and concentrated hydrogen peroxide is called "bombing." This method produces extremely toxic hydrogen cyanide gas and should not be used.

HYDROXIDES such as potassium and sodium hydroxide (caustic soda) are very corrosive to the skin and eyes.

PUTTY (tin oxide) is sometimes used to polish or clean metal. It has no significant hazards except chronic inhalation could cause a benign pneumoconiosis (see page 152).

SOLVENTS used in cleaning are likely to be the glycol ethers (see page 94) which can penetrate the skin and rubber gloves, are toxic, and may be reproductive hazards.

Other common cleaning solvents are the chlorinated hydrocarbons (see Table 5, Common Solvents and Their Hazards, page 89) and these are toxic and usually cancer-causing. In addition, if the chlorinated hydrocarbons are used around heat or ultraviolet light (such as is emitted during welding), they can decompose to emit highly irritating phosgene gas.

SPAREX (sodium bisulfide) is a milder acidic solution that can be used to clean fire scale off hot metal. Like acids, Sparex can damage skin and eyes on contact. Emits irritating sulfur dioxide gases on contact with hot metal.

WHITING (calcium carbonate) is a mild abrasive sometimes used to polish or clean metal. It has no significant hazards.

TABLE 20	Flux, Patina, and Metal Colorant Chemicals

ALIPHATIC AMINE HYDROGEN CHLORIDES are sensitizing and release irritating, sensitizing, and toxic emissions when heated.

AMMONIUM CHLORIDE. With heat, ammonium chloride fume will become airborne. It is moderately irritating. Some of it may break down into highly irritating ammonia and hydrochloric acid gases, especially if over-heated.

ANTIMONY SULFIDE (see antimony in Table 10; sulfides below)

BORIC ACID, POTASSIUM BORATES, AND OTHER BORON-CONTAIN-ING COMPOUNDS are moderately toxic. Boric acid and some other boron compounds can be absorbed through broken skin.

BROMIDES are moderately toxic, but highly toxic hydrogen bromide and other gases may be released when heated.

COPPER SULFATE in some patina formulas will release irritating and sensitizing sulfur dioxide gas.

FERRI- AND FERROCYANIDES are only slightly toxic, but when used with acid or heat, highly toxic cyanide gas can be released.

FLUORIDE COMPOUNDS (potassium bifluoride, boron trifluoride, etc.) are highly irritating and release highly toxic gases. Fluorides can severely damage lung tissue and can cause long-term systemic damage to bones and teeth. Fluxes and patinas containing fluorides should be avoided when possible.

HYDROCHLORIC (MURIATIC) ACID is highly irritating and can damage eyes, skin, and respiratory system.

LEAD ACETATE (see lead, Table 10, Hazards of Metals and Metal Compounds, page 133).

NITRATES (ferric, copper, etc.,) can explode under certain conditions when exposed to heat. They also emit highly toxic nitrogen oxides that can severely damage lungs.

NITRIC ACID is highly irritating and can cause severe skin and eye damage. Nitric acid releases highly irritating nitrogen oxides when it reacts with metals. These nitrogen oxides can cause severe lung damage.

OLEIC ACID AND OTHER FATTY ACIDS are not toxic, but, like all organic compounds, when decomposed by heat, they emit many irritating, sensitizing, and toxic gases and vapors.

ROSIN (colophony) is associated with respiratory allergies and asthma. When burned it releases many toxic gases such as formaldehyde.

SELENIUM COMPOUNDS (except for highly toxic selenium dioxide) are usually only slightly toxic, but in acid-containing patinas, highly toxic and irritating hydrogen selenide gas may be released. Severe lung damage, liver, and kidney damage could result. Selenium also is associated with adverse reproductive effects.

SODIUM LAURYL SULFATE is not toxic, but like all organic compounds, when decomposed by heat, it emits many irritating and toxic chemicals.

STEARIC ACID is not toxic, but, like all organic compounds, when it is decomposed by heat (as during soldering) it emits many irritating, sensitizing, and toxic gases and vapors.

SULFURIC ACID is highly irritating and, in some patinas, it also releases sulfur dioxide gas.

SULFIDES (potassium sulfide, ammonium sulfide, barium sulfide) are irritating to skin and eyes. They emit sulfur oxides when heated. When heated in the presence of water or when reacted with metal, highly toxic hydrogen sulfide gas is released.

THIOSULFATES are usually not toxic, but release highly irritating and sensitizing sulfur oxides when heated.

WETTING AGENTS, SURFACTANTS, ETC., are of varying toxicity and many have not been studied well. Like other organic compounds, they release toxic emissions when burned.

ZINC CHLORIDE. With heat, zinc chloride fume will be airborne. A moderately irritating fume. Very heavy exposures also could cause metal fume fever.

CHAPTER

25 *WELDING*

A ll methods of welding or cutting metal rely upon either heat from burning gas or from electric arc to do the job. Over eighty different types of welding exist and they use these basic heat sources in various ways. But in art, the types most commonly used are oxyacetylene welding, ordinary arc welding, gas metal arc welding (metal inert gas, MIG), and gas tungsten arc welding (tungsten inert gas, TIG). All types of welding can be extremely hazardous.

TRAINING

Safe welding requires knowledge, training, and comprehension of applicable health and safety codes and regulations. Art welders in the United States and Canada should at least be familiar with their state/provincial and federal industry standards.

Learning about these regulations and becoming proficient at welding takes time. The American Welding Society considers 125-150 hours of professional training necessary to qualify for oxyacetylene welding, brazing, and flame cutting. Another 250-300 hours of training are required to qualify for arc welding. Ideally, art welders should obtain this certification.

Instead, most artists pick up welding "by the seat of their pants," by observing other (usually unqualified) welders. In addition, they often weld with old, poorly maintained equipment housed in unventilated spaces, which are located near other activities and are not compatible with fire and electrical requirements imposed by welding.

Those who teach welding certainly should be certified. However, it is not uncommon for universities and art schools to hire uncertified welders to teach this very hazardous craft. (Yet these same schools wouldn't consider hiring art history teachers without degrees.)

In addition to certification, welding instructors should have formal training in welding health and safety. Such courses are regularly scheduled at various locations around the United States and Canada by the American Welding Society (AWS) and the National Safety Council (NSC). They can be contacted at:

> AWS, 550 N.W. LeJeune Road, Miami, FL 33126
> NSC, 444 N. Michigan Ave., Chicago, IL 60611

Right-to-know, Hazard Communication and WHMIS laws (see pages 16-20) now require administrators to provide formal health and safety training for employees, including teachers. Welding surely qualifies and administrators well may want to avail themselves of these outside sources of instruction.

SAFETY PRECAUTIONS

Welding safety is an extraordinarily complex subject, and the safety rules differ depending on the type of welding, the kind of work, and on the shop or on-site conditions. Certain general rules, however, are basic to common types of welding.

GOOD HOUSEKEEPING. Welding shops should be kept scrupulously organized and clean. Only necessary items should be kept in the shop. Combustible materials should be eliminated from the area or covered with fire-proof tarps or other protective materials. The space should be organized to keep floors free of trip hazards because the welder's vision is often limited by face shields or goggles.

ELECTRICAL SAFETY. Most shocks caused by welding equipment are not severe. But under the right conditions they can cause injury or even death. Mild shocks can cause involuntary muscle contractions leading to accidents, and moderate amounts of current directed across the chest may stop the heart. Here are some basic ways to avoid these hazards.

1. Use only welding equipment that meets standards.
2. Follow exactly all equipment operating instructions.
3. Keep clothes dry (even from excessive perspiration) and do not work in wet conditions.
4. Maintain all electrical connections, cables, electrode holders, etc., and inspect each before starting to weld.

COMPRESSED GAS CYLINDER SAFETY. Compressed gas cylinders are potential rockets or bombs. If mishandled, cylinders, valves, or regulators can break or rupture, causing damage as far as 100 yards away.

The different kinds of gases inside the cylinders are themselves hazards. There are three basic types of hazardous gases:

1. *Oxygen.* It will not burn by itself, but ordinary combustible materials like wood, cloth, or plastics will burn violently or even explode when ignited in the presence of oxygen. Never use oxygen as a substitute for compressed air.
2. *Fuel gases.* Acetylene, propane, and butane are some fuel gases. They are flammable and can burn and explode.
3. *Shielding gases.* These are used to shield processes such as MIG and TIG welding, include argon, carbon dioxide, helium, and nitrogen. They are inert, colorless, and tasteless. If they build up in confined spaces such as enclosed welding areas, they replace air and can asphyxiate those in the area.

Some basic rules regarding compressed gas cylinders that all art welders should know are listed below.

TABLE 21	Safety Rules for Compressed Gas Cylinders

1. Accept only cylinders approved by the Department of Transportation for use in interstate commerce. Do not remove or change any numbers or marks stamped on cylinders.

2. Cylinders too large to carry easily may be rolled on their bottom edges, but never dragged.

3. Protect cylinders from cuts, abrasions, drops, or striking each other. Never use cylinders for rollers, supports, or any purpose other than intended by the manufacturer.

4. Do not tamper with safety devices in valves.

5. Return empty cylinders to the vendor. Mark them "EMPTY" or "MT" with chalk. Close the valves and replace valve protection caps.

6. Always consider cylinders as full (even when empty) and handle them with due care. Accidents have resulted when containers under partial pressure have been mishandled.

7. Secure cylinders by chaining, tying, or binding them, and always use them in an upright position.

8. Store cylinders in cool, well ventilated areas or outdoors in vertical positions (unless the manufacturer suggests otherwise). The temperature of a cylinder should never exceed 130 degrees Farenheit. Store oxygen cylinders separately from fuel cylinders or combustible materials.

FIRE SAFETY. Many fires are started by welding sparks. These "sparks" are actually molten globules of metal which can travel up to forty feet and still be hot enough to ignite combustible materials. Welding shops must be planned carefully to avoid combustible materials such as wooden floors, or any cracks or crevices into which sparks may fall and smolder.

Fire extinguishers must be on hand in welding shops because other methods—like overhead sprinkler systems--should not be used. (Imagine the results if an electric arc welder were suddenly deluged with water.) Each welder should have "hands-on" training in the use of the type of extinguishers in the shop. Emergency procedures should be posted and practiced in routine drills.

On-site welding in locations other than the shop requires extra precautions. Included among these are: giving advance notice before welding, curtailing all other activities in the area, removing all combustibles within forty feet of the operation or installing special fireproof curtains and coverings to shield combustibles which cannot be removed, clearing and dampening floors, and assigning a fire watcher with extinguisher at the ready during the welding operation. The fire watcher should remain for half an hour after welding has been completed.

ACCIDENTS. Prepare for accidents and burns by keeping first aid kits stocked with burn and trauma treatments. Post emergency procedures. Ideally, someone on site should have first aid and CPR (cardiopulmonary resuscitation) training.

HEALTH HAZARDS

Hazards to welders' health are less obvious than welding safety hazards, and they vary among different types of welding. In general, the hazards are: radiation, heat, noise, fumes, and gases from welding processes, and gases from compressed cylinders.

RADIATION generated by welding takes three forms: visible, infrared, and ultraviolet.

VISIBLE light is the least hazardous and most noticeable radiation emitted by welding. Although intense light produces only temporary visual impairment, eyes should be protected from strong light.

INFRARED (IR) radiation is produced when metal is heated until it glows. IR can cause temporary eye irritation and discomfort. Repeated exposures can cause permanent eye damage, including retinal damage and infrared cataract. These effects occur slowly, without warning.

ULTRAVIOLET (UV) is the most dangerous of the three types of radiation. All forms of arc welding produce UV radiation. Eye damage from UV, often called a "flash burn," can be caused by less than a minute's exposure. Symptoms usually do not appear until several hours after exposure. Severe burns become excruciatingly painful, and permanent damage may result.

UV also can damage exposed skin. Chronic exposure can result in dry, brown, wrinkled skin, and may progress to a hardening of the skin called keratosis. Further exposure is associated with benign and malignant skin tumors.

HEAT can harm welders by causing burns (from IR radiation to the skin or from hot metal) and by raising body temperature to hazardous levels causing "heat stress."

NOISE can damage a welder's hearing. Fortunately, most welding processes used in the arts produce noise at levels below the level at which hearing is damaged. (Air carbon arc cutting is one possible exception.) If you wear ear plugs, make sure they are fire resistant. Several cases of eardrum damage have been reported when overhead sparks fell into ear canals that were either unprotected or contained a combustible plug.

FUMES AND GASES are produced during the welding process. They sometimes can be seen as a smoky plume rising from the weld. Fumes come from the vaporized metals. Gases can come from gas cylinders or can be created when substances burn during welding. Gases also can form when some types of welding rods are being used. Material Safety Data Sheets on welding rods will identify the emissions expected during normal use.

Many occupational illnesses are associated with substances found in welding fumes and gases, including metal fume fever (see page 131), and a variety of chronic lung diseases including chronic bronchitis. Lung and respiratory system cancer are associated with metal fumes such as chrome, nickel, beryllium and cadmium. Lead poisoning from welding lead-painted metals is also well-documented.

HEALTH PRECAUTIONS
(For safety precautions, see above.)

1. *Obtain Material Safety Data Sheets on all materials* including compressed gases, and welding, and brazing rods. Obtain complete composition of metals to be welded. Avoid materials which will emit highly toxic metals such as beryllium, cadmium, antimony, etc. Never work with metals of unknown composition, painted metals, junk, or found metals unless ventilation is certain to provide total removal of the welding plume.

2. *Provide ventilation* for protection from gases, fumes, and heat buildup. Equip shops with local exhaust ventilation systems such as downdraft tables or flexible duct fume exhausters to capture welding fumes and gases at their source. These local exhaust systems should be combined with dilution systems to remove gases and fumes that escape collection and to reduce heat build up. A simple exhaust fan may suffice for open area welding, while enclosed MIG and TIG welding booths may need floor level dilution systems to prevent layering of inert gases.

Do not rely on working outdoors for protection. Many documented cases of illness have resulted from cutting and welding outdoors, even in windy conditions.

3. *Use respiratory protection if appropriate.* There are respirators sold for welding, but artists should rely primarily on ventilation. For one reason, no single air-purifying respirator will protect wearers from all the contaminants in welding plumes. Metal fume filters will stop fumes, but they offer no protection from gaseous contaminants.

Some air-supplied respirators can provide welders with fresh air, but these are complex pieces of equipment which are expensive, need constant maintenance, and their users need training to use them effectively. For these reasons, they usually are not practical for most artists.

4. *Isolate the welding area.* Isolation keeps other workers from being exposed either to direct or reflected radiation. Walls, ceilings, and other exposed surfaces should have dull finishes such as can be obtained from special nonreflective paints. Portable, fire-resistant, UV-impervious screens or curtains can be purchased to isolate welding areas and to separate individual welding stations.

5. *Use eye protection* such as goggles or face shields to protect each welder for the type of welding he or she does (see figures 4 and 5, pages 58-60). Welders who use methods that leave a slag coating on the weld should wear safety glasses under their shields. A common injury occurs when welders raise their hoods to inspect a weld and the slag pops off unexpectedly.

Face and eye protective equipment should be cleaned carefully after each use and inspected routinely for damage, especially for light shield damage. A scratched lens will permit radiation to penetrate it and it should be replaced.

Visitors and other workers nearby should avoid looking at welding and should wear safety glasses (UV weakened by distance is stopped by ordinary glass).

6. *Protect hearing* by wearing fire-resistant ear plugs, muffs, or other devices if needed.

7. *Wear protective clothing.* Pants and long-sleeved shirts can protect legs and arms. Many welders prefer wool fabrics because they insulate welders from temperature changes and because they emit a strong warning odor when heated or burned. Treat cotton clothing with a flame retardant. Never wear polyester or synthetic fabrics that melt and adhere to the skin when they burn. Pants and shirts should not have pockets, cuffs, or folds into which sparks may fall.

Shoes should have tops into which sparks cannot fall. Wear safety shoes with steel toes if heavy objects are being welded. Hair should be covered, or, at the very least, tied back. Wear gloves when arc welding. Leather aprons, leggings, spats, and arm shields may be needed for some types of welding. Do not use asbestos protective clothing.

8. *Practice good housekeeping.* Control dust by vacuuming with specially filtered vacuums that can trap fume particles or damp mop (being careful not to create an electrical hazard). Sweeping with large amounts of sweeping compound also may be acceptable.

9. *Dispose of waste* metals and other chemicals in accordance with health, safety, and environmental protection regulations.

10. *Arrange for good medical surveillance.* Always be prepared to provide your doctor with information about the materials you use and your work practices.

CHAPTER

26 | *BRAZING AND SOLDERING*

Brazing is the process of filling a joint or coating a metal surface with a nonferrous metal such as silver or copper. Soldering is a method of filling a joint or seam with metal alloys which will melt at lower temperatures than the metals being soldered. Tinning is a special kind of soldering in which areas of metal are covered with a solder surface.

HAZARDS OF BRAZING AND SOLDERING

Brazing alloys can contain an array of metals, some of which are toxic. Silver and copper brazing alloys may contain cadmium, antimony and arsenic. Material Safety Data Sheets for brazing alloys should identify all the metals present in them.

Solders can contain a large number of metals including lead, tin, cadmium, zinc, arsenic, antimony, beryllium, indium, lithium and silver (see Table 10, Hazards of Metals and Metal Compounds, page 133). Solders made for use on copper water pipes and cooking utensils are safer because these alloys must not contain significant amounts of lead. Material Safety Data Sheets which identify all metal constituents should be available on solders.

Prior to soldering or brazing, the metal must be cleaned and degreased. Cleaners and degreasers usually contain toxic solvents, caustics, and/or acids (see Table 19, Metal Cleaners & Degreasers, page 258).

Fluxes are used when soldering and brazing. Inorganic acid fluxes such as those containing zinc and other chlorides are used most widely. Organic solders containing fatty acids will work well on lead and copper. Rosin solders are used primarily for copper electrical work. Rosin fluxes must be activated with toxic bromide compounds in order to work on lead, brass, or bronze (and then only if it is very clean). Fluoride fluxes work very well on many metals and are usually used with tinning solders. However, these fluxes are very toxic (see Table 20, Flux, Patina, & Metal Colorant Dyes, page 259).

During soldering a plume of "smoke" rises, and can be inhaled. The plume will contain a variety of decomposition products from materials in fluxes and metal fumes. These substances can cause eye and respiratory irritation, allergies, and, in some cases, metal poisoning.

The temperature at which brazing or soldering is done affects the amount of toxic materials in the plume. Lower temperatures vaporize less metal. Methods employing soldering guns or electric soldering irons vaporize less metal than methods using torches to heat soldering irons or to fill joints (as in the copper foil method in stained glass). Open pot tinning in which metal objects are dipped in molten solders can product very large amounts of metal fumes.

The heat created during soldering can cause burns. When the metals glow with heat they are giving off infrared radiation which can cause eye damage.

Once the metals are brazed or soldered, the seams are often cleaned of the residual flux chemicals. Cleaning products can contain toxic solvents, acids, caustics, or ammonia. Some cleaning products generate toxic gases when mixed (see Table 19, Metal Cleaners & Degreasers, page 258). Polishing soldered and brazed metals with putty (tin oxide) or whiting (calcium carbonate) is less hazardous.

PRECAUTIONS FOR SOLDERING AND BRAZING

l. Obtain Material Safety Data Sheets and complete alloy composition for all solders and brazing metals. Choose the safest ones for the work to be done. Avoid highly toxic metal-containing alloys such as those containing arsenic, cadmium, and beryllium.

2. Avoid using lead solder. If lead solders are used on the job, employers

must be prepared to meet complex and expensive OSHA Lead Standard regulations in the United States or the OHSA Regulation respecting Lead in Canada.

3. Obtain ingredient information on fluxes. Choose the safest flux for the job. Avoid fluoride fluxes. Do not mix fluxes.

4. Wear goggles that will protect the eyes from infrared radiation and irritating vapors (see figures 4 and 5 pages 58-60). Use gloves when working with solvents, acids, or caustic cleaning agents. Minimize skin contact with fluxes. Wear clothing resistant to heat (see Chapter 25, Welding, pages 267-268.)

5. Have first aid treatment, cool water, and ice on hand for minor burns. Post emergency procedures.

6. Provide local exhaust ventilation for the plume.

7. Braze at the lowest temperatures at which good results are obtained. Use gun or electric soldering iron methods over open flame joining or heating of irons. Avoid open dip pot "tinning" unless excellent local exhaust can be installed.

8. Obtain ingredient information on metal cleaners and degreasers and choose the safest ones. Provide local exhaust for products which emit toxic gases and vapors. Do not mix cleaning agents unless your are sure they cannot react adversely with each other. Use putty or whiting to clean when possible.

9. Practice good housekeeping. Wet mop floors and sponge tables and surfaces to control dust, which may be contaminated with metal fume particles.

10. Dispose of all spent cleaning and polishing materials, fluxes, and metal waste in accordance with health, safety and environmental protection regulations.

11. Always be prepared to provide your doctor with information about the chemicals you use and your work practices. If lead is used, arrange for regular blood tests for lead.

METAL CASTING AND FOUNDRY

Metal casting involves forcing molten metal (by gravity or centrifugal force) into a mold. In the construction of some molds, a positive form of wax or plastic is burned out to leave room for the metal.

Metals can be cast in any size from tiny jewelry pieces to large foundry-cast sculptures. Foundry work is especially hazardous and should not be attempted unless workers are prepared to comply with all applicable occupational health and safety laws and regulations.

The hazards of all types of metal casting include exposure to mold materials, burning out patterns, and working with molten metals.

MOLD-MAKING HAZARDS

CHANNEL MOLDS are made by carving into tufa (a soft porous rock) or investment plaster mixed with pumice. Free silica can be found in investment plasters, and in some pumice and tufa.

CUTTLEBONE MOLDS are made by pressing small shapes (usually jewelry pieces) into cuttlebone (the internal shell of the cuttlefish). The mold is then painted with borax flux and water glass (sodium silicate). Cuttlebone can cause respiratory irritation and allergies; borax is moderately toxic and can be absorbed through broken skin; and some grades of sodium silicate contain some free silica. All of these dusts are eye and respiratory irritants.

SAND MOLDS are made from foundry or casting sand which is usually silica and binders. Some silica mold sands are cristobalite (see page 154). The sands are very hazardous unless they are treated with binding chemicals, which also prevent respirable dust from becoming airborne.

The binders in foundry sands can be a number of organic chemicals such as glycerine and linseed oil. These harden when heated in an oven.

Cold setting high silica sands also are used. The binders in these sands usually are synthetic resins. Many different resins now are used, including urea-formaldehyde, phenol-formaldehyde, urethanes, and other plastics. The resins and the catalysts which set them can be highly toxic and toxic gases may be emitted when the resins burn off during casting (e.g., hydrogen cyanide and isocyanates).

Mold releases may include silica flour, French chalk (talc), or graphite. Some French chalk is contaminated with asbestos. Silica flour is an especially toxic source of silica because of its small particle size.

MOLDS FOR LOST WAX CASTING are made with investment plasters which contain silica flour or cristobalite, plaster, grog (fired clay), and clay. In the past, asbestos was added to this material. Asbestos or ceramic fiber may be used to line investment containers. Shell molds are made with slurries of water and silica, fused silica, or zircon, and sometimes ethyl silicate. The resulting mold is heated in a kiln to form a ceramic-like shell.

Cristobalite, silica flour, and fused silica can cause silicosis (see pages 153-154). Asbestos in any form can be a cancer hazard. Ceramic fiber also may cause asbestos-related diseases (see pages 155-156). Ethyl silicate is highly toxic by inhalation and eye contact. It is an irritant and may cause liver and kidney damage.

BURNING OUT PATTERNS. Patterns for metal casting molds can be made of wax, styrofoam, and other plastics. These materials can be burned out of the mold with a torch or a furnace. Styrofoam often is burned out when the molten metal is poured into the mold.

There are many types of wax including beeswax, carnauba, tallow, paraffin, and microcrystalline wax. When these waxes burn they release many toxic and irritating compounds including acrolein and formaldehyde. Acrolein is an exceedingly potent lung irritant, formaldehyde is a sensitizer and suspect carcinogen.

Wax additives may include rosin, petroleum jelly, mineral oil, solvents and dyes. These organic chemicals will also release carbon monoxide, and other toxic decomposition products when burned.

Burning styrofoam (polystyrene) will produce carbon monoxide and other toxic emissions. Burning out nitrogen-containing plastics such as urethane foam or urea formaldehyde will release hydrogen cyanide gas in addition to other toxic gases.

MELTING AND POURING

Small amounts of metal for centrifugal casting can be melted with torches. Centrifugal casting equipment can be dangerous. If it is unbalanced, metal can be thrown out. Most shields around centrifugal casters probably would not be able to protect bystanders if the arm should break during casting.

Furnaces are needed for larger castings. Furnaces can be heated with

274

gas, coke, coal, or electricity. Fuel-fired furnaces produce carbon monoxide and other combustion gases.

Many metal alloys may be used in casting. The composition of a few common alloys are listed in Table 22. Some of these alloys are hazardous to cast because they give off toxic fumes such as lead, arsenic, nickel, and manganese. For example, nickel fume, which is considered a carcinogen (Threshold Limit Value-Time Weighted Average of 1 milligram per cubic meter, see page 141) is given off when nickel-silver is cast.

Other highly toxic gases also can be released when mold binding chemicals are burned off when the mold is in contact with the hot metal (see above).

Heat from molten metal during pouring of large amounts can cause serious burns. Infrared radiation accidentally caused permanent scarring of an art student who was helping to pour bronze. Infrared can also cause eye damage.

TABLE 22	Composition of Common Alloys

BRASS: copper/zinc alloy with small amounts of lead, arsenic, manganese, aluminum, silicon, and/or tin.

BRITANNIA METAL, PEWTER, WHITE METAL: are of two basic types: tin/lead/copper or tin/antimony/copper.

BRONZE: copper/tin and sometimes small amounts of lead, phosphorus, aluminum, and/or silicon.

GOLD: alloyed with other metals for white, yellow, and other gold jewelry colors.

LEAD: type lead, lead pipe, battery lead, and various kinds of scrap lead have been used for sculpture.

MONEL METAL: nickel/copper alloys with small amounts of carbon, manganese, iron, sulfur, and silicon.

NICKEL SILVER: alloys of nickel/silver/zinc.

SILVER: sterling is silver alloyed with at most 7.5 percent other metals, usually copper. Other silver alloys are usually even less pure.

PRECAUTIONS

1. Be prepared to comply with all workplace occupational safety and health regulations regarding foundry work and metal casting.

2. Obtain Material Safety Data Sheets and ingredient lists for all metals, molds, and pattern materials used. Choose the least toxic products.

3. Choose foundry sands over cold setting sands and resin binders. Replace silica flours and cristobalite with nonsilica materials such as zircon when possible. Do not use asbestos.

4. If ethyl silicate is used, work with local exhaust ventilation and wear eye protection.

5. Provide dust control, ventilation and/or respiratory protection against irritating, sensitizing, and silica-containing mold materials. Dust goggles should also be worn if dust is raised.

6. Use the safest mold release agents such as graphite or asbestos-free talcs.

7. Provide local exhaust ventilation for burn out of any pattern materials. Be especially careful to exhaust the hydrogen cyanide gas generated when burning out nitrogen-containing plastic patterns.

8. Furnaces and ovens for mold-setting, burnout, and melting metal should be equipped with local exhaust ventilation such as a canopy hood. Provide exhaust ventilation for all pouring operations.

9. Avoid alloys containing significant amounts of highly toxic or carcinogenic metals such as arsenic, antimony, cadmium, nickel, or chrome when possible.

10. Avoid casting lead or lead alloys. If lead is used on the job, employers must be prepared to meet complex and expensive OSHA Lead Standard regulations in the United States or the OHSA Regulation respecting Lead in Canada.

11. Wear protective clothing appropriate to the type of casting done. For foundry work, follow protective clothing regulations. Wear infrared goggles whenever working with glowing materials (see figures 4 and 5 pages 58-60). If molten metals may splash, wear a face shield, a long-sleeved, high-necked wool shirt, insulated leggings, jacket, apron, gloves and shoes (steel-toed if heavy materials are being lifted). Tie back hair or wear hair covering.

12. Have first aid treatment, cool water, and ice on hand for burns. Post emergency procedures.

13. Post fire emergency and evacuation procedures and train workers in use of fire extinguishers (sprinkler systems cannot be used in foundries or other places where furnaces or molten metal are used). Hold regular fire drills.

14. When centrifugal casting, make sure the equipment is well balanced and that the protective shield is in good condition.

15. Wear respiratory protection when breaking up and disposing of silica-containing molds. Practice good housekeeping. Wet mop floors and sponge tables and surfaces to control dust which may be contaminated with mold materials or metal dust.

16. Dispose of all mold materials and metal waste in accordance with health, safety, and environmental protection regulations.

17. Always be prepared to provide your doctor with information about the chemicals you use and your work practices. If lead is used, arrange for regular blood tests for lead.

CHAPTER 27 | *SMITHING*

S mithing or forging is the process of hammering hot or cold metals into shape. Blacksmiths work with iron, silversmiths forge silver, and so forth. The tools used in these processes are hammers, mallets, metal blocks, and anvils. Furnaces used for hot forging burn coal, coke, oil, or gas.

HAZARDS OF SMITHING

Percussive hammering on metal produces noise which is very destructive to hearing. Even in the 1700's Ramazini (the father of occupational medicine) observed that tinsmiths went deaf from hammering noise.

Toxic combustion products such as carbon monoxide gas are emitted by forging furnaces. Ventilation systems such as canopy hoods only can provide partial protection from these gases because the bellows used to fan the coals will also blow some emissions from the hood intake area.

Other hazards include infrared radiation given off by furnaces and hot metal, which can damage the eyes and burn the skin. Heavy work in a hot environment can cause heat stress. Some kinds of smithing also use acid pickling solutions to clean hot metal.

Fires are a constant threat. Workers should be trained in fire emergency procedures and the use of extinguishers because other controls such as overhead sprinklers cannot be used in hot forging areas.

Cold forging metals like silver and tin involve hammering metal into or over forms. Small anvils, dapping blocks, and other objects can be used to pound the metal into shapes. Repousse is a special case of shaping by hammering and chasing the metal while it is supported by a bowl of a material made of pitch, plaster of paris and tallow. When shaping is done, the pitch can be removed by a solvent or burned off in a furnace or with a torch.

PRECAUTIONS FOR SMITHING

1. Install fireproof sound-absorbing materials in floors and walls of the shop where possible.

2. Provide good stack exhausts and canopy hood ventilation for forges and furnaces. Additional general shop ventilation will be needed for blacksmithing and other hot forging to reduce heat and to exhaust toxic gases which are blown out of the hood's capture range by the bellows.

3. Plan fire protection carefully. Eliminate all combustibles from areas around forges and furnaces. Do not install sprinkler heads above hot processes. Consult fire marshalls and/or other experts for advice on appropriate fire-fighting systems and extinguishers.

4. Provide bathroom facilities and a separate clean room for work breaks. It is necessary that smiths be able to wash up and retire to a clean area to drink fluids to replace those lost through perspiration, have lunch, and the like.

5. Provide first aid supplies and cold water or ice for treatment of minor burns. Post emergency procedures. Water also should be available to drink frequently, to quench metal, etc.

6. Obtain ingredient information on all materials used in the work and use proper precautions. For example, if solvents are used, as for removal of pitch from repousse, follow all solvent safety rules (see pages 87-89).

7. Practice good housekeeping. Wet mop or sponge floors and surfaces. Never allow trip hazards in the work area.

8. Wear ear plugs or other suitable hearing protection.

9. Wear goggles to protect eyes from infrared radiation (see figures 4 and 5, pages 58-60).

10. Wear protective clothing: long-sleeved, closewoven cotton or wool shirts; leather gloves, and safety shoes. Tie back hair or wear hair covering. Leave clothing in the shop to avoid tracking dusts home. Wash clothes frequently and separately from other clothes.

11. Wear gloves and goggles when handling acids, caustics, or solvents. If hot metal is dipped or cleaned in acid or Sparex, provide gloves, goggles, protective clothing (e.g., rubber aprons), and ventilation to exhaust gases rising from the bath.

12. Dispose of all spent acids, metal waste, and other materials in accordance with good hygiene and waste disposal regulations.

13. Always be prepared to provide your doctor with information about the chemicals you use and your work practices.

28 *WOODWORKING*

Virtually any type of wood may end up in art, including hard and soft wood, exotic woods, plywood, composition board, and so on. Often art studios and school shops are filled with the sounds of noisy machines and clouds of sawdust.

WOOD DUST HAZARDS

Many artists consider wood dust as nothing more than a nuisance. It is far more than that. Wood dust has caused countless fires and explosions. A spark or static discharge is sufficient to detonate fine airborne sawdust. In addition, some wood dusts cause allergies, some are toxic, and others contain highly toxic pesticides, preservatives, flame retardants and other treatments. Some trees deposit significant amounts of toxic silica in their heartwood. It has also been established that certain types of cancer are related to wood dust exposure.

DERMATITIS. There are two common types of wood-related skin diseases. One of these is *irritant dermatitis*. It is caused most often by exposure to the sap and bark of some trees. It will affect artists if they cut trees, saw raw timber, or work with unusual woods such as cashew.

The other major wood-related skin disease is *sensitization dermatitis*. It results from an allergy to sensitizing substances present in some woods. The symptoms may start as redness or irritation, and may proceed to severe eczema, fissuring and cracking of the skin. The condition may arise anywhere on the body that the sawdust contacted.

Some exotic woods even have caused dermatitis in persons exposed only to the solid wood, not to its dust. Rosewoods are one such type. Prolonged contact with rosewood musical instruments, bracelets, or knife handles has been known to cause sensitization dermatitis. Should you suspect that a skin problem is caused by a particular wood, a doctor can conduct a patch test on your skin. Although one can become allergic to almost any wood, those woods most likely to cause this condition are shown in Table 23.

RESPIRATORY SYSTEM EFFECTS, such as damage to the mucous membranes, and dryness and soreness of the throat, larynx, and trachea can be cause by some woods, especially sequoia and western red cedar. These effects may proceed to nosebleeds, coughing blood, nausea, and headache. Eye irritation usually occurs as well.

Lung problems—like asthma, alveolitis (inflammation of the lung's air sack)—affect a minority of workers exposed to irritant sawdusts. However, these are serious diseases and a few woods, such as sequoia and cork oak can cause permanent lung damage. The symptoms may not appear until several hours after sawdust exposure, making diagnosis difficult. Any persistent or recurring lung problems should be reported to a physician familiar with wood dust hazards.

Types of wood associated with lung problems are listed in Table 23.

CANCER.The most prevalent cancer related to wood dust is cancer of the nasal cavity and nasal sinuses. Early symptoms of nasal sinus cancer may include persistent nasal dripping, stuffiness, or frequent nosebleeds.

A recent twelve-country survey showed that an astonishing 61 percent of all such cancer cases occurred among woodworkers. Hardwood dusts are definitely associated with cancer, and early results from studies on workers exposed to soft woods indicate that both woods are implicated.

Most artists are exposed to much less dust than the professional woodworkers in the study, so their risks are lower. They need not give up wood as a material, but they must reduce their sawdust exposure to a minimum.

TOXIC EFFECTS. Some woods contain small amounts of toxic chemicals that may be absorbed through the respiratory tract, intestines, or occasionally through skin abrasions. These chemicals may cause headache, salivation, thirst, nausea, giddiness, drowsiness, colic, cramps, and irregular heart beat. In exceptional cases, poisoning has occurred from food containers, spoons, or spits made from woods such as yew or oleander.

If you suspect that your symptoms are related to a particular wood, inform a physician and have the wood identified. See Table 23 for list of toxic woods.

WOOD TREATMENTS

Almost every imported wood and most domestic woods in the United States and Canada have been treated with additives, pesticides, and/or preservatives. These chemicals can vary from relatively safe to highly toxic pesticides. The most hazardous pesticides are usually applied to wood intended for use in contact with the outdoor elements.

It is usually difficult to find out exactly what chemicals had been used on wood. Three common outdoor use wood preservatives are Pentachlorophenol (PCP) and its salts, arsenic-containing compounds, and creosote. These three types of preservatives are associated with cancer, birth defects, and many other hazards. Art workers should avoid wood treated with them. There are many other more suitable preservatives on the market.

PLYWOOD AND COMPOSITION BOARDS

Many health effects also can be caused by wood glues and adhesives. Plywood, pressboards, and many other wood products contain urea-formaldehyde or phenol-formaldehyde resins. These glues release formaldehyde gas which is a strong eye and respiratory irritant and allergen. Formaldehyde is also a suspect carcinogen known to cause nasal sinus cancer in animals.

Some manufacturers are turning to other adhesives such as urethane plastics. It is hoped these binders will be more stable and less hazardous.

MEDICAL SURVEILLANCE FOR WOODWORKERS

1. Prevent wood dust-related diseases by avoiding toxic or allergy-provoking woods, or woods treated with PCP, arsenic, creosote or other highly toxic chemicals when possible.

2. For occupational health problems, consult a doctor who is board certified in occupational medicine or one who is familiar with wood-related illnesses.

3. Have base-line lung function tests done early in your woodworking career. Then have your physician compare this test with subsequent pulmonary function tests done in your regular physical examinations in order to detect lung problems early.

4. Have your physician pay special attention to your sinuses and upper respiratory tract. Report symptoms like nasal dripping, stuffiness or nose-bleeds.

5. Know the symptoms and diseases your woods can cause. If these symptoms occur, report them immediately to your physician.

6. Be able to give your doctor a good occupational history. Always be prepared to provide your doctor with information about the chemicals you use and your work practices. Keep records of recurring symptoms and chemical/wood exposures.

7. Suspect that a health problem may be related to your work if the problem improves on weekends or during vacations.

8. Should symptoms or illness occur and persist even after treatment, seek a second opinion.

WOOD SHOP REGULATIONS

EXPOSURE STANDARDS. Workplace exposure to wood dust is regulated in both the United States and Canada. The exposure limits (Permissible Exposure Limits and Occupational Exposure Limits, see pages 32-33) are 5 mg/m^3 for all woods except Western red cedar which is set at 2.5 mg/m^3 in recognition of the severe allergies it causes. It is expected that other sensitizing woods will be assigned this lower limit as health data accumulates.

Other chemicals present in some sawdusts also are regulated. For example, the silica standards will apply if the wood contains it. Formaldehyde exposure limits also may be enforced if plywood or other composition materials are used.

VENTILATION. Essentially, the wood dust regulations make it necessary to equip all woodworking machines with local exhaust. The preferred dust control method involves a central collection system to which each machine is connected. These systems work best if the air they draw from the machines is expelled from the shop (not filtered and recycled). For shops unable to afford such systems, portable collectors that can be moved from machine to machine may suffice.

Good housekeeping and hygiene also must be practiced if woodshops are to meet the regulations.

RESPIRATORY PROTECTION may be used in some cases to reduce employee exposure to wood dust. However, respirators provide very limited protection and ventilation methods are preferred. If respirators are used, follow all rules for proper use (see pages 71-79).

MACHINE GUARDS. United States and Canadian standards require guards on woodworking equipment. Yet machines in art schools and studios commonly are found unguarded.

People who use guarded saws for the first time may find them awkward. However, workers accustom themselves quickly, and soon would not be without them. It takes much longer for artists to adjust to using hands with less than ten fingers.

OTHER REGULATIONS include lockouts to prevent the start up or release of energy during maintenance or repair of machines, central power switches to shut down all machinery in emergencies and many other rules. Artists should get copies of applicable regulations from their local occupational health and safety offices.

OTHER WOODSHOP HAZARDS

SOLVENT-CONTAINING PRODUCTS such as finishes, adhesives, paints, paint removers, and the like may contain solvents. All solvents are toxic and most are flammable (see Chapter 9, Solvents).

GLUES AND ADHESIVES. Many skin conditions and allergies can be caused by wood glues and adhesives. See Table 14, Hazards of Common Adhesives, page 172 for hazards of these materials and precautions.

In general, polyvinyl acetate (PVA) emulsion glues or white glues are exceedingly safe in comparison to many other types of wood glue. These glues require longer setting times than some of the solvent adhesives and epoxies, but you should used them as often as possible.

Safe use of more hazardous adhesives requires avoiding skin contact, sparing and careful use, keeping containers closed as much as possible during application, and good general shop ventilation.

FIRE HAZARDS. Woodworking shops harbor many fire hazards. As previously mentioned, fine wood dust in a confined area can explode with tremendous force if ignited with a spark or match. Combining wood dust, machinery, and flammable solvents greatly increases the hazard.

Fire prevention authorities agree that adequate ventilation is the best way to curb the risk of fire. Ventilation should be combined with safe solvent handling, good housekeeping, and regular removal of dust and scraps.

VIBRATING TOOLS. A significant number of persons who use vibrating tools now are known to be at risk from a more permanent condition commonly called "white hand," "dead fingers," or Vibration syndrome. This disease can lead to severe pain, ulcerations, and even gangrene in some cases. (See page 37).

NOISE. Saws, planers, routers, sanders, and the like can easily produce a cacophony of ear-damaging sound waves. Poorly designed ventilation systems also can produce hazardous amounts of noise (see pages 35-37).

Prevent hearing loss by purchasing well-engineered machines that run quietly. Some machines also can be purchased with dampering equipment such as mufflers and other sound-absorbing mechanisms. All machines will run more quietly when they are well-oiled and carefully maintained. Mounting machinery on rubber bases will reduce vibration transmission and rattling.

If noise levels are still high in your shop, wear ear protection. For lighter noise, special and readily available ear plugs can suffice (do not improvise with cotton or other materials). Use the protectors that look like ear muffs for heavy noise exposure. A physician should evaluate people with preexisting hearing loss before they are exposed to noise which may cause further impairment.

GENERAL PRECAUTIONS FOR WOODWORKING

1. Prevent fires by providing good shop ventilation, dust collection and control, sprinkler systems or fire extinguishers, emergency procedures and drills, and by banning smoking.

2. Obtain Material Safety Data Sheets on all wood products, glues, and other materials. Choose the safest ones.

3. Try to purchase wood from suppliers who know a good deal about the kinds of wood they sell, where it is from, and how it was treated.

4. Avoid wood treated with PCP, arsenic, or creosote. Some of the arsenic-preserved woods can be identified by their greenish color and avoided.

5. Equip all woodworking machinery with local exhaust dust collection systems. Ideally, these systems should vent to the outside rather than return air to the shop.

6. Prevent hearing damage by purchasing quiet machines using damping equipment such as mufflers or rubber mounts. Keep machines well-oiled and maintained. Use ear plugs or muffs if needed. Have a base line hearing test and periodic hearing tests as often as your doctor suggests.

7. Prevent Vibration Syndrome by using tools that are ergonomically designed and produce low amplitude vibrations, working in normal and stable temperatures (especially avoiding cold temperatures), taking ten-minute work breaks after every hour of continuous exposure, and not grasping tools too hard.

8. Wear dust goggles and a NIOSH-approved dust mask when dust cannot be controlled easily such as during hand sanding. Follow all laws and regulations regarding goggles and respirator use.

9. Wear protective clothing to keep dust off your skin. Wear gloves or barrier creams when handling woods known to be strong sensitizers.

10. Practice good hygiene. Wash and shower often. Keep the shop clean and free from sawdust. Vacuum rather than sweep dusts.

11. Follow all rules for use of solvents when using solvent-containing paints, glues, etc. (see pages 87-89).

12. Be prepared for accidents: know your blood type and keep up your tetanus shots. Keep first aid kits stocked. Post and practice emergency procedures.

13. Follow all Medical Surveillance Rules for wood dust exposure above.

TABLE 23	Some Woods and Their Health Hazards

KEY

Commercial Name(s). Different commercial names often are given to the same species or to different species within the same family. These names may be misleading. For example, redwood and California redwood are not related by family. For some woods, not every commercial name is listed.

Family and Origin. To completely identify wood, the family, origin, and exact species may be required. Scientific species names are not given in this table. Samples of wood can be completely identified by the Forest Products Research Laboratory in Madison, Wisconsin.

Health Effects

D = Dermatitis
C-R = Conjunctivitis-rhinitis (inflamed eyes and runny nose)
A = Asthma (inflammation of the bronchial tubes in the lungs)
Al = Allergic alveolitis (inflammation of the lung's air sacs)
T = Toxic effects (systemic poisoning)

Commercial Name(s)	Family	Origin	Health Effects
Maple	Aceraceae	——	D
Cashew	Anacardiaceae	America	D
Birch	Betulaceae	——	D
Gabon mahogany	Burseraceae	——	D C-R A Al
blue wood (spruce), purple heart	Caesalpinaceae	America	T
redwood	Caesalpinaceae	America	D T
Virginian pencil cedar, eastern red cedar	Cupressaceae	America	D C-R A T
White cedar, Western red cedar	Cupressaceae	America	D C-R A T

White cypress pine	Cupressaceae	Oceana	D C-R A
Chestnut, beech, oak	Fagaceae	——	D C-R A
Walnut	Juglandaceae	——	D C-R A
American whitewood, tulip tree	Magnoliaceae	America	D
Red cedar, Australian cedar	Meliaceae	America/Asia/ Oceania	D C-R A
Mahogany (m), Honduras m.,Cuban m., American m., Tabasco m., baywood	Meliaceae	America	D C-R A Al T
White handlewood	Moraceae	Oceania	D T
Iroko, yellowood, kambala, African teak, tatajuba	Moraceae	Africa/America	D C-R A Al
Alpine ash, yellow gum, mountain ash	Myrtaceae	Oceania	D C-R A
Ash	Oleaceae	——	D
Ebony, rosewood, blackwood, jacaranda, foxwood	Papilionaceae	Africa/Asia/ America	D C-R A T
Pine	Pinaceae	——	D C-R A
Douglas fir, red fir, Douglas spruce	Pinaceae	America	D C-R A
New Zealand white pine	Podocarpaceae	Oceania	D C-R A
Cherry, black cherry	Rosaceae	——	D C-R A
Boxwood	Rutaceae	America	D C-R A

| Poplar | Salicaceae | —— | D C-R A |
| Sequoia, California redwood | Taxodiaceae | America | D C-R A T |

Footnote: This table was developed from information derived from the International Labour Organization's *Encyclopaedia of Occupational Health and Safety,* Vol. 2, third edition, Geneva, 1983. pages 2308-2316.

CHAPTER 29

PHOTOGRAPHY AND PHOTOPRINTING

U nfortunately, many art photographers work in unsafe conditions. Art schools and universities often teach photography in improperly vented areas and without proper protective equipment. And many photographers develop and print in converted bathrooms, kitchens, and other inadequate spaces in their own homes. Health and safety hazards abound in these under equipped, poorly vented darkrooms.

HEALTH HAZARDS

Vast numbers of substances, many of them very complex organic chemicals, are involved in photographic processes. Many of these are known to be hazardous, while the hazards of many others are unknown and unstudied. In addition, new photochemical products are developed frequently.

For these reasons, it is impossible in the scope of this book to discuss all photochemicals. Instead, it is easier to look at the effects of photochemical exposure.

DISEASES ASSOCIATED WITH PHOTOCHEMICALS

Photochemicals are particularly associated with skin diseases and respiratory allergies. It is not uncommon to know of photographers who have had to change careers because they have developed these occupational illnesses.

SKIN DISEASES. Many types of dermatitis have been seen in photographers including:

1. irritant contact dermatitis and chemical burns from exposure to irritating chemicals such as acids and bleaches,

2. allergic contact dermatitis from many developer chemicals such as metol and p-phenylenediamine,

3. hyper- and hypo- pigmentation (dark and light spots) from exposure to developing chemicals such as hydroquinone,

4. lichen planus (inflammatory condition characterized by tiny reddish papules that may darken and spread to form itchy, scaly patches and ulcerations) thought to be caused by some color developers, and

5. skin cancer from exposure to ultraviolet light sources such as carbon arcs. (There also is a potential for cancer to develop in lichen planus.)

RESPIRATORY DISEASES. Photochemical baths emit substances which are recognized as the typical darkroom odor. These substances also may be responsible for many of the respiratory diseases associated with darkroom work. Table 24 lists some of these airborne substances and their hazards.

TABLE 24	Common Darkroom Air Contaminants	
Chemical	Major sources	Primary hazards
acetic acid	stop baths	irritant
formaldehyde	hardeners and preservatives	sensitizer, irritant, and animal carcinogen
hydrogen sulfide	emitted by some toners	highly toxic to nervous system, irritant
sulfur dioxide	breakdown of sulfites in baths	respiratory irritant and sensitizer
various solvents	color chemistry and film cleaners	irritants, toxic to nervous system, see Table 5 hazards of specific solvents.

Darkroom chemicals can cause a variety of respiratory diseases. Low doses of irritating chemicals can cause slight damage to respiratory tissues that may leave photographers more susceptible to colds and respiratory infections.

Heavy exposures to irritating chemicals may cause acute bronchitis or chemical pneumonia. Such serious effects are most likely to occur if highly irritating substances such as concentrated acid vapors are inhaled, or if significant amounts of the dusts from dry chemicals are inhaled. Many photochemicals in the dry, concentrated form are powerful irritants and sensitizers.

Chronic diseases from years of exposure to darkroom chemicals can lead to chronic bronchitis and emphysema. In fact, these diseases are seen frequently among darkroom technicians.

Allergic diseases such as asthma and alveolitis may result from exposure to sensitizing substances such as sulfur dioxide, formaldehyde or from dust inhaled while mixing powdered developers.

Many experts believe that respiratory system cancers also may be associated with exposure to formaldehyde. Photographers who smoke are certainly at risk for lung cancer and are at greater risk for most of the other diseases associated with photochemicals.

SYSTEMIC DISEASES. Some photochemicals also are toxic to other bodily systems. For example, if significant amounts of some photochemicals are inhaled or ingested, they can cause methemoglobinemia. This is a disease in which the chemical damages the blood so that it can no longer carry sufficient oxygen. Exposure to bromide-containing chemicals and solvents may harm the developing fetus. Material Safety Data Sheets should alert users to these kinds of hazards.

Photochemical products that contain extremely toxic substances should be replaced with safer materials. Some extremely toxic chemicals include: chromic acid bleaches; lead toners; mercury vapor (Daguerreotype); mercury intensifiers and preservatives; uranium nitrate toners; and cyanide reducers and intensifiers (not ferri- or ferrocyanides, which are safer).

GENERAL PRECAUTIONS

1. Provide darkroom ventilation (at a rate of roughly twenty room exchanges per hour for small darkrooms, ten room exchanges per hour for very large gang darkrooms) for black and white developing. Provide local exhaust systems such as slot hoods or fume hoods if toners, intensifiers, color process, or solvent-containing products are used. Purchase photo processors equipped with factory-built local ventilation systems.

2. Replace dry chemicals with premixed chemicals when possible. When powders must be used, handle and mix them in local exhaust ventilation such as a fume hood or with respiratory protection. Avoid skin contact and clean up dust and spills scrupulously.

3. Obtain Material Safety Data Sheets on all photochemicals and select the safest materials. Do not use extremely toxic chemicals such as those containing chromic acid, lead, mercury, uranium or cyanide.

4. Provide and use protective equipment including an eye-wash fountain, gloves, chemical splash goggles, tongs, and aprons.

5. Provide additional protection if concentrated photochemical solutions and glacial acetic acid are used including a deluge shower, and face shield. Dilute or mix these chemicals in local exhaust ventilation such as a fume hood. Always add acid to water, never the reverse.

6. Gloves and tongs always should be used to transfer prints from baths. Barrier creams can replace gloves if only occasional splashes of black and white chemicals are expected. (Note: barrier creams may smudge prints if they are handled.)

7. Store photochemicals in the original containers when possible. Never store photochemicals in glass bottles which can explode under pressure.

8. Prepare to handle spills and breakage with chemical absorbents and/ or floor drains and hose systems (if regulations permit).

9. Practice good housekeeping. Clean up all spills immediately. Never work when floors or counters are wet with water or chemicals. Eliminate trip hazards and clutter.

10. Clean up and wash off immediately all spills and splashes on the skin. Do no allow splashes on clothing or skin to remain until dry. Instead, remove contaminated clothing and flush skin with copious amounts of water. After washing off caustic materials, use an acid-type cleanser.

11. Keep first aid kits stocked and post emergency procedures.

12. Prevent electrical shocks by separating electrical equipment from sources of water and wet processes as much as possible. Install ground fault interrupters on darkroom outlets.

13. Follow manufacturer's recommendations and governmental regulations when disposing of photochemicals. If chemicals may be put down drains, dilute and flush with large amounts of water. Be sure the water treatment facility into which the chemicals will drain can handle them. Never flush into septic systems.

14. Do not allow heat or ultraviolet (UV) light (from carbon arcs or the sun) to affect photochemicals. For example, ferri- and ferrocyanides can release hydrogen cyanide gas if exposed to heat or UV.

15. Replace carbon arc light sources which emit dangerous UV, highly toxic gases and metal fumes. Use halide bulbs, quartz lamps, sunlight, or other high intensity lights. Avoid direct eye contact with all intense light sources.

16. Follow all rules for flammable and/or toxic solvents (see pages 16-19) if solvent-containing products such as film cleaners and color photochemicals are used.

17. Always be prepared to provide your doctor with information about the chemicals you use and your work environment.

PRECAUTIONS FOR SPECIFIC PHOTO PROCESSES

BLACK AND WHITE PHOTOCHEMICALS. Most common black and white photochemicals can be used safely if they are purchased premixed and diluted with care, and if the precautions above are followed. Especially provide good general dilution ventilation (see Precaution 1 above).

TONING. Almost all toners require local exhaust ventilation systems. Most of these chemicals are highly toxic and emit toxic gases during use. For example, sulfide toners produce highly toxic hydrogen sulfide gas and selenium toners produce large amounts of sulfur dioxide.

COLOR PROCESSING. Color processing employs many of the same chemicals that are used in black and white processing. In addition, they contain dye couplers which are associated with serious skin problems. Formaldehyde also is present in many color processing products and some products contain toxic solvents such as the glycol ethers (see pages 86).

Mixing of color processing chemicals and open bath color processing requires local exhaust ventilation, gloves, and goggles. Small hand tank developing can be done with dilution exhaust, gloves, and goggles.

Automatic color processing requires local exhaust ventilation. Today, most automatic color processors are made with local exhaust hoods built into them, or the manufacturers offer exhaust equipment accessories. However, many salespeople do not make it clear to buyers that these machines should be connected to exhaust fan extraction systems.

PHOTOPRINTING. Many photographic processes have been adapted to printmaking uses. Included are photo lithography, photo etching, and photo silkscreen processes. These processes use similar chemicals and require similar precautions.

High intensity light sources are needed for these processes and carbon arc lamps should be avoided (see Precaution 15 above).

Photo etching relies on solvents to etch plastic. Some of these photo etching solvents are highly toxic and may include the glycol ethers (see Table 5, Common Solvents and Their Hazards, page 89). Photolithography uses solvents and dichromate solutions.

There are two types of photo-silk screen processes: direct and indirect emulsion processes. Direct emulsions usually use ammonium dichromate as the sensitizer. Indirect emulsions use presensitized films which are developed by concentrated hydrogen peroxide and cleaned of emulsion with bleach.

The chemical ingredients used in each of these processes fall into four groups listed in Table 25.

NON-SILVER PROCESSES:

BROWN PRINTING (VAN DYKE PROCESS) employs ferric ammonium nitrate, tartaric acid (or oxalic acid), and silver nitrate. These chemicals are mixed with distilled water and applied to paper. The paper is exposed to light and developed with a water/borax mixture and fixed with sodium thiosulfate solution. Oxalic acid and silver nitrate are especially hazardous and require extra care to avoid eye and skin contact, and inhalation of the dry materials. Developing can be done with dilution ventilation.

GUM PRINTING (GUM BICHROMATE) involves coating paper with an emulsion of gum arabic, water, pigments, and ammonium dichromate. After exposure to light, it is developed in water and hung up to dry. Multiple printings can be done by changing the pigments.

Hardening and clearing are done in a solution of potassium alum and water or in a dilute solution of formaldehyde. Mercuric chloride, thymol, and other hazardous biocides may be used to preserve the solution.

Avoid solutions containing mercuric chloride or any other highly hazardous biocide. Dichromates are very toxic and are potent sensitizers. Local exhaust such as a fume hood should be used when working with powdered dichromates, dry pigments, and formaldehyde solutions.

CYANOTYPE (BLUEPRINTING) is similar to brown printing except that ferric ammonium citrate and potassium ferricyanide are used. (See Precaution 14 for hazards of these chemicals.) Ordinary dilution ventilation should suffice for cyanotype.

SALTED PAPER PRINTS use silver nitrate as the major component. Silver nitrate is especially hazardous and requires extra care to avoid eye and skin contact with the solution. Ordinary dilution ventilation should suffice.

TABLE 25	Precautions for Photoprint Chemicals

SOLVENTS used in photo printmaking have varying hazards (see Chapter 9, Solvents, pages 83-96) and ventilation requirements will depend on the toxicity of the solvent and the amount that becomes airborne. Some are the glycol ethers, which have reproductive hazards and are absorbed by skin. Provide good ventilation and avoid skin contact or use special gloves (usually nitrile gloves will provide protection).

CONCENTRATED HYDROGEN PEROXIDE AND BLEACH can cause severe eye and skin damage and gloves, goggles, and local exhaust ventilation should be used. When used to remove emulsions, bleach emits chlorine gas which also requires local exhaust ventilation.

DICHROMATES are very toxic and sensitizing. Gloves and local exhaust ventilation such as a fume hood should be used when working with powdered dichromates.

PHOTO EMULSIONS usually are sensitizers and skin contact with them should be prevented.

298

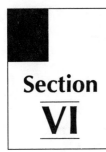

Section
VI

*Teaching
Art*

30 CLASSROOM HAZARDS

Teaching art safely requires special consideration of the hazards of art materials. Hazardous materials jeopardize not only students' health, but the liability of teachers and/or schools. To protect both health and liability requires 1) a safe classroom and 2) proper instruction.

1. The safe classroom is one that is free of hazards and that it is suitable for the chosen activity. For example, the room must be without fire and electrical code violations, possess proper ventilation, safety equipment, and so on.

2. Proper instruction requires teachers to:

> a. fully and accurately inform students about the hazards;
> b. thoroughly train students to work safely;
> c. enforce safety rules; and
> d. provide an example of proper conduct (i.e. teachers must practice faithfully all the precautions they have instructed students to follow).

These rules apply only to students who are able to understand fully the information and training. Children or students who are intellectually or psychologically impaired must not be given any materials that could harm them, even if large amounts would have to be eaten or if they would have to abuse the material in some way. (See Table 28 for materials suitable for these students.)

AIR-QUALITY STANDARDS FOR STUDENTS

If all students were healthy adults, we might use or modify the air-quality standards developed for the workplace (see pages 32-33). There are two reasons this cannot be done. First, the students are not employees and legally have not accepted the risks associated with workplace standards. Second, the workplace standards were developed for healthy adults. Many students are neither healthy nor adults and are at greater risk.

In order to evaluate classroom hazards and plan curricula, we must first understand the needs of these high risk students.

IDENTIFYING "HIGH RISK" STUDENTS

"High risk" students are those who are more likely to be harmed by chemical, biological, or physical agents than average healthy adults. Some high risk groups are listed in Table 26.

CHEMICAL EFFECTS ON HIGH RISK GROUPS

CHILDREN. Children are especially sensitive to toxic substances because they are still growing and have a more rapid metabolism than an adult. They absorb and incorporate toxic materials more readily. Their brain and nervous systems are still developing and may more easily be harmed by neurotoxic chemicals. Their bodily defenses are not as developed and their lower body weight puts them at risk from smaller amounts of chemicals than if they were heavier adults.

Children are also at risk from psychological factors. For instance, a child under twelve cannot be expected to understand toxic hazards or to carry out precautions consistently or effectively. Even adults have difficultly understanding the need for caution, so it is unreasonable to expect that children will.

In addition, children have certain behavior patterns that may put them at increased risk of exposure. For example, young children go through a stage where they put things into their mouths. Even older children may

TABLE 26	Who Is at Higher Risk?

ALL PEOPLE AT CERTAIN TIMES OF LIFE SUCH AS:
- CHILDREN TWELVE AND UNDER are at greater risk. The younger the child, the greater the risk.
- THE PREGNANT WOMAN AND THE FETUS both are at greater risk. The fetus is at greatest risk.
- THE ELDERLY who have lost resistance to physical damage or chemical exposure with age.

PEOPLE TEMPORARILY IMPAIRED SUCH AS:
- THE SICK. For example, a respiratory infection could put one at higher risk from chemicals which damage the lungs.
- THE CONVALESCING after surgery or physical injury.
- THOSE UNDER EXTREME STRESS from emotional trauma, chronic anxiety or pressure.
- THOSE ABUSING ALCOHOL OR DRUGS.

PEOPLE CHRONICALLY IMPAIRED INCLUDING:
- THE CHRONICALLY ILL such as those with chronic bronchitis, heart disease, liver impairment, and the like.
- MENTALLY RETARDED.
- OTHERS NEUROLOGICALLY IMPAIRED such as those with multiple sclerosis, cerebral palsy or epilepsy.
- THE PSYCHOLOGICALLY DISTURBED.
- SEVERELY ALLERGIC INDIVIDUALS.
- THE VISUALLY IMPAIRED.
- THE HEARING IMPAIRED.
- THOSE WITH SOME KINDS OF PHYSICAL DISABILITIES.
- THOSE TAKING CERTAIN MEDICATIONS.

have high hand-to-mouth contact behavior or "pica," a disorder of the appetite in which nonfood substances are craved.

PREGNANT WOMEN. A pregnant woman's blood volume increases by 30 to 40 percent, making her anemic. This anemia makes her more susceptible to blood-absorbed toxins such as carbon monoxide (carboxy hemoglobin) and solvents.

Pregnant women also inhale more air to provide for the increased oxygen needs of the fetus. This means that they will be more susceptible to inhaled substances. Wearing respiratory protection may not be recommended because of the breathing resistance caused by wearing a mask or respirator. Pregnant women should consult their doctors before wearing respiratory protection.

Even after pregnancy, some toxic substances are concentrated in breast milk. Examples include heavy metals, solvents, and many pesticides.

THE FETUS. Many metals such as lead, manganese, antimony, and selenium, and many pesticides, drugs, and solvents are known to affect the fetus adversely. The effect of many solvents, for instance, is similar to that of alcohol.

It is difficult for women to know when they have been exposed to amounts of chemicals that can cause harm to the fetus. This is because some toxins can cause severe damage, even fetal death, at amounts which are so small that they produce no symptoms in the mother.

Even substances to which the mother was exposed before conception may cause harm to the fetus (see cumulative toxins, page 22). For example lead stored in the mother's body may affect the fetus months after she stopped working with it. Women working with cumulative toxins should consult their doctors when planning pregnancies.

Unfortunately, a great many chemicals used by artists have never been studied for their reproductive effects. Since pregnancy is of limited duration and the outcome so important, it is prudent to avoid chemical exposure as much as possible.

THE PHYSIOLOGICALLY LIMITED. People who are physically limited in their ability to expel or resist chemicals will be more damaged by exposure than someone who is unimpaired. For example, people with emphysema cannot expel an inhaled toxic gas from their lungs as fast or efficiently as someone without emphysema.

Similarly, people with damaged livers are more susceptible to chemicals which must be metabolized by the liver, people with dermatitis will absorb more skin-penetrating chemicals, people with anemia are more susceptible to chemicals which affect hemoglobin in the blood, heart patients may not be able to tolerate the irregular heartbeats often caused by solvent exposure, and so on.

MEDICATED STUDENTS. Some medications are known to interact adversely with chemicals in the body. For example, ingesting barbiturates and alcohol together can seriously threaten life. Similarly, barbiturates taken while inhaling alcohol vapors from shellac would have an identical interaction.

Some predictable medication/chemical interactions or additive effects might include the following:

1) medications which depress the central nervous system are likely to interact with or exacerbate the effect caused by chemicals which also are depressants, such as solvents and some toxic metals;

2) medications which interact with alcohol in ways not related to central nervous system depression;

3) medications containing catecholamines or amphetamine derivatives that could sensitize the heart (to epinephrine) making it more susceptible to solvent-induced cardiac arrhythmias (irregular heart beats);

4) medications that cause photosension of the skin, which could exacerbate effects of ultraviolet radiation on the skin (e.g., during welding);

5) mood-altering amine oxidase-inhibiting drugs that cause adverse reactions in individuals exposed to amine epoxy catalysts or amine solvents (e.g. ethanolamine);

6) manic depressive patients on lithium carbonate therapy affected by additional exposure to lithium carbonate in some ceramic glazes or metal enamels.

SENSORY-IMPAIRED STUDENTS. Those who have impaired abilities to see, hear, smell, feel, or otherwise sense the presence of chemicals are also at greater risk of being over-exposed than unimpaired people. For example, the visually impaired may paint with their faces held extraordinarily close to their work and consequently may inhale far more paint vapors than someone working at a greater distance. The visually impaired also may not notice spills, may have more frequent accidents, or may not see well enough to clean up well.

Just as obviously, those who cannot detect odors may inhale large amounts of toxic gases and vapors without being aware, those who cannot sense pain may be injured when exposed to chemicals which burn the skin, and so on.

306

NEUROLOGICALLY IMPAIRED STUDENTS. People whose brains and nervous systems are damaged are likely to be more susceptible to chemicals which also damage the nervous system. For this reason, those with cerebral palsy, Parkinson's disease, multiple sclerosis, and related diseases are likely to be at greater risk from exposure to solvents and toxic metals such as mercury, lead, and manganese.

Exposure to these neurotoxic chemicals is even more devastating to the retarded because these solvents and metals can impair their already compromised mental acuity. Further, the retarded are even more at risk because they also 1) may not be able to understand the hazards of the chemicals, 2) may not be capable of learning to take proper precautions, 3) may have habits, such as hand-to-mouth contact, which exposes them to greater amounts, 4) they may not know when they have been overexposed, and 5) they may not be able to clearly describe their symptoms to doctors or to others from whom they would seek help.

For these reasons, it is unconscionable to place these individuals in programs that employ toxic chemicals such as ceramics programs using lead glazes, or painting and graphic arts programs in which solvent-containing materials are used.

ALLERGIC STUDENTS. There are many chemicals in art and craft materials that are well-known sensitizers, such as many dyes, pigments, plastics chemicals, natural substances such as turpentine, rosin, and gum arabic, and metals like chrome and nickel. People with serious allergies such as contact dermatitis and asthma, or who have had incidences of urticaria (hives) or anaphylactic shock, should avoid exposure to strong sensitizers.

BIOLOGICAL HAZARDS

Microorganisms such as viruses, bacteria, rickettsia, fungus, molds, mildew, and yeasts can cause infections and allergies. There are many sources of these biological hazards in art and craft materials.

HOW PEOPLE ARE EXPOSED TO MICROORGANISMS. In order for microorganisms to harm people they must be 1) inhaled, ingested, or skin-absorbed into the body, 2) the organisms must be of a type that can cause disease or allergy in the exposed individual, and 3) they must be present in numbers large enough to overwhelm the individual's defenses.

Most microorganisms are harmless, which is reassuring since they are everywhere including in the air, in water, and on people. Airborne mold, mildew, yeasts, and bacteria will contaminate any art material left uncovered. For example, diluted acrylic paints left standing at room temperature will give ample evidence of microorganism's presence by their offensive odor. Inhalation of spray or airbrush mist from these contaminated materials could cause a variety of illnesses, depending on which microorganisms were established in the material.

Even microorganisms that are considered harmless may cause allergies in some individuals, or may cause disease in individuals who are immune deficient. Table 27 lists the kinds of people who are at greater risk from biological hazards.

People can be a source of microorganisms as well. For example, United States hospitals have OSHA guidelines to prevent transference of diseases such as AIDS and hepatitis B. Yet many teachers of craft and occupational therapy programs for these patients do not consider these guidelines when planning their activities, clean-up, and accident procedures. In some cases, teachers are not told of students' illnesses. In this case, both the student and the teacher may be at risk.

TABLE 27	Those at High Risk From Biological Hazards

A. People with Compromised Immune Systems Due to:

   1. Inherited Immune Deficiency or Acquired Immune Deficiencies from:

- AIDS and other diseases which affect immune response
- leukemia and other diseases affecting bone marrow
- defense systems that are engaged in fighting other diseases
- being physically run down, malnourished, etc.
- being under extreme stress

   2. Certain Chronic Illnesses (for example, people with chronic bronchitis are more susceptible to organisms that cause respiratory infections).

   3. Taking Immune-Supressive Drugs or Treatments

- cancer patients on some types of chemotherapy and/or radiation
- organ transplant recipients

---

4. Exposure to Chemicals that Affect the Immune System

  • benzene and other chemicals that damage bone marrow
  • other chemicals, now suspected of affecting the immune system in various ways.

B. People at Elevated Risk from Biological Allergens

  1. People who are Asthmatics

  2. People with Dermatitis

  3. People who have a History of Hives or Anaphylatic Shock

CONTROLLING EXPOSURE TO BIOLOGICAL HAZARDS

The ingredients necessary for microorganisms to prosper are 1) a warm temperature (those ranging from room temperature to warm tap water temperatures are optimal), 2) moisture, 3) organic matter for food (can be almost anything such as acrylic polymer in paints or minute amounts of vegetable matter in clay), and 4) introduction of the microorganisms into the system.

The ways to reduce exposure to microorganisms is: 1) to control temperature and humidity, 2) remove sources of food for microorganisms by keeping materials covered, cleaning up spills, and good housekeeping, 3) avoid practices that contaminate materials or hands with microorganisms, 4) kill microorganisms with soaps and disinfectants. This later practice requires caution, since some disinfectants and soaps also have toxic properties or cause allergies.

In other words, maintaining a comfortable environment, working neatly, and practicing good personal hygiene will go a long way toward reducing danger from microorganisms.

PHYSICAL HAZARDS

Physical hazards consist of: hazards from exposure to physical phenomena such as noise, vibration, heat, or radiation; and safety hazards such as accidents or overuse injuries.

NOISE. Noise of ear-damaging intensity is produced by many art processes (see pages 35-37). Hearing-impaired people should not be exposed to noise unless it is determined that it will not further damage their hearing. This determination should be made by an otologist since it requires understanding the exact diagnosis of the cause of each individual's hearing loss.

Some experts feel that it is not acceptable to expose hearing-impaired people to noise, even if further damage to frequency receptors will not affect their ability to hear. They reason that new methods of restoring hearing may be developed, which will rely on intact frequency receptors.

It may be possible for the hearing-impaired to work in noisy environments if their ears are protected from the noise. Here again, an otologist should be consulted to match the kind of protection to the type of noise in the environment and the individual's particular needs. Contrary to common opinion, merely turning down a person's hearing aid may not protect hearing. Aids with vented ear-pieces or ear-pieces which do not fit tightly may transmit significant amounts of noise.

Those planning programs that involve noise must be aware that there may be some participants who are not aware that they have hearing losses or who choose not to make their hearing loss known to others. This is especially true in programs for the elderly.

Noise may also cause increased blood pressure and stress-related illnesses. The elderly and others with high blood pressure or conditions exacerbated by stress should be protected from noisy environments.

Hearing-impaired students also should not participate in activities in which hearing warning calls can be crucial to their safety, such as in theatrical rigging and lighting.

VIBRATION. Vibration, such as that transferred to users of hand held tools, can also be harmful (see page 37). There is no data on physiological response to vibration in people whose circulation is impaired for other causes, such as aging or heart disease. However, prudence dictates exposure to vibration should be limited for such individuals.

Even less is known about whole body vibration such as that encountered on buses or trucks. Whole body vibration is suspected of causing sleep disturbances, tremors, and general nervous upset. Program planners might want to consider the possibility that whole body vibration also may affect some participants adversely.

IONIZING RADIATION. Ionizing radiation such as X-rays and radioactivity can cause harmful biological effects including cancer. These forms of radiation are rarely encountered in arts and crafts unless uranium-containing pottery glazes or metal enamels (see page 38) are used. People who already have had X-ray therapy or radiation treatment would be at even greater risk from the additional exposure.

NONIONIZING RADIATION, including visible light and ultraviolet and infrared radiation con be hazardous to high risk individuals.

   LIGHT. It is well-known that inadequate lighting, glare, and shadow-producing direct lighting can cause eye strain and accidents. Poor lighting is even more likely to be harmful to visually impaired individuals. Conversely, special lighting can be used to aid some visually impaired to better use their limited sight. Careful attention to lighting is crucial for many art and craft programs for the visually impaired.

   ULTRAVIOLET (UV) AND INFRARED (IR) RADIATION. UV sources include sunlight, welding, and carbon arc lamps. UV is known to cause eye damage and skin cancer in welders (see page 38).
   Eye-damaging amounts of IR are produced whenever metals or ceramic materials are heated until they glow. IR radiation can cause conjunctivitis, dry eye (decreased lacrimation), cataracts and other effects. Everyone, especially those with visual impairments, should wear protective goggles whenever IR or UV radiation is present (see Tables 4 and 5, Filter Lens Shades and Selection Chart for Eye and Face Protectors, pages 58-60).

VIDEO DISPLAY TERMINALS (VDTs). Many forms of harmful radiation are associated with these devices (pages 38-39). It is suspected that they may be most harmful to the fetus and to young children.
   In addition to radiation, VDTs are associated with eye strain, overuse injuries, and stress. When high risk individuals such as those with musculoskeletal or visual problems use these devices, lighting should be carefully planned, desk and chair arrangements should be comfortable, the users vision should be periodically checked, and frequent work breaks should be planned.

OTHER RADIATION. There are Threshold Limit Values for other forms of radiation hazards such as heat stress, cold environments, laser radiation, microwaves, and more. In general, comfortable environments, which preclude exposures to these forms of radiation, should be maintained for most high risk individuals.

ACCIDENTS. Statistics bear out the fact that accidents do not occur without a reason. This means they also can be prevented by eliminating the causes. A few common causes of accidents in the workplace that can be remedied include 1) faulty or poorly maintained equipment and tools, 2) poor condition of walking surfaces, 3) unguarded machinery, and 4) poor lighting.

When high risk individuals work where these conditions are present, accidents are even more likely. Visually impaired people are less likely to notice that equipment is damaged and hazardous, people unable to judge distances accurately would be at greater risk of accidents if lighting is inadequate, people with balance problems especially need well maintained walking surfaces, and so on.

Attention to safety hazards is especially crucial in programs for high risk individuals.

OVERUSE INJURIES. Overuse injuries are most often associated with repetitive motions or with heavy work such as lifting. While learning to lift properly and taking frequent rest breaks during repetitive tasks may be important for all people, it is crucial for many high risk individuals. In fact, in many cases, lifting may be precluded by certain illnesses, injuries, or musculoskeletal problems. Some research indicates that older workers are more likely to sustain overuse injuries.

It is imperative that each individual be medically evaluated before placement in programs involving physical effort or repetitive tasks. Physical therapists may also be needed to assist individuals in learning to do tasks safely.

STRESS. Stress refers to an internal response to a demanding situation. Studies show that chronic stress is the most damaging and is associated with hypertension, peptic ulcers, heart disease, and many other illnesses.

Many high risk individuals already are managing stress from dealing with their handicaps. Programs for high risk individuals should be designed to preclude added stress. Some strategies include placing only realistic demands on participants, providing pleasant and peaceful working conditions, and providing individuals with ways to make their needs known and met.

PLANNING PROGRAMS FOR HIGH RISK INDIVIDUALS

EMPLOY QUALIFIED TEACHERS. All too often, general teachers, volunteers, professional artists or craftspeople, and others without formal training in special education are urged to teach high risk students.

Teaching most types of high risk individuals requires special training. To protect the students and the schools' and teachers' liability, teachers should have generally accepted qualifications for teaching the kind of students in the school or someone qualified should be supervising teachers.

RESEARCH THE LOCATION. When setting up a new program, be sure that the students have easy access to the facility. Equally important, be sure emergency egress for the handicapped is equally accessible.

Schools and institutions must have comprehensive emergency plans and hold regular drills. Other emergency equipment that should be available include a communication system in each activities room to summon help, first aid equipment, and fire protection equipment (extinguishers or sprinklers, smoke detectors, etc.).

In addition to emergency response equipment, it is important to see that the classroom is equipped to maintain appropriate ventilation, temperature, and relative humidity. Higher than normal temperatures may be desirable to provide comfort for elderly or ill students. Good control of humidity may be helpful in controlling biological hazards.

Sanitation and proper clean-up of materials must also be provided. Sinks and running water for washing hands and tools are a must. Custodians should provide clean-up methods appropriate to the materials used. For example, wet mopping should be used in rooms where dusts such as clay and plaster must be controlled.

CHOOSE SAFE MATERIALS AND ACTIVITIES. Know the potential hazards of the products that will be used in the activities. This may require research, since merely reading product labels will not be sufficient. Obtain Material Safety Data Sheets and any additional ingredient information possible. Table 28 lists products and activities acceptable for children and other high risk individuals.

If there is any question about the safety of a product, contact a toxicologist and/or the product's manufacturer. Some reputable manufacturers will release more complete ingredient information to teachers of high risk students.

When moderately toxic materials are used with students that are capable of handling them, follow Material Safety Data Sheet recommendations for ventilation, protective equipment, and the like. Keep in mind that the precautions listed on the Material Safety Data Sheets are for healthy adult workers. More stringent precautions are required to protect high risk individuals.

EVALUATE THE PARTICIPANT/STUDENT. Secure all available background information about each student. This information may be obtained through interviews with parents or guardians, doctors, therapists, previous teachers, and when possible, the students themselves. Unfortunately, some educators feel that the students' privacy is violated by such inquiries. However, the students' safety and health may be jeopardized unless teachers are familiar with their students' physical and psychological limitations, the effects of medications they are taking, the emergency procedures which would be necessary in a crisis, and the like.

Some educators also feel that teachers who know about their students' intellectual or psychological handicaps will treat them unfairly or will not sufficiently challenge the student to learn. If this were true, the answer would not be to know less about a student's handicap, but to give the teacher even more information and education.

If there are nonhandicapped students in the class, it may be necessary to educate them about the handicap as well.

OBTAIN ADVICE FROM OTHERS. Once the information about the student and the activity have been gathered, obtain advice from parents, therapists, physicians, previous teachers, and other interested parties. Schools and institutions often find that organizing review panels works well in coordinating such information and making decisions.

SPECIAL PROBLEMS OF HOMEBOUND PROGRAMS

Homebound art and craft programs utilize materials and equipment in the home. Homes are not proper settings for practicing some arts and crafts. Projects which create toxic solvent vapors are especially hazardous since the homebound spend long hours exposed to them. And if fine toxic dusts contaminate the home, they are likely to be a hazard to the occupants for a long time, perhaps years.

Avoid projects which employ toxic materials such as solvents, lead, other toxic metals, and two-part plastic resin systems such as polyester.

Also avoid projects that create dusts or fumes such as sanding and clean-ing ceramic greenware, using soft pastels, and soldering or casting metal.

Instead, select materials that do not need special ventilation, which will not cause injury on skin or eye contact, which don't involve high heat or burring processes, and generally meet the criteria for safe materials (see Table 28).

Homebound students also must be counciled not to employ equipment for projects that also is used for other purposes. For example, kitchen ovens should not be used to harden or cure plastics, inks, clay, or simi-lar materials. Dye pots should not later be used for food.

TABLE 28	Art Materials and Projects Suitable for Children and Other High Risk Individuals

Teachers of children under age 12, the intellectually and physically disabled, the chronically ill, the elderly, and others at elevated risk from exposure to toxic chemicals can replace toxic materials with safer ones as follows:

DO NOT USE	SUBSTITUTES
SOLVENTS & SOLVENT-CONTAINING PRODUCTS	WATER-BASED & SOLVENT-FREE PRODUCTS
Alkyd, oil enamels, or other solvent-containing paints.	Use acrylics, oil sticks, colors, water containing paints, or other water-based paints containing safe pigments.
Turpentine, paint thinners, citrus turps, or other solvents for cleaning up or thinning artist's oil paints.	Mix oil-based, solvent-free paints with linseed oil only. Clean with baby oil followed by soap and water. Choose paints containing safe pigments.
Solvent-based silk screen inks and other printing inks containing solvents or requiring solvents for clean up.	Use water-based silk screen inks, block printing, or stencil inks with safe pigments.
Solvent-containing varnishes, mediums, and alcohol-containing shellacs.	Use acrylic emulsion coatings, or the teacher can apply it for stu-dents under proper conditions.

DO NOT USE	SUBSTITUTES
Rubber cement and thinners for paste up and mechanicals.	Use low temperature wax methods, double sided tape, glue sticks, or other solvent-free materials.
Airplane glue and other solvent-containing glues.	Use white glue, school paste, glue sticks, preservative-free wheat paste, or other solvent-free glues.
Permanent felt-tip markers, white board markers and other solvent-containing markers.	Use water-based markers.

POWDERED OR DUSTY MATERIALS	DUSTLESS PRODUCTS/PROCESSES
Clay dust from mixing dry clay, sanding greenware, and other dusty processes.	Purchase talc-free, low silica, pre-mixed clay. Trim clay when leather hard, clean up often during work, and practice good hygiene and dust control.
Ceramic glaze dust from mixing ingredients, glazing, and other processes.	Substitute with paints or buy glazes free of lead and other toxic metals which are premixed, or mix in local exhaust ventilation. Control dust carefully.
Metal enamel dust.	Substitute with paints. Even lead-free enamels may contain other very toxic metals. Avoid enamels also because heat and acids are used.
Powdered tempera and other powdered paints.	Purchase premixed paints or have the teacher mix them. Use paints with safe ingredients.
Powdered dyes for batik, tie dyeing, and other processes.	Use vegetable and plant materials (e.g. onion skins, tea, etc.) and approved food dyes (e.g. unsweetened Kool-Ade).

DO NOT USE	SUBSTITUTES
Plaster dust.	Have the teacher premix the plaster outdoors or in local exhaust ventilation. Do not sand plaster or do other dusty work. Do not cast hands or other body parts to avoid burns. Cut rather than tear plaster impregnated casting cloth.
Instant papier mache dust from finely ground magazines, newspapers, etc.	Use pieces of plain paper or black and white newspaper with white glue paste, or other safe glues.
Pastels, chalks or dry markers which create dust.	Use oil pastels or sticks, crayons, and dustless chalks.

AEROSOLS AND SPRAY PRODUCTS LIQUID MATERIALS

Spray paints, fixatives, etc.	Use water-based liquids which are brushed, dripped, or splat tered on or have the teacher use sprays in local exhaust ventilation or out doors.
Air brushes.	Replace with other paint methods. Mist should not be inhaled and air brushes can be misused.

MISCELLANEOUS PRODUCTS SUBSTITUTES

All types of professional artist's materials.	Use only products approved and recommended for children when teaching either children or adults who require very special protection.
Toxic metals such as arsenic, lead, cadmium, lithium, barium, chrome, nickel, vanadium, manganese, antimony, and more.	These are common ingredients in ceramic glazes, enamels, paints, and many art materials. Use only materials found free of highly toxic substances.

DO NOT USE	SUBSTITUTES
Epoxy resins, instant glues, and other plastic resin adhesives.	Use white glue, library paste, glue sticks or other safe adhesives.
Plastic resin casting systems or preformed plastic materials.	Do not do plastic resin casting or use any plastic material in ways that release vapors, gases, or odors.
Acid etches and pickling baths.	Do not do projects that use these.
Bleach for reverse dyeing of fabric or colored paper.	Do not do projects using bleach. Thinned white paint can be used to simulate bleach on colored paper.
Photographic chemicals.	Use blueprint paper to make sun grams or use Polaroid cameras. Be sure students do not abuse Polaroid film or pictures which contain toxic chemicals.

MISCELLANEOUS PRODUCTS SUBSTITUTES

Stained glass projects.	Do not do projects using lead, solder or glass cutting. Use colored cello phane and black paper or tape to simulate stained glass.
Industrial talcs contaminated with asbestos or nonfibrous asbestos minerals used in many white clays, slip casting clays, glazes, French chalk, and parting powders.	Always order talc-free products.
Sculpture stones contaminated with asbestos such as some soapstones, steatites, serpentines, etc.	Always use stones found free of asbestos on analysis.
Art paints and markers used to decorate the skin (e.g., clown faces).	Always use products approved for use on the skin (e.g., cosmetics or colored zinc sun screen creams).

DO NOT USE	SUBSTITUTES
Scented markers.	Do not use with children. It encourages them to sniff and taste art materials. They are acceptable for older visually impaired students for distinguishing colors.
Plants and seeds.	Check identity of all plants to be sure no toxic or sensitizing plants are used (e.g., poison oak, castor beans).
Donated, found, or old materials whose ingredients are unknown.	Do not use these materials unless investigation identifies the ingredients and they are found safe.
Products with possible biological hazards.	Use clean, unused materials. Products used with food or other animal or organic materials may harbor bacteria or other hazardous microbes (e.g., washed plastic meat trays may harbor salmonella).

APPENDIX

THE RIGHT-TO-KNOW LIBRARY

The following books and periodicals are recommended for those developing a professional quality health and safety library for their Right-to-Know program. Of course, THE ARTIST'S COMPLETE HEALTH AND SAFETY GUIDE is also suggested for this purpose.

ACTS FACTS, Arts, Crafts and Theater Safety, New York. A monthly newsletter updating health and safety regulations and research affecting the arts. Available from ACTS, Attn: M. Rossol, 181 Thompson St., #23, New York, NY 10012.

Art Hazards News, Center for Safety in the Arts. A newsletter published 10 times a year on various topics related to health and safety in the arts. Available from CSA, 5 Beekman St., 10th floor, New York, NY 10038.

American Conference of Governmental Industrial Hygienists, 6500 Glenway Ave., Bldg. D-7, Cincinnati, OH 45211-4438. 1-513-661-7881. publications 1 and 2 updated yearly.

> **1.Threshold Limit Values and Biological Exposure Indicies.**
> **2.Industrial Ventilation: A Manual of Recommended Practice.**
> **3.The Documentation of TLVs and BEIs.**

Best's Safety Directory, A.M. Best Company, 2 Volumes, Ambest Road, Oldwick, NJ 08858. 1-201-439-2200. Sources safety equipment and supplies. Updated yearly.

Clinical Toxicology of Commercial Products. 6th Edition, Gosselin, Robert E., Et al., Baltimore: Williams and Willkins Co., 1987. Updated regularly. Available in the technical section of many book stores.

Dangerous Properties of Industrial Materials, 7th Edition, Sax, N. Irving and Lewis, Richard J. Sr., Van Nostrand-Reinhold Co., New York, 1988. (Also available from the ACGIH. Call 1-513-661-7881 for publications catalog.)

Encyclopaedia of Occupational Health and Safety, 3rd Revised Edition 2 vols. International Labour Organization, New York: McGraw-Hill, 1983. (Also available from the ACGIH. Call 1-513-661-7881 for publications catalog.)

Hawley's Condensed Chemical Dictionary, 11th Ed., Hawley, Gessner, revised by Sax, N. Irving and Lewis, Sr., Richard, Van Nostrand Reinhold Co., New York, 1987. (Also available from the ACGIH. Call 1-513-661-7881 for publications catalog.)

Hazardous Substance Fact Sheets, New Jersey Department of Health, Trenton, NJ 08625. 1-609-984-2202. These are excellent fact sheets on individual chemicals. Around 900 chemicals are covered.

"How to Read a Material Safety Data Sheet," The American Lung Association of San Diego and Imperial Counties, 1988. A five page data sheet which defines MSDS terms. Contact your local American Lung Association for information on obtaining it.

Industrial Hygiene and Toxicology. Vol. II, 3rd edition, Part A, (1980), Part B, (1981), Part C, (1982), Patty, Frank, (ed.), Interscience Publishers, New York. (Also available from the ACGIH. Call 1-513-661-7881 for publications catalog.)

National Fire Protection Association, Batterymarch Park, Quincy, MA 02169. 1-800-344-3555. Obtain catalog of the 270 codes. Choose pertinent codes such as NFPA #30. Flammable and Combustible Liquids Code.

Registry of Toxic Effects of Chemical Substances. National Institute of Occupational Safety and Health, US Department of Health and Human Services, 1981-2 Edition plus yearly supplements. Reproduced by the National Technical Information Services, Port Royal Road, Springfield, VA 22161.

The MSDS Pocket Dictionary, J.O. Accrocco, Ed., Genium Publishing Corporation, Rev., 1988. A dictionary of terms used on Material Safety Data Sheets. Contact Genium Publishing at 1145 Catalyn Street, Schenectady, NY 12303-1836. 1-518-377-8854.

The WHMIS Handbook, Corpus Information Services, 1450 Don Mills Road, Don Mills, Ontario M3B 2X7. 1-416-445-6641. A well-written, page-tabbed guide to WHMIS.

The WHMIS Pocket Dictionary, Jon Mayo, Ed, Genium Publishing Corp.,1988. Contact Genium Publishing at 1145 Catalyn Street, Schenectady, NY 12303-1836. 1-518-377-8854.

Ventilation: A Practical Guide. Clark, Nancy; Cutter, Thomas; McGrane, Jean-Ann; Center for Safety in the Arts, New York,1980. Available from CSA, 5 Beekman St., New York, NY 10038.

Art workers and administrators should also call their local Department of Labor to obtaining publications and information on the general occupational safety and health regulations applicable to their workplace.

INDEX

The Sea Among The Rocks

Travels in Atlantic Canada

Harry Thurston

Pottersfield Press, Lawrencetown Beach, Nova Scotia, Canada

National Library of Canada Cataloguing in Publication

Thurston, Harry, 1950–
        The sea among the rocks: travels in Atlantic Canada / Harry Thurston
        Expanded version of his earlier work entitled: Atlantic Outposts.
ISBN 1-895900-54-9
1. Atlantic Provinces – Description and travel. 2. Atlantic Provinces – Social life and customs. 3. Atlantic Provinces – Environmental conditions. I. Title.
FC2004.T483 2002   971.5'04   C2002-903593-7

Book cover design by Dalhousie Graphics

Pottersfield Press acknowledges the ongoing support of the Nova Scotia Department of Tourism and Culture, Cultural Affairs Division. We acknowledge the support of the Canada Council for the Arts which last year invested $19.1 million in writing and publishing throughout Canada. We also acknowledge the finanacial support of the Government of Canada through the Book Publishing Industry Development Program for our publishing activities.

Pottersfield Press
83 Leslie Road
East Lawrencetown, Nova Scotia, Canada B2Z 1P8
Web site: www.pottersfieldpress.com
To order, phone 1-800-NIMBUS9 (1-800-646-2879)
Printed in Canada

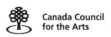 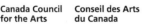 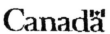

Contents

In memory of
Kenneth MacCormack
(1950-2001)
dear friend and sgeulaiche

Preface

THESE STORIES OF ATLANTIC CANADA span four decades, from 1979 to 2000. My hope is that they are a valuable record of time and place, especially in light of the rapid pace of change that is eroding a way of life here.

Many of the early stories were published in the sister magazines, *Harrowsmith* and *Equinox*, founded by publishing wizard James Lawrence in the late 1970s and early 1980s. A generation of journalists like myself found a kindred spirit in the editorial philosophy of these two magazines. They fearlessly addressed important environmental issues, presenting an alternative to the corporate agenda of consumerism and the damage it has wrought upon the natural world and the integrity of traditional communities.

Many of the stories presented here (from a variety of magazines) might be grouped under the term environmental journalism. It is a relatively new species of journalism that has been viewed warily by both the traditional journalistic community and the public-at-large as promoting a point of view rather than presenting a "balanced perspective."

But in assessing the question of balance, perhaps it is well to keep in mind the words of Teya Ryan, former senior producer of Turner Broadcasting's *Networth Earth*: "Let me first submit to you that, with respect to the environment, advocacy journalism is a misnomer. Think a minute: Who do you know who is against the environment?"

Ryan goes on to point out that covering the environment is "about empowering people." It does no good to simply adopt "the duelling perspectives approach," which ultimately leaves the reader confused and, worse, apathetic. As my editor at *Audubon*, Gary Soucie, used to say: "For every PhD there is an equal and opposite PhD." By simply writing the two-handed story, you distort the complexity of the issue and, more importantly, the state of knowledge surrounding it. Instead, it is vital to report the consensus view, rather than presenting both sides of a story as if they had equal credence. For this writer, arriving at that consensus viewpoint, and therefore credibility and fairness, demands an open mind and exhaustive research.

The earlier stories often centred on human communities, where people still maintain a working relationship with their surroundings – in the backwoods and mines, on islands and the water. In small towns and villages scattered throughout the region, from northern Labrador to southwestern Nova Scotia, I found men and women who quietly follow the old ways: cutting in sauerkraut, separating cream on the farm, teaming oxen, keeping sheep on islands, and building and sailing wooden boats, because for them there is pleasure and dignity in simply doing something right.

The stories, old and new, also address the bounty, wanton destruction, and tardy attempts at conserving what remains of our natural heritage, in the belief that the well-being of communities is inseparable from the health of the environment – a fact that might seem patently obvious if it was not so often ignored by policy makers. The tragic collapse of the North Atlantic cod stocks and its devastating impact on the 500-year-old fishing culture of Newfoundland is the most dramatic example of this principle, and all the more tragic because we now know that it was avoidable.

I have taken the title for this collection of Atlantic stories, *The Sea Among The Rocks*, from the writings of Evelyn Richardson, one of the first, and still most important, of the region's writers on nature. I pay homage to her legacy in the last story presented here. Although she and her husband legally owned Bon Portage Island, where they kept the light, Richardson was wise enough to know "the spots of earth we call our own . . . never actually belong to any of us." Quite the opposite, we belong to them.

These stories, then, are about belonging – to a place I humbly call home.

Harry Thurston

July 2002

1. A Memory of the Wind

A Memory of the Wind
Lunenburg, Nova Scotia

I WAIT PATIENTLY as a woman places her order at Ye Olde Towne Meat Market in Lunenburg, Nova Scotia. The shop is spotless, which should come as no surprise. In Lunenburg, order is a civic virtue.

The well-stocked meat cases display great coils of the local delicacy known as Lunenburg pudding, or sausage. When the butcher heads off to retrieve a special cut from the freezer, the woman draws her woolen sweater around her and says to me with a shiver: "I was down on the shore gathering seaweed. I'm not really cold now, it's just a memory of the wind." A memory of the wind. Everywhere I went in Old Town Lunenburg I was stirred by memories of a time when Nova Scotia's fortunes rode on the sea and the wind. Nowhere has this been more true than in this quintessential east coast fishing port.

In 1753, the winds of colonial war between France and England brought Lunenburg its original settlers from three areas: the German Palatinate, the Montbeliard region of France, and Switzerland. Today, their descendants are called "Lunenburg Dutch," derived from Deutsch (German). During the nineteenth century, winds of fortune filled the sails of Lunenburg's famous

Grand Banks fishing fleet – as well as the coffers of local merchants. Winds then swept the schooner *Bluenose* across the finish line ahead of all challengers, not just once, but at every International Fishermen's Trophy race between 1921 and 1938. "The Queen of the North Atlantic" brought lasting fame to her birthplace. Now the winds of change are swirling through Lunenburg in the wake of collapsing Northwest Atlantic fish stocks.

The town that fish built has turned to tourism. Walk along its streets and you will understand why students from Harvard's School of Architecture make pilgrimages here to soak up the town's heritage, why film crews come in search of ready-made historical sets and why, in December 1995, Lunenburg's Old Town was declared a UNESCO World Heritage Site.

Nowhere in North America will you find a collection of vintage wooden architecture so intact. Blue and red chandleries face the sea, and spires of Gothic churches – among the oldest in Canada – pierce the sky. Colourful Victorian and Georgian houses march up the hillside from the harbour like "little Dutch toys," in the words of nineteenth-century writer Captain William Moorsom. Lunenburg bumps, the ornate windows and porches that "bump out" into the street, give the town its prosperous profile.

Frugality has preserved this maritime treasure, but Lunenburgers will be the first to assure you that their home is not about to become a museum or Disney-style attraction. Lunenburg is lived in. It may be mystic, but a practical heart still beats here. Every day, scallop boats emerge from the fog, their holds filled with a succulent take. Foundry workers transform molten metal into gleaming propellers; and sailmakers diligently stitch together the sails that billow in yachters' dreams. The din of shipbuilders at work reverberates up from the waterfront to the rooftop widow's walks, from which sea captains' wives once kept watch for their husbands' homecoming.

Montague Street, one block from the waterfront, is like a mermaid – half human and half aquatic – with one end lined by boutiques, galleries, craft shops and the other by a row of traditional marine suppliers. I venture through the open doors of one of these seaport emporiums. There is no sign on the storefront, but etched into the back window of a truck parked outside is this catch-all label: "Anything Marine since 1945, Bruce Parsons, Marine Consultant-Researcher." The license plate reads SEADOG.

By way of greeting, proprietor Bruce Parsons, appropriately nautical in a navy blue sweater, drops a needle onto a record album and cranks up the volume on a rousing rendition of *A Life on the Ocean Waves* by the Royal Marine Band. The music brings to life a room overflowing with antique marine equipment – Make 'N Break engines, marine lights and radios, even handmade birch brooms. It looks as though a tidal wave had swept clean Davy Jones' locker and deposited its contents here in this old red store.

The salty music swells through the open door. "People say you'll hear this place before you see it," says Parsons, who proudly describes himself as "an outspoken curmudgeon"; others affectionately call him "a modern-day buccaneer." He specializes in finding large wooden boats, especially schooners, for clients on both sides of the Atlantic. He scours the docksides and even the sea bottom for classic boats. "If someone wanted the last steam tug in the world, I'd know where to get it," he boasts.

Parsons and Lunenburg seem a perfect match of place and personality. With its collection of sailmakers, marine blacksmiths and boat builders, Lunenburg is a prime destination if you're looking for anything nautical. "You never know who will walk through that door next. The cross-section of people is incredible. I meet nearly all the 'round-the-world sailors, not to mention yachtsmen from around the globe." Before I leave, Parsons shows me a photograph. I recognize the shop, but it takes me a moment to identify the guy in a T-shirt and dark glasses and the tall beautiful woman as Billy Joel and Christie Brinkley, arms around one another in happier days.

Most visitors to Lunenburg swing through the cavernous, bright red chandlery that dominates the waterfront. The Fisheries Museum of the Atlantic was once home to Zwicker & Co., established in 1789, the same year Paris mobs stormed the Bastille. Live cod swim in the aquarium – an ironic tribute given the commercial extinction of northern cod stocks. Master ship carpenter Edward Mosher can be seen fashioning classic wooden boats, and men like Captain Matthew Mitchell, who worked 20-hour days hand-lining and "dressing" fish, will tell you about dory fishing. "Tourists like talking to us guys. They like to get it from the horse's mouth. I show them how to bait a trawl," says Mitchell, a soft-spoken man whose speech retains the lilt of his Newfoundland roots. As proof, Captain Mitchell proudly produces a framed photograph of First Lady Hillary Clinton watching him work while visiting Lunenburg in June 1995 during the G-7 leaders' conference in Halifax.

Many come to Lunenburg hoping to find *Bluenose II* in port. The replica of Canada's most famous tall ship was built in 1963 by Lunenburgers who, to this day, preserve the shipwrights' secrets. Captain Wayne Walters and I stand on the Museum dock watching the 48-metre *Bluenose II* ride gently on the harbour chop. Walters bears a remarkable resemblance to his grandfather, Angus, the legendary captain of the original *Bluenose*. Although Angus discouraged his family from going to sea, considering the work too dangerous, at sixteen, Wayne shipped aboard a freighter carrying dynamite to the Caribbean. "That was it for me. I was bitten by this going-to-sea-on-ships thing," he says. "My grandfather was really upset. But I guess I inherited his stubborn streak." In 1982, Walters became the first Canadian in forty years to earn a Sailing Master's ticket, which allows him to sail a tall ship like the *Bluenose* anywhere in the world. "I think if he were here today to see me taking her out of the harbour, he would be pleased," says the quiet-spoken Walters.

Increasingly, people from both sides of the Atlantic are arriving in Lunenburg with the idea of docking here permanently. So it was with Murray Creed and Joan Watson, who retired to a classic Cape Cod house in the newer part of Lunenburg a few years ago. Creed had worked on CBC Radio's Fisherman's Broadcast in the early 1950s and found Lunenburgers to be "the most friendly group of people I have encountered across Canada – very outgoing but in a quiet way." He has been welcomed back by old friends and accepted by new ones, despite his CFA – Come From Away – status.

For Watson, the former host of CBC's national consumer affairs program *Marketplace*, coming to Lunenburg has also been a homecoming of sorts. She grew up in the coastal town of Weymouth and in Halifax: "I was looking for some of the things that made my childhood memorable," says Watson. "It was amazing to come back here and find that the Nova Scotia I remembered was still here. Normally, it's dangerous to return somewhere because things change. But here, every walk I take reinforces my memories – the sounds, and the smells, and the people – and I just slipped into it all very easily."

This is what happens in Lunenburg. One simply slips into the past like a boat into water. Here, nostalgia is stirred around every corner. Those memories – of the sea, wind and ships – are enough to make one shudder with delight.

The Magic of Wooden Boats
Petite Rivière, Nova Scotia

IT IS FOUR IN THE MORNING, somewhere in the South Pacific, 2,000 kilometres from Peru, the nearest landfall. I take the helm from my shipmate Terry Halcrow, a native of the Shetland Islands who, at thirty, is sailing around the globe for the second time. "Steering 180, Ha'dy," Halcrow commands in his thick Scottish brogue.

The dawn watch is my favourite. At 2 a.m., when it begins, the Southern Cross, the sky's brightest constellation, is just rising from the inky waters of the Pacific, off the port bow. Due south from us, I can see the Magellanic Clouds, galactic clusters of faint stars, which shine diffusely through the mainmast shroud.

I take the helm gladly, feeling the ship respond to the slightest touch of the wheel. Under full sail, we are doing fifteen kilometres an hour, powered by brisk southeast trade winds. The ship is almost steering herself, heading up into the wind, then falling off, her bow plunging through the broad swells. Although I have been at sea for four days now, it is still hard to believe that I am living out a lifelong dream of shipping aboard a Nova Scotian-built sailboat.

The *Tree of Life*, as she is called, is a classic 30-metre schooner built in 1989 at the Covey Island Boatworks in the little village of Petite Rivière on Nova Scotia's south shore. With her sails catching the steady trade winds, we are making about 220 kilometres a day on a 3,700-kilometre passage between the Galapagos Islands, off the coast of Ecuador, and Easter Island, possibly the most isolated inhabited scrap of earth on the planet. This is the longest leg of an around-the-world voyage undertaken by the *Tree's* owner and captain, Richard "Kelly" Kellogg of Alexandria, Virginia, a retired builder and man of independent means who sails the oceans because, as he says, it's what he does best.

Halcrow, my stand-by, dozes in the wheelhouse behind me, ready to lend a hand in case of complications. The other crew members are asleep below. At night, under steady winds and clear skies, I have time to think about what I'm doing here and the history that has spawned such boats as this.

GROWING UP IN YARMOUTH, N.S., one of the world's great seaports in the 19th century, I was steeped in the romance of the sea. And, like most Nova Scotians, I have the sea in my blood. Two family members had followed the sea. Their fates were starkly different – one exotic, the other tragic – and as such were typical, I suppose, of the many Nova Scotians who went down to the sea in ships.

The exotic was represented by my great-uncle Charles Thurston of Yarmouth, who went to sea in 1884 at the age of fourteen. He crossed the Atlantic several times and was shipwrecked twice before setting his sights on the Pacific Ocean. In 1889, he reached Hawaii on the barquentine *W.H. Diamond* and settled on the island. He worked in the customs services there and subsequently joined the Honolulu Fire Department.

Tragedy lay in the fate of my grandfather Jeremiah Reede, a Cape Island fisherman who shipped aboard a schooner not unlike the *Tree* and was lost at sea in 1922 off Lockeport, Nova Scotia, when a winter storm stirred the ocean into mammoth waves, swamping his dory before he could row back to the mother ship.

On nights such as this, with my hand on the helm, I sense these men are with me, evoking the spirit of Nova Scotia.

It seems appropriate that I should realize my sailing dream in 1996, for this has been designated the Year of the Wooden Boat by the Nova Scotia government. Communities across the province are celebrating Nova Scotia's undisputed prowess as a producer of wooden boats. In the village of Jordan River, on the province's south shore, residents are recalling their native son Donald McKay, who designed the famous clipper ship *Flying Cloud*, the fastest vessel afloat in the mid-19th century. And sailing aficionados are making pilgrimages to Westport, Brier Island, the childhood home of Joshua Slocum, the first person to sail around the world alone. It is a celebration of the province's golden age, when the prosperity of Nova Scotia rode on the marriage of wood, wind and sail.

Nearly every Nova Scotian coastal town and village can trace its development to shipbuilding. Unfortunately, in numerous communities, all that remains to remind us of this seagoing heritage is the great wooden houses, many with widow's walks, from where anxious wives of sea captains kept watch for the sight of familiar sails.

It's said that every harbour, cove or beach along Nova Scotia's sea-girt coast witnessed the launching of at least one tall ship. It was from the little Bay of Fundy village of Maitland that the *William D. Lawrence* was launched in 1874. Nearly eighty metres long, the "great ship," as it was dubbed, was the largest wooden sailing ship ever built in Canada. Every year in Maitland, the launching of the *William D. Lawrence* is re-enacted.

But ships for long-distance voyaging were not the only vessels to be designed in Nova Scotia. Inshore fishers designed an array of small wooden boats suited to their specialized purposes and local sea conditions. Writing in *Small Wooden Boats of the Atlantic*, Marven Moore, manager of collections at the Maritime Museum of the Atlantic, observes: "Their construction reflects the skills and traditions of generations of boat builders and seafarers whose craftsmanship and ingenuity enabled them to confront successfully the often hazardous marine environment." Thus were born the Lunenburg dory, the Bay of Fundy shad boat, the St. Margaret's Bay trap skiff and the Tancook schooner.

Today, Nova Scotia is perhaps best known for the modest but eminently serviceable Cape Islander, a turn-of-the-century fishing boat designed by the Cape Island boat builder Ephraim Atkinson. The Nova Scotian writer Evelyn Richardson compared its revolutionary hull shape to a seagull's wing. Though the tall ships have all but vanished, brightly coloured Cape Islanders can still be seen daily going to sea from hundreds of small fishing villages throughout Atlantic Canada and New England, an enduring testament to the province's maritime genius.

How did Nova Scotia achieve such nautical distinction? As the novelist Ernest Buckler noted of his peninsular province, Nova Scotia is "nearly an island." Nowhere are you more than sixty-five kilometres from the sea. It was only natural, therefore, that early settlers turned to the sea for their livelihood and that it became a highway for trade. With a ready supply of timber from the Acadian forest, it made sense for Nova Scotians to build their own vessels.

In the days of sail, Nova Scotians were involved in every aspect of maritime industry, from building ships to insuring them. People often cut the timber on their own woodlots, built the boats and then sailed them themselves. "People here had a part in the whole process," says the marine historian Conrad Byers, a former curator of the Age of Sail Heritage Centre in Port Greville, on the Bay of Fundy. "They all had a vested interest in making it work. Generally, it was an extremely efficient operation, and that's why Nova Scotians could compete with the big boys in New York and Clyde [Scotland]."

There is no more dramatic example of Nova Scotians adapting to the sea than that of the settlers of Lunenburg County. Landing on a rock-strewn coast in 1753, they were farmers from the German Palatinate, from the Montbeliard region of France and from Switzerland. Finding the glacial soils rocky, they had, within a generation, turned to the sea. They constructed the first offshore fishing fleet of schooners, the famous Grand Bankers, which brought their owners fortunes from cod. The most famous of this black-hulled fleet, the *Bluenose*, became a Canadian icon.

This year is the seventy-fifth anniversary of the launch of the *Bluenose* at the Smith and Rhuland Shipyard in Lunenburg. To many, her birth marked the pinnacle of Nova Scotia's tradition of wooden boat building. Designed by the Halifax marine architect William A. Roue, with her sleek hull, towering masts and the world's largest working sails, she was both a commercial vessel and a racer and acquitted herself honourably in both capacities. Her lasting claim to fame was her unbeaten record in the hotly contested International Fishermen's Races between Nova Scotian and New England fishing schooners – an alternative event to the America's Cup, which the masters of working schooners openly scorned. Her success, however, had much to do with the men who sailed her and especially her captain, Angus Walters, a diminutive man who embodied all of the grit for which Nova Scotia's sea captains were famed.

Walters was what is known in fishing trade as a "highliner," a captain who consistently brings home the largest hauls of fish. His crew respected him not only for this but for his judgment and seamanship. In 1926 the *Bluenose* was caught in a storm off Sable Island, the graveyard of the Atlantic, which that August night claimed eighty men and two other Lunenburg schooners. Having lost her anchor, the *Bluenose* was being driven by gale force winds between two of Sable's fatal sandbars. Walters ordered his crew to lash him to the wheel. Sending his men below, he braved the storm alone, guiding the ship to safety throughout the long night. Clement Hiltz, a 13-year-old crew member at the time, recalled later, "The captain just took it in his stride, just one of those things . . . . Yes sir, wonderful ship, wonderful man."

Unfortunately, 1996 also marks the fiftieth anniversary of the loss of the *Bluenose* on a Haitian reef. She had been cut down (her topmasts removed) and ended her career as a cargo vessel in the Caribbean. Her death symbolized the end of an era for Nova Scotia.

Most tall ships – brigs, barques, barquentines, square-riggers, and clippers – had been replaced by faster steamers by the turn of the century. Schooners, however, continued to move bulk cargoes such as coal and pulpwood along the Eastern Seaboard and to the Caribbean until the outbreak of the Second World War. These so-called coasting vessels could compete simply because the cargoes were not perishable, and therefore speed was less critical.

There are a few men and women who can remember this twilight era of Nova Scotia's golden age of wooden vessels. One is Captain James Richards, who, with his wife Marlene, and the writer Eric Hustvedt, set down the life and times of his grandfather, Captain Andy Publicover, in *The Sea in My Blood*. I visited the Richardses in the little fishing village of Dublin Shore, Nova Scotia, at the mouth of the LaHave River. Publicover, a diehard wooden boat sailor, owned the last four-masted schooner, the *Lillian E. Kerr*, to sail out of Nova Scotia on business.

"Everybody took their families on the coasting vessels in the summertime," James Richards recalls. "And I remember, in the early years [in the late 1930s], we'd be in port over in New York and New Haven in company with some of the other vessels from the Maritimes. The families would be visiting back and forth. That's the way I grew up the first ten years of my life."

Young James's idyllic childhood was soon to be marred by tragedy. In October 1942, having announced his retirement, Andy Publicover watched the *Lillian E. Kerr* leave LaHave Harbour with his son Bill in command and his son-in-law John Richards – James's father – as second mate. It was the last time that Publicover was to see the vessel or her crew. A ship in convoy, running without lights under wartime regulations, collided with the schooner in the Bay of Fundy. She sank in three minutes. John Richards was picked up an hour later, clinging to a smashed timber, but died soon afterwards. "All hands lost" was again entered in Nova Scotia's annals of tragedies at sea.

Despite the loss of his father, James clung to the notion of going to sea. At age seventeen he shipped aboard an Imperial Oil tanker and eventually earned his Master's Certificate. Determined to follow in his grandfather's footsteps, he bought an old fishing dragger when he was twenty-two, with the ambition of going into the coasting trade in Newfoundland.

"My grandfather tried to talk me out of it," he says. "He could see that coasting vessels were going out, but I couldn't see it. This was in my blood, and I just couldn't get it out." The venture failed, and Richards later worked as second mate on the Prince Edward Island ferry, eventually becoming superintendent of Nova Scotia's ferry system. Listening to him recount his grandfather's adventures, I sensed his disappointment at not having lived the seagoing life.

Books like *The Sea in My Blood* are helping to keep alive memories of a time when Nova Scotian wooden vessels were afloat on all the world's oceans and have helped revive interest in the recreational wooden boats that still cruise the coast and find refuge in Nova Scotia's many harbours.

Since 1990, Mahone Bay, near Lunenburg, has hosted an annual wooden boat festival, during which more than a hundred historic and traditional vessels fill the picturesque, island-stippled harbour. The festival attracts more than 30,000 visitors to watch such events as a schooner race and traditional boat launchings using teams of oxen.

As well, every year tall ships from around the world call at Lunenburg to take advantage of the unique concentration of marine services for wooden vessels still found there – from sail and block making to a dry dock and foundry.

Last year, Lunenburg shipwrights once again proved their mettle, restoring the *Bluenose II*. The replica was built by the Oland family in 1963 in the same Lunenburg shipyard – and by some of the same people – as the original *Bluenose*. She was sold to the province of Nova Scotia for one dollar in 1971 and since has acted as Nova Scotia's goodwill ambassador, making voyages to Canadian and U.S. ports to promote tourism and trade. When the Nova Scotia government threatened to tie her up permanently, claiming it would cost nearly $1 million to repair her, Nova Scotians sprang to her defence. Under the direction of Snyder's Shipyard of Lunenburg County, local shipwrights made her seaworthy again at half the estimated cost. And, in a seeming stroke of historical justice, the newly founded Bluenose II Preservation Trust appointed as the ship's captain Wayne Walters, grandson of the captain of the original *Bluenose.* "Repairing the *Bluenose II* showed the world that we can take care of our sailing ships," says Walters.

And then there's the vessel on which I am sailing. It is a prime illustration of the fact that the death knell of the wooden-boat-building tradition in Nova Scotia was sounded prematurely. Voted by *Sail* magazine as one of the one hundred greatest yachts in North America, the *Tree of Life is* a fine example of what age-old skills and modem technology can create – a boat both beautiful and capable. She is a tribute to the Lunenburg County craftspeople – shipwrights, carpenters, sail makers, blacksmiths and foundry workers – who built her.

A DAY OUT OF THE GALAPAGOS, I am up at six in the morning to relieve Halcrow at the helm. The sun has just risen, and the sea is silken smooth. Five hundred metres to starboard, white-sided dolphins are cavorting, hurling their bodies free of the water, then splashing down, completing perfect, sun-spangled parabolas.

I grew up with the notion that someday, like my great-uncle before me, I might sail away to exotic destinations. That I have actually been able to realize such a romantic fantasy leaves me wondering at my good fortune.

At home, the romance of Nova Scotia's sailing history is permanently portrayed at museums such as the Maritime Museum of the Atlantic in Halifax and the Fisheries Museum of the Atlantic in Lunenburg. My favourite, however, is the Yarmouth County Museum, which has been honoured by the American Association for State and Local History and which, in 1989, was given the Canadian Parks Service Heritage Award, being described as "one of the finest community museums in North America . . . a real gem."

To enter the grey granite building is to walk into the past – into the 19th-century parlour of one of Yarmouth's many sea captains. The museum has the third largest collection of ship portraits in Canada – 110 of them. Nearly all the vessels portrayed were registered in Yarmouth or commanded by Yarmouth captains. My favourite display is a glass case of treasures from around the world collected by Captain Fred A. Ladd, who commanded Yarmouth's last square-rigger, the *Belmont,* until 1915. There is an ivory backscratcher from Shanghai, a cigar case woven from peacock quills from Java, and an ant-egg necklace from South Africa, to name a few.

I always leave the museum with mingled emotions of pride and sadness. The days of sail created the only prolonged period of prosperity that Nova Scotia has known. At the time of Confederation, Nova Scotia wasn't a poor cousin in the Canadian family, but a wealthy uncle. Perhaps more important than financial rewards, wooden boats created a culture that was extraordinarily cosmopolitan and outward looking. They spread Nova Scotia's name around the world, and their crews returned home intoxicated with images as exotic as those narrated by the seaman in Joseph Conrad's *Youth.*

A century later, for many Nova Scotians like me, the magic of the wooden boats endures.

Outport Renaissance
Petit Forte, Newfoundland

THERE IS NO ROAD into Petit Forte. Rounding the light at Easter Point, the red roof of the church draws the eye toward the inlet where the community is sequestered. The long harbour faces south and is enclosed by the calipers of a rugged and barren range of mountains. It is not until you pass the natural breakwater of Hayden's Point that you view the village in its entirety; at the water line, the sombre coloured fish stores propped on weathered and spindly spruce pole wharves called stages; the houses in a semicircle behind, by contrast white and trimmed in Christmas colours, but also erected on spruce pylons, levelled and facing the sea. This is "The Harbour" and it sits in the lap of a precipitous bluff, simply called "The Look-Off." From its peak, on a clear day, you can see the breadth of Placentia Bay to the Cape St. Mary's headland, some sixty-five kilometres away. This morning, fog was hanging on the mountaintops in billows backlit by the sun. Petit Forte was illuminated in the deceptively intense light that filtered through its prisms.

Ten years ago, in 1971, Petit Forte's future was shrouded in uncertainty and the face it presented was considerably less bright, as Newfoundland's notorious resettlement program threatened to empty another outport harbour.

At first sight, the peacefulness of the place masked its current vitality. The sleepy appearance was heightened because it was noon – the men were at sea, the women and children in their houses. Even the stages where the old men busy themselves were idle. As we drew opposite the public wharf, Billie Synard wheeled sharply to port and cut the engine at precisely the same moment, so that we drifted to a dead stop at the stage ladder.

Petit Forte lies at the mouth of Paradise Sound, an arm of Placentia Bay which cuts deeply into the eastern shore of the Burin Peninsula. On the two-hour trip from its head at Monkstown, I saw only one place where Billie Synard's 12-metre longliner could put in along the fjord-like coastline. A stream divided a thin strip of beach, and over the eons had cut a gulch through the mountains which flank both sides of the sound. At the crest of the beach was an acre or so of grass, where a handful of houses might have clustered, though nothing man-made remained to confirm that this was ever so. I pointed out the haven to Billie Synard. He cast his quick blue eyes from the wheelhouse. "Darby's Harbour," he shouted above the inboard diesel's steady din. After that, wherever I saw a clearing carved out among the alder, blueberry and spruce, I felt that it was safe to assume that people once wrested a living there. It seems that on "The Rock," as Newfoundlanders affectionately call their island, man must settle for a landfall, a place to rest between the sea which provides for him and the land which broods at his back.

When Newfoundland joined Confederation in 1949, many of its 1,500 rural communities were located on islands or along inaccessible reaches of its 10,000-kilo-metre coastline. These were the outports. Life was based on salt sun-cured cod, as it had been since the first colonists followed the excursions of Basque and Bristol fishermen who had harvested the riches of the Grand Banks as early as the fifteenth century.

Throughout Canada, the post-War period was marked by a rural to urban population drift. In Newfoundland, however, the phenomenon took place on a community-wide scale. In 1953, Premier Joey Smallwood undertook what has become known as the resettlement, or centralization, program. As the cost of providing services to many outports was considered prohibitive, entire remote communities were relocated to government approved "growth centres." The program continued until the early 1970s. More than two hundred outports were evacuated, but far fewer than the original government goal of six hundred. Some planners conceded that the mass rural depopulation program would work to the detriment of many adults, but justified it in terms of the potential benefits to their children. For the first time, a generation of Newfoundlanders was to have access to modern education facilities and alternatives to a life of fishing.

ALL REGIONS OF NEWFOUNDLAND were affected by resettlement, but none more profoundly than the Burin Peninsula. Boot-shaped like Italy (though of a less foppish turn), the Burin juts out into the Atlantic from the southwest corner of the island. Off its toe lie the islands of St. Pierre and Miquelon, the last vestiges of France's New World empire. The Burin's proximity to the Grand Banks attracted settlers to the many islands and snug harbours along its ragged coast. The harsh and lonely environment bred a people whose life Newfoundland novelist Harold Horwood has described as "hard, cruel and dangerous, with limitless scope for heroism and resourcefulness." Resettlement displaced them to growth centres like Marystown (population 5,915), which offered employment in the fish processing plant and shipyard and the amenities rural Canadians everywhere have come to expect of a service town.

Petit Forte, however, refused to be rationalized, cajoled or lured into oblivion. It stood, as the origin of its French name suggests, "small but strong" in the midst of a sea change of events.

"Resettlement was a mistake; it didn't make the country better," Mike Walsh says with an authority befitting a man older than the century. Although he thinks joining Confederation was the right move, for Mike and many like him, "the country" is, and always will be, Newfoundland. He introduces me as "the gentleman from the Dominion of Canada" to his wife.

29

Mike and Ida Walsh's house stands at the bottom of the harbour. Like an elderly statesman, it seems to greet and bid farewell to all visitors to Petit Forte. It is the paragon of a type: a two-storey, square structure with a shed roof – no frills except for the white picket fence that sets it off.

Mike is the patriarch of Petit Forte, and at eighty-seven is fit enough to have roofed his house last summer. He believes that resettlement put many people of his generation in the grave before their time. He remembers a trip on the coastal boat, which makes a weekly run along Newfoundland's south coast between Argentia and Port-aux-Basques. That day, an old woman embarked at Red Island. She was leaving her lifetime home to resettle in Placentia, a town of 2,209, on the Avalon Peninsula. "I thought she was going to sink the boat from crying – it's sentimental stuff but it's true, boy."

After World War II, overseas demand for salt fish fell off dramatically, and prices plummeted to as low as $1.25 per quintal (112 pounds dry weight). It is no wonder that some welcomed resettlement, if only as a chance to get clear of the fishery.

"There were a lot of people moving out," Alfred Pearson remembers. "There was nothing to be done here, only go fishing."

However, you need only experience the desolation of one of the abandoned communities – collapsed roofs, black-eyed windows staring vacantly out to sea, the look of a place that has been bombed out or ravaged by plague – to understand the bitterness that many outport Newfoundlanders still bear against the program.

Despite my outlander status, I soon felt at home at Eugene and Geraldine Jones', and became accustomed to the constant crackle of the Citizens' Band radio. The boats clear the harbour before dawn and may not return until after dark. CB radios connect the fishermen to their families and to one another. The set might bring mundane news from "The Jiggin' Cove" – "The squids was jiggin' when we first got here, but they're not jiggin' at all now" – or a drama that threatens to bring life to everyone's worst fears, as happened on my last day in Petit Forte: "She won't sink altogether, will she?" came a woman's plea. Eugene was one of those who helped tow Albert Heffernan's burning longliner into the safety of her home harbour of South East Bight.

Eugene says nothing of the exploit when he returns home. A man who spends the best part of his days on the water knows well that the spectre of drowning is constantly leering over his shoulder, and that he can't afford bravado, certainly not for the benefit of strangers. The work is inherently dangerous and necessarily hard, but not so hard as it used to be, when men shipped off St. Mary's and the Labrador coast in schooners and handlined all day from dories.

I was surprised at the size of the boats used by the Newfoundland fishermen today. Most fish from open punts, which average eight metres in length, small boats compared to the Northumberland Strait and Cape Island models preferred by Nova Scotian inshore fishermen, and seemingly fragile craft, considering they are fishing in North Atlantic waters.

Squid jigging is an institution in Newfoundland. Many fishermen still use trawl lines, and you need squid to bait the trawl hooks. Squid jigging, as anyone will tell you, can be one of two things: boring or dirty.

The two nights I went out, the squid were not jigging. For two hours, we sat bobbing the jigger, wearing the scar made by the jigging line deeper into the boat's gunnels. It's like in the famous A.R. Scammel song:

> There's some standin' up and there's some lyin' down;
> While all kinds of fun, jokes and tricks are begun,
> As they wait for the squid on the squid jiggin' ground.

It is best to take along a bottle of beer, an illegal act, but one of the freedoms outport Newfoundlanders enjoy and would be loath to relinquish. Like all refuse, beer bottles are unceremoniously pitched into the sea. "Let her go, boy," I was admonished, when caught trying to stow a bottle in the bottom of the boat where someone might just trip over it.

If there are no squid, you might be lucky, as I was, to pass the time watching a pod of pothead whales, or spot two bald eagles take flight from their perches on the sheer bluffs which rear up from the water line.

For more than ten years, Eugene was forced to leave home after the summer fishing season to find work on freighters out of Nova Scotian ports. It is a pattern Burin men have been repeating for longer than most care to remember. In 1950, more than half of the work force of the Burin Peninsula was away from home for most of the year, either employed at the U.S. air force and naval bases in St. John's and Argentia, or, like Eugene, shipping out of mainland harbours.

Eugene is one of an expatriated generation of "Petit Forte Boys" who has returned to claim his birthright.

"Well, boy, I been on the boats all these winters, and all I saw was hard work. And you were always working for somebody else. I found after going around as much as I did that I was just as well off or better in Petit Forte as I would be anywhere else, so I built this house, got married and stayed here ever since."

Eugene built a modern bungalow for his bride, and, like many outport couples, the Joneses moved in on their wedding night. There are six new bungalows under construction. Architecturally bland – the ubiquitous Canadian house – they are nevertheless important symbols of a brighter future for Petit Forte, which teetered on the brink of extinction for a decade.

Eugene remembers when he left home in 1969: "First when I left it didn't look very good, because resettling was on then. It went down to seventeen households and it looked for a while that they were going to go too."

In its initial form, the program required, as a precondition for government assistance, that the whole community agree to resettle. Many must have felt that they had no choice, for those who held out did so at the risk of angering their neighbours. It made "bad friends."

The incentive was hard cash, more than most outport Newfoundlanders had ever had in their pockets before: a basic $1,000 grant plus $200 for each member of the family up to a maximum of $3,200. It proved, however, to be barely adequate to begin a new life in the growth centres.

"There are people who made it better, quite a few," admits Eugene Jones, adding quickly, "There were an awful lot of people who made it worse, too." Many discovered to their dismay that they had to return to their old homes in the summer to make ends meet. "They know nothing, only fish. What are they going to do in St. John's? Nothing," was the way one Petit Forte fisherman summed up the predicament of many who resettled.

Earl and Bride Hickey have been coming back to Petit Forte every summer since they resettled in the late 1960s in Southern Harbour, a town with a population of 759, which received people from Bar Haven, Davis Cove, Red Island, Port Royal, St. Anne's, St. Joseph's, and Gladys Harbour, all outports from the Placentia Bay area. At seventy-one, Earl still fishes, though more to please himself, and he cuts his own firewood. He's quick to point out that he can't do either in Southern Harbour.

"I never earned a dollar since I got down there. We didn't really realize what we were up against until we got there. They were saying the coastal boat was going to be taken. They were going to take the school, we'd be left with nothing. They were more or less drivin' you out. Now it's better than it ever was."

In the late 1960s, the community's morale reached a low point. Those who stayed were unsure whether they would be able to hold out much longer. The houses and stages began to show signs of needing maintenance. By the early 1970s, however, those who had persevered began to feel that their instincts had been correct. They could see what was happening to those who had left.

Then, in 1974, the Smallwood government was overturned, and the growth centre concept was phased out in favour of a grass-roots approach to rural development. Small communities throughout the province organized and incorporated as regional development associations. They now determine their own needs, then lobby government. The government provides funds for the hiring of a full-time co-ordinator for each association and sponsors leadership training courses. "We're offering self-help," says George Green of the Department of Rural, Agricultural and Northern Development. Petit Forte was a charter member of the Placentia West Development Association, which now represents ten communities.

Eric Hayden is vice-president. Two years ago, at age thirty-nine, he dissolved his successful survey business in Labrador City and returned to the ancestral place, Hayden's Point, to fish.

Eric is rediscovering the private comforts of a small place – "Here I have no bad friends" – and he emphasizes that the community projects often entail a personal sacrifice: "I know in a lot of instances people went to work here and lost money, as they could stay home and draw fairly good unemployment. But they went to work because they knew what they were doing was for the good of the community."

The past few winters, for Canada Works' minimum wage, the men have upgraded the fish storage facility, built a new government wharf, and last year erected the community's pride, a medical clinic, which is visited biweekly by a doctor who helicopters in from Come-by-Chance.

There are thirty households and 120 full time residents in Petit Forte today, half as many as before resettlement, but the number is growing modestly every year. Another nearby outport, South East Bight, like Petit Forte, hung on through resettlement, and is now undergoing a revival. And a handful of families are once again overwintering just across the sound in neighbouring Little Paradise, which, in fact, did resettle.

All three communities now belong to the Placentia West Association. President Henry Moores of Rushoon says, "Every community is behind each other. That makes everything fall in place. I don't know, boy, it's almost too good to be true."

The renaissance that Petit Forte has experienced to date has gone hand in hand with a remarkable upswing in the inshore fishery, which itself was occasioned by Canada's declaration of a 200-mile fishing limit. Nevertheless, Neil Murray, editor of *The Union Forum*, the house organ of the Newfoundland Fishermen, Food and Allied Workers Union, warns, "The Union has found that a lot was false expectation. There are still a limited number of people who can make a living." In fact, the Union's position is that the present number of people in the fishery cannot be sustained without government price support, and, at the Union's urging, there are currently tight restrictions in place on the issuing of new licences. That worries Eugene Jones: "That's one of the things that's going to make it bad for these places, if a young fellow comes out of school and can't get a licence. If he's gotta go and find a job, you don't know if he's going to come back or what he's going to do."

The inshore fisherman's average net income is $8,000 to $9,000 for a season that extends from April to October. During the off-season he is eligible to collect unemployment insurance. It seems little enough, but a man's standard of living in an outport like Petit Forte is higher than the raw figures would indicate. It must be remembered that he does not have car expenses nor, in most cases, a mortgage. He hunts, fishes and cuts his own firewood. He is a self-styled carpenter, plumber and electrician, and if the job requires more than two hands, the neighbours can be counted upon. There's not a young couple here that doesn't have a few thousand in the bank.

"THE ROAD" IS A FOOTPATH, really, that at its widest can accommodate three men abreast – if they don't swing their arms. It circles "The Harbour" between the stages and the houses, beginning at Hayden's Point and petering out, a kilometre away, among the rocks. I found that I never reached my destination without first stopping for a yarn with those I met.

The Road's one sidebranch ambles up Church Hill and along Jones Cove. Just past the church, a new punt, its hull half planked in, rests its keel in a yard. It is Mike Lake's first effort as a boat builder and he admits to being heartened by the approving nods – no more – of the old-timers.

Mike grew up in Rushoon, a nearby resettlement centre which now boasts a population of seven hundred. His father fished, but there is little fishing done there now. Most of the young men settle for seasonal work on "The Track," laying rail line for the Canadian Pacific Railway in western Canada. They stay long enough to collect unemployment insurance, then return home for the winter.

Next year, he hopes to launch his 8-metre boat and, where it now rests, to build a new home for his family, his wife Evelyn, a native of Petit Forte, and their infant son, Michael.

"First time I came down here, I was talking to people same as if I knew them a long time," Mike remembers. "This is home to me now. I wouldn't move."

In Petit Forte, people are proud that their doors are left unlocked – "You goes out to someone's house and no knocking, you walk in. Here we find it strange for someone to knock on the door. You think, 'Is someone dead or what?'"

Doors open into kitchens. Most are appointed with two stoves, a wood-burning Enterprise or Fawcett and an electric range. You can see your face reflected in their chrome. And in the women's eyes, grandmother and girl-child alike, a clarity shines out, as if the order of their home was a reflection of some inner sanctuary.

Monday: Bread is rising on the warming oven. Through the window I can see rows of wash flapping in the sea breeze. A crucifix hangs on the lintel. The icons of Catholicism have their station in each Petit Forte home as surely as do family portraits. If it is an old house like this one, there is a couch next to a window, the exposed ceiling beams are generously coated with white gloss paint. I accept the customary offer of a drink.

"I didn't want to come home," recalls Maureen Pearson. "I more or less figured that we'd get back in Petit Forte and I'd be stuck in the house all the time with nothing to do." Maureen is now post mistress.

The children, too, have adjusted to outport life. "The children love it here," their mother says. "It's not like in Labrador City where we lived on a busy street. Now they have their breakfast and they're gone, and you don't worry about them."

"The children are some keen now," their grandmother chimes in. "But if they grow up here, they know the simpler things too."

The simpler things: climbing the hills which, to a child, must seem of mythic proportions; trout fishing or handlining for tomcods and cunners which cruise around every wharf where they eagerly devour whatever offal is thrown their way; or taking a Sunday boat ride with the family to Port Anne or Paradise, where someone is sure to get out an accordion or harmonica.

Aubrey Pearson had a well-paying job as a millwright in Labrador City when he and Maureen came back to Petit Forte in the spring of 1978 to wait out the strike. They put their house in Labrador City on the market, not expecting it to sell. When it did, they decided to stay in Petit Forte, an option that had not been open to either of them as teenagers.

Aubrey left home in 1965 to work on a freighter: "Joey (Smallwood) was on the go. You haul up your boats and burn them. There was going to be no more fishery. At the same time, there wasn't too much future here."

Maureen did what most girls of her generation were obliged to do, leave home to finish high school. (Many still do, although the two teachers in Petit Forte are qualified to graduate high school students.) Maureen believes times have changed for the better: "In Lab City, Aubrey was making a lot more money than we do here but I find we can save more and get whatever we want in Petit Forte. Most of the young people who are growing up now, they're not going to be leaving, they'll stay here."

If they do there may once again be houses on "The Other Side," as the shore opposite the harbour is known. As at Darby's Harbour, a clearing at the water's edge is the only sign that people once lived there.

"That would be nice," Maureen says, with a longing in her voice, "to look over at night and see the lights again."

The light source wouldn't be kerosene, as it was before resettlement. Five years ago, electricity came to Petit Forte, supplied by three 180-horsepower generators. Two years ago, telephones were installed. "We got a little slice of everything that was going," says Eugene Jones, who credits the Development Association.

The chief object of conjecture these days is the road that would connect Petit Forte to the rest of the island. It would have to penetrate twenty-five kilometres of dauntingly rugged terrain.[1]

THE CN COASTAL BOAT, *Hopedale*, pulled out of Petit Forte at 5:00 a.m. under cover of heavy fog.

There was freight aboard to be unloaded in Monkstown. As I looked, with the same awe-struck humility, at the shoreline I had passed just a few days earlier with Billie Synard, I thought of what his wife said to me of their resettlement from Port Elizabeth on Flat Island to Baine Harbour: "The place you're born, you can't forget."

During the 1950s and 1960s, when resettlement was taking place in Newfoundland, a whole generation of Canadians were, similarly, being deracinated by the trends in society which made people more mobile – and that mobility one-directional, toward the cities and towns. In Newfoundland, the phenomenon was more remarkable because the government showed its hand – often a heavy one.

Whether in Newfoundland or elsewhere in Canada, the essence of the small place was community spirit. It existed, quite simply, because people needed each other. Nowhere, perhaps, has this been more evident than in outport Newfoundland. The environment demanded that people stick together, to maintain a hold on that narrow place which the sea and land had surrendered to them. It wasn't only a matter of surviving the elements, however. You made your own fun too, you celebrated together. They still do in Petit Forte, whether by seeing the sun up at a wedding party or just dropping in for "a little argument, a few cards and a drink."

In Petit Forte, the extended family is alive and well; there's a genuine neighbourliness, a graciousness toward strangers and a rugged individualism

---

1. In April 1990, the road was approved for completion in fall 1991.

which needs the presence of others to define itself. For those of us who left such a place, it is a vital example of what we thought only existed in memory, and it approaches the ideal sought by the counter-culture generation that fled the cities.

None of the talk of resettlement prepared me for the desolation of Big Paradise, once a vibrant neighbour to Petit Forte. There, as had occurred on my entry into Petit Forte harbour, the first thing to catch my attention was the church. The steeple of the Big Paradise church is red also, but there all similarity ends. You see that the roof is collapsed, that the rafters only support the low ceiling of an impassive sky. The gay colours that were once someone's fancy are fading from the walls. Soon the houses will be the colour of the winter sea, the colour of rock. They sit mouldering, abject, at land's end.

Little Paradise is separated from its counterpart by a rocky point. We made anchor in the deep harbour, while a motorboat came out to meet us with passengers bound for Argentia. Some people return here in the summer to fish. And the last few years, a handful of families have overwintered. I recall Maureen Pearson's simple history of Petit Forte and its own recovery from Smallwood's resettlement: "A few people, they were stubborn, they wouldn't leave because their friends were staying or their family. . . . Now there's people coming back." She is right, and I now understand the proud, stubborn gleam that came into her eye as she said it.

End of the Trail
Advocate, Nova Scotia

THIS IS A FORGOTTEN SHORE and that's a shame. For nowhere in Nova Scotia will you pass through white clapboard villages with a better prospect of the sea than along the Chignecto peninsula, north of Parrsboro. With the great blue bulk of the Minas Basin stretched out by your side, the road dips, climbs and switchbacks through lonely vistas of hardwood which clothe the Cobequid Mountains. Through V-shaped mountain slots, you can sight Cape Split and Cape Blomidon, headlands worthy of their place in Mi'kmaq tradition as the seats of power of the man-god Glooscap. The sheer basalt of Cape Split rises defiantly from the water line to its 122-metre, anvil-top, overlooking the whirlpools and torturous currents of the Minas Channel which foam with the fury of the Bay of Fundy's comings-and-goings.

It never ceases to surprise me that so few Nova Scotians are familiar with this 32-kilometre stretch of shoreline, known as the Parrsboro Shore. Residents proudly call it "The Little Cabot Trail." Chauvinism aside, it is well-named, for it offers up the most spectacular Nova Scotian seascape west of Cheticamp.

The village of Advocate Harbour stands at the end of this yet-to-be discovered tourist route. It is flanked by two mountainous headlands of its own, Cape d'Or and Cape Chignecto – cradling the sister communities of East and West Advocate – and faces the eminence of Isle Haute. The houses of the three communities, locally called Advocate for short, form a continuous string like colonies of white barnacles hugging the shoreline. The dramatic setting impresses with an almost unearthly quality as if it had been laid out on the easel of a nineteenth-century romantic landscape painter.

The harbour is protected at its mouth by a natural breakwater of driftwood that has piled up along a 6-kilometre-long sandbar. The narrow difficult entrance to this snug berth was well known to the coastal trade. Also, Advocate men followed the sea in locally built ships with names as exotic as their destinations – like *Calcutta* and *Amazon*.

According to the historian Frederick J. Pohl, Advocate Harbour was the stopping place of Prince Henry Sinclair, the Earl of Orkney, one hundred years before Columbus's voyage of discovery. Pohl makes a convincing case for the Earl's New World explorations, and believes Sinclair built a new ship in Advocate Harbour in 1398 to return to the Orkneys.

There are clear and indisputable records of Samuel de Champlain's exploits here in the seventh century. He came to Advocate Harbour, which he called Port of Mines (the name later given to the greater basin), in search of copper. With a navigator's keen eye, he described his cautious introduction to the harbour: "To enter one must lay down buoys, and mark a sandbar which lies at the entrance, and runs along a channel parallel with the opposite coast of the mainland. Then one enters a bay about a league in length and half a league in width. In some places the bottom is muddy and sandy, and vessels can there lie aground. The tide falls from four to five fathoms."

Today there are a half-dozen fishing boats beached by the side of the wharf, waiting to be refloated by the tide. For now, the famous Fundy tide has retreated, turning the harbour into a muddy lagoon.

The fortunes of the town also seem to be on an ebb. People here have always de-pended on the fishery and the forests but these once bountiful resources have been severely depleted in recent years. Local fishermen claim that the fishing's been bad ever since Polish factory ships anchored off Cape d'Or several years ago and scooped up the spawning herring stocks. Now, many residents fear that Scott Paper's 30-year onslaught on the Cape Chignecto timber stands is reaching its inevitable conclusion. Some people in town say that the next decade could see the community's largest employer pull out.[1] And all the talk about tourist potential is just that: talk and potential.

Advocate is facing up to these grim prospects in what seems an unusual, even novel, way in these times of increasing dependence on government initiative. They have formed a good old-fashioned self-help group. The Advocate and District Action Organization got its start in 1979 when a local farmer's barn burned down. Bernard Elliot was in his early sixties, had no insurance and, it looked to him, no option but to abandon farming.

Byron Hefferon, the United Church minister at the time, called a community meeting to deal with Elliot's plight and eventually his neighbours raised $2,500. Scott Paper donated free stumpage; volunteers cut, trucked and sawed the logs. The new barn went up in a week. It was the first barn building bee in the community's living memory, and people frankly surprised themselves with what they had accomplished. In fact, the notion of community self-help looked too good to just let it drop.

Since then, the Action Organization has replaced a home for a family that was burned out and met other day-to-day emergencies, by supplying milk and home heating fuel to families whose unemployment insurance had been cut off.

Walton Rector, a retired car salesman, was the first president of the group and is now the area's county councillor. He's seen the changes in attitude that the self-help model produced: "A lot of young people gained confidence and have come to realize that you can do something if you are willing to co-operate and work together."

CO-OPERATION IS ONE THING, tackling the economic ills that afflict the community as a whole quite another proposition. However, the action group has begun to turn its attention to community works – in effect, to act as a

---

1. Scott Paper closed their Parrsboro sawmill and lumber operations in 1991.

village council – and recently it undertook its most ambitious project, the construction of a recreation complex to meet current local and projected tourist needs.

They have laid out a ball field, replete with bleachers, dugouts and an outfield fence, the latter scrounged from a derelict outdoor hockey rink. Tying the project together will be a log recreation centre, which is being funded by a government grant. Rector insists, however, that it is not just another make-work project with no hope of paying returns on the taxpayer's investment. He sees a cottage craft industry in the recreation centre's basement, and eventually, log cabins and a motel for tourists, a camping area, and perhaps even a tennis court in the old gravel pit.

"That's my vision," Rector says, casting his eyes over the now idle acres at the back of the village. "It's reasonable, and let's say, I have high hopes."

Rector pauses, then adds in an exasperated tone: "That goddamned road is the whole key."

That road is now a broken line on the province's highway map; in reality, a dirt track that connects Advocate to Joggins, Nova Scotia, and completes the loop around the Chignecto peninsula.[2] Advocate stands at the apex of the triangular peninsula where it juts into the Bay of Fundy like the prow of a ship. Rector maintains that tourists avoid the unpaved section "because they don't like gravel roads and they don't like backtracking." As a consequence, most never reach Advocate to see what it has to offer: Fishing, hunting, beachcombing, but mostly, magnificent solitude.

Rector doesn't want handouts, just incentive to allow the area to be its own ambassador: "I feel that if the highway is opened up, tourism will gradually develop on its own through the private sector."

However, the Action Organization's perennial petitioning of government to pave the road so far hasn't paid off. It is not so surprising, for the area is a political barren. With the exception of New Salem and Apple River, there are only lumbering ghost towns between Advocate and Joggins.

---

2. The final section of the road was paved in 1992-93.

Local tourism boosters argue, perhaps rightly, that the backwoods ambience is just the tonic the Trans-Canada and city-weary traveller is seeking. There is an irony at the heart of this virtue, however, for the area's unsullied beauty is the last natural resource with which people can bargain with the outside world.[3]

Burnell Reid is seventy. Like his father before him he operated a sawmill. He remembers when he could hear the whistles of three other locally owned mills every morning. In 1967 his own became the last to close. Now there is only a pile of rotting sawdust to mark where it sat on the beach at West Advocate, and a colour snapshot in his kitchen to remind him of what it looked like.

Reid saw the writing on the wall. He was not going to be able to compete, either for the best woodsmen or access to the best timber, with Scott Paper Maritimes Ltd., which had established a large sawmill in Parrsboro. "So," he recalls with resignation, "we got out before we had to get out."

The closing of Reid's mill also signalled the passing of a time-honoured approach to forest management. Reid was of a generation of local lumbermen who would not cut a tree that was less than a foot in diameter at the butt. It was a practise that ensured a wood supply for the future. "But when the big companies came in and when they put a road through, they wanted everything cut that was there," Reid explains, "because they could move out of here and not come back for a hundred years."

Reid's speculation has the unsettling ring of prophecy. In recent years, Scott has mounted a reforestation program, but Reid is not alone in thinking it may be too little too late.

"A few years ago, before they came in on this clear cut, they said they were going to farm our woods, replant and farm, and that our woods were all going to come back. They were going to show *us* how to produce lumber.

---

3. Community volunteers developed the Cape Chignecto Provincial Park, at 4,200 hectares, the largest in Nova Scotia. It opened in 1997.

"But before they got done – just go and take a picture. The destruction! There'll be no more cutting for maybe 125 or 150 years," Reid insists.

To make matters worse, the reforestation program itself runs contrary to Reid's lifetime experience of the Acadian forest: "One thing the people resent the most of anything is this replanting and then spraying to kill off all the hardwood. It's natural for our forests to have spruce and hardwood. And if you change the thing, it's not going to work.

"Oh, it might work for one generation," Reid concedes, "but then the land's going to run out."

With the timber resource promising a slow recovery at best, and the fishery in apparent decline, what does it augur for Advocate's future? "It's a good place for retirement, old age pensioners, and that's what we're going to have the most of," Reid says sadly.

STILL, THERE ARE YOUNG PEOPLE willing to stake their future in Advocate.

One of them is Gerry Field. "I was one of the first to break the chain of young guys leaving." After finishing high school, Gerry cut pulp for Scott Paper, which is often the only employment option open to the community's young men. He found that the work not only jarred his bones but rankled his principles, too. "I helped them slaughter the land," he says with regret. "If it wasn't for the need of money, I wouldn't have done it."

For the past two years, he's turned his back to the woods and looked to the sea for a living. At the same time, he erected a 9-metre tower that commands a view of the tide-rip off Cape d'Or, and the blue finger of land on the horizon that is the Annapolis Valley's North Mountain range. The tower, his self-built home and the acre of garden that surround both stand as stubborn symbols of Field's newfound independence, his determination to make subsistence farming and part-time fishing a way of life, much as Advocate's early settlers did.

The fishing, however, hasn't been as good as he would like. "It used to be," he says, with the air of an old salt, "you could fill a boat off there, but now you don't know whether you'll get enough for a meal."

Like most fishermen, Field is always hopeful. His optimism that the fish will return is shared by Mike Fraser. The two young men plan to fish together this summer.

Fraser, nineteen, could be found this spring in a boatshop that belongs to his granduncle, Captain William Morris, at eighty, one of the last of a generation of Advocate men to distinguish themselves as sea captains. While Fraser worked feverishly, fitting his Cape Islander with a new keel and replacing worn out planking, Captain Morris watched admiringly: "I couldn't do that at his age – I couldn't do that now."

Fraser doesn't have illusions about the standard of living that fishing can provide. He says that he'll be happy if he can net $10,000. Although there's always risk associated with making a living from the sea – particularly, given the area's precarious stocks – it's as reliable, perhaps more so, than work in the woods.

"There's never been steady work here. You never know whether it's going to snow and you'd be thirteen or fourteen stamps short to qualify for unemployment insurance. Then you'd have no money all winter," Fraser explains.

This uncertainty has bred a deep-rooted fatalism in many young people. "Pogey" is as much an accepted way of life in Advocate as it is in other small, isolated Maritime towns where the work is seasonal. The recent nine-month Abercrombie plant strike against Scott Paper shut down the woods and removed even that economic crutch. It provided a disturbing glimpse into what might be in store for the community if Scott Paper ever did pack its bags: Idleness and tension spilled out in acts of vandalism. "What is there for young guys to do but drink and raise hell?" rationalized one disenchanted youth.

Jet Robinson's General Store was a target of the discontent. "It gives a guy a funny feeling to come in and find the window blown out like that,"

Robinson says, pointing to his office window which bears the unmistakable pattern of a shotgun blast.

"You go home at night and see the tide coming and going, and you think it's such a peaceful place; then you have ridiculous things like that happen."

Robinson, who left a dairy farm in Connecticut and followed a "Land for Sale" ad in *Field & Stream* to Advocate, is philosophical about what could easily be interpreted as local bigotry. He points out that he hasn't been the only victim, and that business has actually picked up since the incidents started.

"I was rather impressed with how well we were received by the town, and especially after we took over the store. Small town people – I think they're a warmer type of person."

The doctor comes in and Robinson promptly plunks a fresh halibut down on the counter: "This is for you." Someone, wishing to remain anonymous, has left it as a gift, in the tradition of small town gratitude for a service.

That same week, Dr. Maurice Meyers was planning to leave his post as the only doctor at the rambling farmhouse that has served as the community hospital since 1945. Advocate's relative isolation makes having its own hospital a necessity, especially to cope with woods' accidents and obstetrical emergencies.[4] Older patients like it because it's homier, but the staff has to adjust to antiquated equipment, such as the 40-year-old U.S. Army field unit x-ray which, Meyers points out, is identical to the model Klinger used on *M*A*S*H*. "A fellow straight out of medical school would have quite a problem," he says.

Meyer, who served in Canada's North, was attracted by the professional and personal independence that Advocate's rustic isolation offered. However, after four years, he began to recognize the creeping signs of rural doctor burnout: "In the old days," he reflects, "you had somebody to drive your

---

4. Advocate opened a new 10-bed hospital in October 1989.

horse, now you have to drive yourself." Meyers was the fourteenth doctor to serve Advocate in the last thirty years. He plans on semi-retirement, but will return to the area to spend time at his cottage.

The area seems to hold a special attraction for individualists like Meyers. Notable among them was playwright and actor Sam Shepherd. Shepherd was a 1960s cohort of Allen Ginsberg and Bob Dylan, but gained a modicum of academic respectability by copping the coveted Pulitzer Prize for drama in 1979 for his play *Buried Child*. "Sam was deep," remembers a neighbour.

Shepherd hasn't been back to Advocate in two decades. While living there he owned the house that once belonged to Captain Joshua Dewis. Dewis was the builder of what just might be the world's most famous sailing ship, the *Mary Celeste*. Christened the *Amazon*, she was launched in neighbouring Spencer's Island in 1861. In 1872, the ship was found abandoned in the mid-Atlantic. The crew's food was on the table, but no trace of them was ever found. Their fate remains a mystery to this day.

Joshua's grandson, Rhodes Dewis, still lives in Advocate. He remembers his grandfather's common sense version of events. The *Mary Celeste* was carrying a cargo of alcohol. Spontaneous combustion took place, blowing the hatch off: "He said all that happened was they panicked. They jumped ship and didn't attach a line, and the ship drifted away from them – they just made a stupid move."

Dewis is now in his seventies. As a boy he remembers playing in what is now his grassy beachside yard, among the ribs of vessels shaped by the hands of some of the world's best shipwrights. Between 1820 and 1920 nearly seven hundred wooden ships were built and launched from the Parrsboro Shore. During that era, Advocate was neither isolated nor inward-looking but almost cosmopolitan, and as evidence Dewis produces from the parlour a ceramic jam jar that his grandmother brought back from a trip to Bombay in 1882. He fears that such proud ancestral memories will be lost with his generation: "It's only the last few years that people have been writing the history down."

Don Gamblin, a young teacher at the Advocate District School, has been doing his part to keep alive memories of Advocate's more halcyon days, when it boasted a furrier, photography salon and several hotels. He's been getting his social studies class to assemble a scrapbook of old photographs. They show a prosperous sawmill in the ghost town of Eatonville, mining row houses at the abandoned Cape d'Or copper mine, sailing ships in Advocate harbour, decks piled high with deal. In every photograph, proud men – in some cases, the children's grandfathers – stand before the camera sure of their small but important place in history.

Some ask, "What happened?"

Gamblin recounts the familiar story of the demise of wooden ships that ravaged local economies. However, he still sees the resourcefulness in the Advocate people that accounted for their entrepreneurial past.

"People from this area have their own unique character," Gamblin maintains. "If you look at the people in this area and their ability to do things on their own, they have a lot of natural resources to draw on. I learn from them all the time. If I want to fix something or, say, build a patio deck, I don't buy a book; I go and ask one of my buddies."

This innate resourcefulness has helped residents survive the bad times. The recession of the early 1980s forced many young people to return to the area. As one young man, who had spent a few years in Alberta, told me: "You can pick up odd jobs – nobody starves around here." At least in Advocate they have the support of family, or as recent history has shown, of the community if circumstances warrant it.

Action Organization President Arthur Fillmore spent fifteen years in the services before moving back home. He believes, "If the economy stays the way it is, I think people are better off in a community like this one rather than in a larger town or city."

However, Fillmore acknowledges that there is little future if the tourist potential isn't developed to offset the loss of jobs in the forest and fishery. He's confident that it can be: "I've been over the Cabot Trail and, I think, it's every bit as pretty here. It's just not as long, that's all."

Right now, many tourists who come to Advocate get there quite by accident by taking a wrong turn at Parrsboro. "Once they are here," says William Morris, proprietor of the Harbour Lite restaurant, "they can't understand why there are so few people around."

II. The Fat of the Land

The Fat of the Land

Tatamagouche, Nova Scotia

THE LAST OF OUR CALVES that I remember was born weak. It was not the first time that it had happened. The barn was all but empty, our herd reduced to two cows from the usual complement of eight. The calf had not been tongued dry by its mother when I first saw it. I kept vigil with my mother, sharing her anxiety and sense of helplessness, during the first few days of the newborn's life. The calf did not survive. All the stanchions were soon idle, the rituals of separating the cream and churning the butter were things of the past. My brothers and I argued over who would mix the packet of food colouring into the ghastly vegetable lard which replaced our homemade butter at the table.

Bang's disease, the cause of the abortions and weak calf syndrome, dealt the final blow to the farm. But the move was inevitable. For twenty years the farm had pro-vided a meagre income – never enough for a new coat of house paint, but always enough to keep us warmly clothed and well fed. Milk, butter, eggs, vegetables and pork for the table came from the farm. We sold surplus from our market garden locally, cut pulp, exported a few crates of blueberries on the Boston boat, and, in later years, my father worked part-time as a carpenter in town. In short, we made do in a mixed way.

Always, however, the mainstay was the cream cheque. Without it the farm had no future. It was 1960.

In 1960, 8,000 cream shipping farms were scattered from Cape Breton Island to the southern tip of Nova Scotia, where I grew up. Today [in 1981], there are fewer than 300.[1] Most of these are concentrated along the North Shore of Nova Scotia, in proximity to the three creameries which still accept farm-separated cream for the manufacture of butter. There were once twenty-seven. Located in small towns and villages, the creameries were an integral part of the local economies. Why cream producing farms have been ravaged numerically and, in some circles, held up to ridicule, has as much to do with social changes external to the farm as on-the-farm common sense.

In 1967, a Milk Industry Inquiry concluded that three-quarters of all dairy farms in Nova Scotia were "uneconomic units." Although the Inquiry Committee stopped short of recommending that the small shipper (of cream and milk) be legislated out of existence, effectively, he was being asked to hang it up or be squeezed out. It was proposed that cream shippers undertake the capital intensive transition to whole milk production, or withdraw.

Between 1963 and 1967, more than 3,000 cream producers had gone out of production and the verdict of "The Inquiry," as it is still known, seemed to place the capstone on a dying industry. It predicted a future for the cream producers that was discouraging at best, with "pressure resulting from land consolidation, increased costs of production and increased costs of pickup and transportation" all working against the small dairymen.

The cream producer separates his own milk on the farm, selling the cream for butter production and retaining the skim milk for conversion into a product for which there is a demand: pork, veal or poultry. Cream producers believe that they should occupy a special niche in the dairy industry and that there are convincing arguments for the preservation of their place in an increasingly hostile bureaucracy.

The decline in their numbers, in fact, has abated in recent years. There has been an infusion of new blood. This so-called "new wave" of cream shippers has revived the defunct Cream Producers' Association. The biggest

---

1. By 1994 there was only one cream farm, which has since gone out of business.

challenge facing them is to convince the government that they are not an anachronism.

The perception of the cream producer as someone who is less than a professional dairyman persists. The stereotype: a man over fifty who milks a few cows in summer when they are on pasture. In winter he dries the herd off. He may, but just as likely not, feed the skim milk to hogs or veal calves. His greatest asset is the land he sits on. It is paid off, and when he tires of farming, he will sell it for non-agricultural purposes and have a tidy nest egg for retirement. In the eyes of government he is apathetic and inefficient, a hobbyist who farms as a lifestyle, not a business.

That the image is not without example does little to convince the government that they should provide incentive to the cream sector. For the new wave of cream shippers, it makes their way all the more an uphill struggle.

ONE OF THE NEW WAVE is David Butlin. He and his wife, Nina, arrived in Nova Scotia in 1975. For several years, they had homesteaded in partnership with six other couples on 113 hectares, near Hundred Mile House, BC. "It was difficult for us," Nina recalls. "We wanted to farm and it wasn't the ideal place to be farming. We would have required as much capital to clear land as to buy a farm." Then, David came across a fateful article about cream shippers in Nova Scotia. "We had the idea that here was a market we could hit," says David, "and we were interested in dairy."

The Butlins came to Nova Scotia with other convictions: They wanted cleared, arable land with a house on it – they didn't want to clear or to build again. And, if they were going to live in Nova Scotia, they wanted to be near the water. After a nine month tour of the province, they settled on Tatamagouche. It was not only on the Northumberland Strait – it had a creamery. "Things began to gel."

One day in December, when the first winter storm was blowing itself out, I decided to walk the long unploughed driveway to Crackwillow Farm. It had been a year since I last visited the Butlins. Nina was in the kitchen. Stainless steel buckets of tallow were rendering slowly on the blacktop furthest from the firebox. I found David in the basement at the cutting table, where a side of beef was in the stages of becoming hamburger, roasts and steaks. The other half of the cull cow was hanging in the cool air.

At supper, David was justifiably proud of the good taste of his organically raised Guernsey beef. To top things off, there was heavy, golden cream for the coffee. It was fare that I was to share in every household, while making my rounds in pursuit of the economics and lifestyle of cream shipping: home-raised meat and heavy cream which makes money in your cup, if not always for the farm ledger.

The Butlins' is still known locally as the "Willie Arthur place." David and Nina valued local opinion in making their choice of a farm. "People told us that Willie Arthur raised a cracking fine family off that place. It was renowned. If any place should produce, it should be this place, we thought." David's laugh is tinged with irony.

On arrival in Nova Scotia, they also sought out advice at the Nova Scotia Agricultural College on what kind of farming they were recommending. The flat answer was nothing. "I imagine the answer is still nothing," says Nina. "To me that's the wrong answer."

David goes on: "There doesn't seem to be enough attention paid to givens in farming, to climate, soil, and the type of land that you have and what it is capable of producing. If you look at these factors and limit yourself to the type of farming that is suited to what you're given, then you don't come up with trying to grow corn in Nova Scotia. You come up with a forage-based farming. Cream shipping fits the bill."

The Butlins were undeterred by the chilling negativity of the experts' answer. They had to wait a year before there was quota available, but with one cow (aptly named Butterscotch), a milk pail and less than $10,000 up front, they started producing. "It's an opportunity that is rare in Canada and in Nova Scotia," says Nina."I don't think that it's appreciated how rare it is."

The stakes were soon raised by what David calls the animal inflation factor. As the return per animal decreases due to inflation, more animals must be acquired to make ends meet. The Butlins' herd has doubled in the last year, to fifteen milking cows. Even so, at less than $10,000, the personal draw for the family is substandard. And that meagre return is contingent upon things working out on the farm as they do on paper. Still, Nina says, "Cream shipping is no worse than anything else in agriculture. It's no more marginal than other commodities, and it's only thing you can do as a beginning farmer in Nova Scotia and get an income right away."

"Cream shipping hinges on idealism," David says. "Underlying it all is the strong conviction that the principles behind mixed farming – farming that is geared to the supply of local needs and doesn't contribute to overproduction, and is ecologically sound, therefore is not a monoculture type of existence – must one day prove themselves right."

The next morning begins inauspiciously. It is bitterly cold. The last cow in the milking line must be cajoled, kicked and dragged to her feet, only to discover that she has a swollen stifle joint – another veterinary bill. The line to the tractor radiator breaks as David is ploughing the lane. And as we are about the load the cream for market, we discover that the back door to the station wagon is frozen shut.

To balance the ledger: The weaners are spry, the pigs will soon be ready for market, and the milk-fed calves are bearing out their good breeding.

It is eight kilometres from Crackwillow Farm to the Tatamagouche Creamery, which Nina describes as an "island in the storm." David talks as we manoeuvre the icy dirt road. "It's tremendously satisfying to know that you are providing a need for the community. As the price of transportation increases, the importance of locally produced food is going to increase. Butter is one of the most underproduced commodities in Nova Scotia. With the new generation of cream producers, who are looking at it with a lot more emphasis on management and production, presumably we can produce butter as competitively as it can be imported."

The Tatamagouche Creamery now operates at only one-third capacity, even though the province imports 80 percent of its butter. When we arrive, cream cans are being unloaded from the Valley Truck. Once a week, cream is shipped over 320 kilometres from the few remaining cream producing farms in the Annapolis Valley to Tatamagouche. In the '40s, six 3-ton trucks were kept busy, every day except Sunday, picking up cream roadside in the local area. For the past ten years, farmers have had to transport their own cream to market, for which they receive a provincial transportation subsidy of ten cents per pound.

The numbered cans are weighed on the Toledo scale and a small sample ladled from each for sweetness and butterfat tests, the two indices which determine the creamery premium paid to the producer. Like most new shippers, David transports his cream in five-gallon plastic buckets, as the traditional cream cans are no longer available. Replacement parts for separators are equally hard to come by. The closest supplier is in Calgary, Alberta. Today, you are more likely to see a separator gracing a suburban front lawn than to see it in use on a farm.

As David's cream is being weighed in, a fellow shipper confides that he may not be in business for much longer. His application for construction of a new barn has just been turned down by the Farm Loan Board. A few days later, with the dejected look of the unsuccessful applicant still clear in my mind, I questioned loan counsellor Bob Adams about the FLB's alleged prejudice against small farms. He answers that there is no policy at the FLB to discourage small farms in general, or cream shippers in particular. He notes that the cream shipper can carry only half the debt load that a shipper of fluid milk (fluid is the milk we drink) can, and that they must advise against overcapitalization: "The last thing we are here for is to get people into trouble."

David has had to overcome his conditioning, as a child growing up in postwar England, that credit is the ruination of a person. He has accepted money as another tool, like a tractor or a spade. For the Butlins, it has been a year of major commitments: an addition to the old barn, acquisition of quality breeding stock and expansion of their land base.

David received one of only two FLB loans made to cream shippers in 1979. He says," Our experience with the Department has been very good, certainly not antagonistic. We've always been surprised at the support we've unearthed when we presented our case. They just don't think about it. Cream shipping is an idea that has to be promoted."

In Tatamagouche, the Butlins have found the traditional society which they were seeking for themselves and their two preschool children. Also they have close bonds with a community of newcomers. The hundred strong North Shore Organic Growers' Association provides a ready market for David's organically raised beef and home cured pork. Looking back at B.C., Nina says, "It was nothing like being a farmer. You didn't feel like you were going to be carted off at any minute. Our vision has always included some kind of apocalypse in our lifetime, when everything falls apart. And the best place to be is on some land, which hopefully won't be taken away from you."[2]

CHARLIE ORR IS A ZEALOUS SUPPORTER of cream production. He was a prime mover in the formation of the Cream Producers Association and its first president. He argues that Nova Scotia is ill-suited for large agribusiness type farms, whereas cream production "fits into the scale of things."

I've heard it murmured in bureaucratic quarters that his logic is "insidious." His approach, however, reflects the scientist's objectivity. Upon examination of his credentials, this is not surprising: BA, University of Glasgow, Scotland; MA, University of Guelph, and PhD, post-Doctoral, in Biochemistry, Johns Hopkins, Baltimore. How an RNA-researcher from the venerated halls of Johns Hopkins ended up championing the cause of the small farmer requires several giant steps in the telling.

Charlie's talk is spiced with his native Scots brogue and a healthy dose of humour. About his undergraduate training in agriculture, he quips, "God knows how I got into agriculture in the beginning. It had something to do with no parental guidance. I thought that I wanted to be out in the fresh air, so I went into agriculture." Far from getting him out in the fresh air, it led him on the path of a professional student. When the research purse strings tightened in 1972, he decided it was time for a change.

To the horror of his academic colleagues, Charlie and his wife Jennie, who was a Research Assistant at Johns Hopkins, headed for the Wild West. The scheme, abetted by the Wyoming Department of Agriculture, was to

---

2. The Butlins abandoned farming; David now builds boats.

grow pedigree legume seed on the banks of the Grey Bull River. When the movie makers and television crews arrived, Charlie repented, "If I was going to make a pure ass of myself, I wanted to do it quietly." The Orrs retreated to the East, then to Scotland, where Charlie resumed teaching and bought and refurbished a derelict 1640 cottage, to raise another stake. Within three days of coming out to Nova Scotia to reconnoitre farming prospects, Charlie became the owner of an abandoned North Shore farm. Their troubles were only beginning.

The first year, the Orrs raised sheep but soon found that the cash flow was insufficient for a family of six. A cream cheque seemed the only option. They bought Jerseys "because any bigger cow would have been standing in the gutter." They were getting set up when, on Christmas Day, 1974, the old Cumberland barn burned to the ground. They lost their tractor and all of their hay and grain. Fortunately, the animals were saved. The cows were dispersed to neighbouring barns, and the pigs took up residence in the cellar of the house for a noisy, smelly tenure. In the face of financial ruin and the February cold, Charlie began to rebuild, saddled with a second FLB loan.

The time since has been spent bringing back the land, improving breeding stock, and most importantly fine-tuning the use of the skim milk for the feeding of the hogs. In sharp contrast to the willy-nilly methods attributed to the old-time shippers, Charlie has approached the use of his skim milk (which he describes as an almost perfect pig feed) with the discipline learned studying cell membranes. His on-the-farm experiments may serve as a model for other cream shippers. Certainly, they fill the vacuum which currently exists in cream production research in the Department of Agriculture.

"What is difficult is to have the pig numbers tied in with the number of milking cows, so that at all times you have an adequate supply of skim milk. When that's working, I can produce pigs cheaper than anyone in the province," he claims.

But Charlie and Jennie are familiar with the animal inflation factor. Cream shipping farms are small and are likely to remain so, unless there is a quantum leap in the state of the art. The manual separation of the cream and hand feeding of the skim is labour intensive. There is also a limit to the amount of skim milk that can be handled without creating a rancid mess. The Orrs are working toward a 28-cow milking herd, in order to provide an income for their teenage family and to keep creditors off their back. Such a herd size would give the Orrs the option (with the one proviso the quota is available and affordable) to make the switch to fluid. If it were a matter of livelihood, they would[3]; however, they remain determined to demonstrate that cream shipping is "as profitable as any other dairy enterprise." They also are committed to the mixed farming concept.

"It's the only dammed way to farm," says Charlie. "Basically, you've got to make the ground produce for you and the only way you can do that is to produce shit.

"I feel quite strongly about this old, tired land here. I'm fundamentally opposed to inorganic fertilizers, because I'm sure that they are destroying the health of our soils. I'm sure the bacteria cannot survive that localized acidity.

"If you destroy that health in your soil, you are basically just farming hydroponically. You've got a dead substrate out there. You have to let nature help you. The ground is the legacy we have to look after."

Charlie admits that finding new caretakers of the land will not be easy: "There's no glamour associated with being a cream shipper and that's a major drawback. But the glamour comes when it's shown that it's profitable.

"It doesn't seem to be a mental block for a young fellow to assume a debt of $150,000, but then he hasn't assumed that kind of debt before. It's bandied about rather freely in the agricultural bureaucracy that it's the kind of debt one can handle – it's an intolerable burden."

The cows are milked, the hogs fed. Jennie has separated the cream, attended to the calves and her personal pride, two handsome Brown Swiss heifers that she brought into the herd from Connecticut. She excuses herself, it's 9:30, bedtime. Charlie and I sit beside the kitchen stove for a last round of tea. The muscled forearms, projecting from the frayed ends of his long-sleeved undershirt, are of a man far removed from the lecture theatre and the glass world of the lab. My question probes his day's end tiredness, for any tag end of regret.

---

3. The Orrs briefly switched to fluid production but opted for a small farm in Maine.

"It's a great family operation. These kids have learned one hell of a lot more than if I had been a prof. They are different kids, smarter kids. They understand the value of a dollar, which I never did at their age. And they've seen life and death, which is hard at first.

"The family is always working together. It can't work if there's any friction or problem there. You soon know whether the relationship is sound or not. You have to be totally dedicated – otherwise you're not going to make it."

CHARLES AND JUDITH HUBBARD are also immigrants. Reluctant converts to cream production, they are now steadfast supporters. Their farms are near Northport, Cumberland County. On one side of the road is a garishly orange, steel-sided barn: This is Charles' domain, a modern farrow-to-finish operation. Opposite, on the home side of the road, is the big weathered barn where Judith houses her herd of Jerseys. Their setup offers a rare opportunity to compare, side by side, modern agribusiness practice with the traditional small farm philosophy.

Born in England, their honeymoon in a Welsh cottage led to their becoming farmsteaders on a 16-hectare holding. A neighbour in the all Welsh-speaking community christened Charles' first sow "Mother Hubbard." They bought several cows, and the pigs increased over time. Also the family grew. Judith recalls, "The arrival of four children, one after another, limited my usefulness in the barn." Finally, their ambition outgrew the homestead potential. Returning to England, they had to settle for an even smaller holding of two hectares and an affiliation with a cooperatively owned hog artificial insemination unit. The unit prospered, but the Hubbards still dreamed of their own land base.

When they arrived on Nova Scotia's North Shore in the late 1960s farms were for sale "two for a penny." The purchase of 324 hectares satisfied their yen for land, but for new farmers, it was disconcerting to find themselves stepping into a vacuum. "There was no one to follow," says Charles. "There were very few people here doing anything." His contacts in England helped to get them started. Today, Charles is considered one of Nova Scotia's premier swine breeders, and his gross income places him in the ninety-fifth percentile of provincial producers.

The more modest cream side of the balance sheet came about at the behest of a neighbour. Pat Darragh was a retired dairyman who worked for Charles. "He told us that we'd never be able to put the farm on its feet unless we had cattle. Of course, he was right," says Judith, "because we had the land – and all those stupid pigs over there – and were not using it. We began to listen to him, and we decided eventually to go into cream production and have Jersey cows, which, in fact, was what I always wanted."

After defending his "stupid pigs," Charles continues: "When we got the cows, we were able to use the grain we were growing. You can look at it from the point of view that it is the cows now that we are using as a converter of pork meat from grass."

Charles' side of the road has remained tied into the use of imported, pelleted grain. However, there is an interchange between the two farms. Judith's barn has become an infirmary of sorts. "We bring over his disaster cases," Judith says. "And we can very often save their lives."

Charles picks up on the point and the humour: "It's just incredible. It seems silly to say it, because all we're doing is repeating what great-grandfather would have said sixty years ago. But so many of these modern people have forgotten what great-grandfather said.

"We brought twenty pigs over – we literally brought them over, because they were unable to travel under their own steam. The first lot we brought over, none of them died. Within a short time, they were in pretty good shape. In fact, one day when we came down the hill from the church (Judith had left the door open) the whole darn lot were running all over the place. You never would have believed that they were the lot who couldn't even walk here."

In addition to its medicinal value, Charles believes that the skim milk increases the margin per cow by 50 percent. "Some would say that the value of the skim is ten or fifteen cents per gallon. That is not the way to look at it. The end product is fifty cents worth of meat – that's what you get paid for."

The cows have made it possible for the Hubbards to put into practice the principles of their European grounding in agriculture: Production must be founded on its land base. There must be a direct relationship between livestock units and acres involved. Charles does not see these principles being practised in Nova Scotia.

"Some of our finest units are based on acres from the West. In essence, the majority of the livestock units are manufacturing units. They are not farming units in the traditional sense.

"The stupid form of thought says that the only type of production is based on cheap energy and the quantity per unit. None of this is related to the amount of production per acre, which is the way they teach things in Europe. That's why we feel the cows and work that Judith is doing is so important, as much as it's a totally different system. Of the two, the cream side will last longer. I'm not worried about profits, but about principles. And as things change this side, (the cream) will be in existence much longer."

The signs of change cannot be ignored: skyrocketing energy, fertilizer and machinery costs and the tenuous production of those Western acres, where the organic matter of the soils is being depleted by monoculture. Nevertheless, Charles is given the well-intentioned advice to worry about nothing except the pigs and their production per unit. And Judith must endure the patronizing attitude that she is dabbling in cream production as an amusement, one she can afford because of the other side of the road. "Little do they realize," says Charles, who is weathering the bottoming out of the pork market, "that the only money we're living on at the moment is the cream money." When pork prices are better, the Hubbards continue to sacrifice their bottom line to build up a complete farm.

Charles views the status quo as a kind of Tower of Babylon, with the farmer as the column supporting an outsized superstructure. "On the far side of the road, being highly capital-intensive and very largely dependent upon borrowing monies, we are in practice supporting an awful lot of people in one form or another. On this side of the road, we are supporting very few people.

"The farms would be all right but the system would break down if we all reverted to this [cream] side of the road. All those who are dependent on the present system, which is based on cheap energy, would suddenly find themselves flat on their faces. You can see where the vested interests are."

Charles gets incensed about cost of production figures and meaningless statistics, like the one which classifies his side of the road as a "Superfarm." He has calculated that his working wage is less than that his 19-year-old son can make at a summer job in the nearby town of Amherst. To compound the irony and insult, Charles alone produces enough pork to supply half of the demand of Amherst's 9,000 inhabitants.

"Someone has to say to these idiots, 'Look! One man cannot look after more than a certain amount, and while we're insisting on a relatively reasonable society, which involves certain standards, therefore, holidays or leave or number of hours worked, then stop fooling around with these things, because the only reason for doing so is to try to come up with a cost of production per unit.' They should be decent enough to put these criteria into the cost of production formula, and not continue to assume one man can do more and more in a given time. There are limits which, overreached, will cause the whole system to collapse, where the next generation will not take over the family farm – then you will have expensive foods."

For the consumer, Charlie believes that there is security only in farm numbers. "For the North Shore, the farming of the future will be compact little units, which probably one man can handle – no more than thirty cows or thirty or forty sows – with its acreage behind it feeding that unit and machinery innovations to adapt to its climate."

The school bus has arrived. The Hubbard children (there are seven) pour into the back porch, pausing only long enough to deposit their lunchboxes and to grab their skates. Charles disappears to his duties across the road. There is time for a brief tour. The barn is well lit and clean, the Jerseys surprisingly diminutive, when one is used to a milking line of Holsteins. Kittens and spotted pups roll about in the hay.

Judith and I stand at the back door of the barn. The children, who look like little figures in a Breughel painting, are skating where a depression in the pasture has made a natural rink. Horses and ponies canter about the field. The brow of the hill is ploughed in rippling rows, ready for next year's grain. I remark on the sombre beauty of Nova Scotia, which, as a native, I am congenitally attached to. "I didn't think so at first," Judith rejoins, "but yes, it is beautiful."

MOST PEOPLE NATIVE TO the North Shore have cream shipping in their background. Those old enough witnessed the emigration from farms, precipitated and accelerated by World War II. Of the young men who came back from overseas, many did not return to the farms. Many who stayed on the farm during the war were shunted into war-related industries, such as the Pictou shipyards and the Trenton carworks and gun shop. Better industrial wages continued to lure people off the family farm in the '50s and '60s. Today, thousands of acres of land that once produced cream lie idle, at the mercy of alder and pasture spruce, and consequently there is a dearth of father-son cream shipping farms.

One is Blockhouse Farm, which takes its name from Fort Franklin, built on the site in 1763 to guard the entrance to Tatamagouche Bay. A Golden Guernsey sign hangs at the roadside. Looking down the long lane, one would guess that this is a prosperous farm, though it is far from ostentatious. The large hip-backed house has a new coat of white paint with red trim. The outbuildings and barn are painted to match. The straw stubble, bristling through a light cover of snow, adds to the general impression of tidiness and comfort.

Baillie Ferguson's father bought the 80-hectare farm in 1919. At age twenty-two, Baillie's only son, Keith, is assuming more responsibility on the place. He will be the third Ferguson generation to ship cream to the Tatamagouche plant.

The redolence of deep-frying doughnuts wafts from the kitchen when Baillie comes to greet me on the back porch. For the past few months he has been convalescing from major surgery. When well he plies his carpenter's trade part time (as did my own father). "I had to get sick to have a vacation," he says, as we sit down at the kitchen table.

Baillie is forthright. He wonders out loud how new farmers can undertake rapid expansion and finance the purchase of purebred cows. When he started into farming, he says, "I didn't have money to invest and I wasn't going into debt. I always figured that I was going to own my own little manure pile and if I wanted to quit, I could quit, and call everything my own."

Because of the debt load, he has never entertained a changeover to fluid. Before there was a government support for butter, the fluid shippers were "besting" him, but today, he can say, "I figure that we're as well off as milk shippers, because we don't have as big an overhead to carry. The stuff we can get by with, we can come out at the end of the year with as much to show as the milk producer."

Of large farms, he says, "It's not as rosy as it looks." The Fergusons have a ready market for their weaners and veal, grow their own grain and, as Keith says, "The cows give enough to fill the pail." Unlike the new shippers that have had to start from scratch, Keith will not have a debt load on his shoulder. Like his father, he will be able to farm to suit himself. [4]

As we're drinking coffee over a plate of Mrs. Ferguson's delicious doughnuts, a neighbour drops in to ask after Baillie's health. He is introduced as a one time shipper. As for so many, there was no one who wanted to take over the farm.

Baillie leans forward, his arms resting on the table: "I often wonder who is going to do the farming after the generation of my age is done. They're still not getting many young fellows encouraged. There's not the profit in it for them, that's the trouble. I've preached that for years, that they can't let the land go back to the woods because the population is increasing and the farmers are getting less."

He reflects for a moment, "I may never see it, but there's going to be nothing to eat."

---

4. After Baillie's death, the Fergusons sold Blockhouse Farm which is now the site of a Tim Hortons summer camp.

Exhibition Time in Ox Country
Bridgewater, Nova Scotia

IN THE 1950s, when I was a member of a 4-H Club, I got a week off school in September to attend Exhibition. Since then, whenever I return to agricultural fairgrounds, I am seized by a sense of time stolen, of delicious leisure. This feeling is heightened by the fact that while the world has changed dramatically, exhibitions have remained very much the same.

The familiarity is reassuring: a larder of prize-winning pickles and baked goods is, alas, as inviting to the palette as to the eye; yards of handcrafts have been stitched, quilted, knitted, crocheted, tatted, hooked, then embroidered, smocked and appliqued into a lamé of colour and practical design; and familiar patterns like Log Cabin are draped beside such modern mutants as Urban Sprawl. There are piglets and ponies – always a delight – as well as poultry in an improbable array of colours, shapes and exotic plummages. There are the livestock barns: cow barns; horse barns (light and heavy); sheep and swine barns and ox barns.

Three decades after my introduction to this festival of rural culture, I find myself on the fairgrounds of the South Shore Exhibition in Bridgewater, Nova Scotia. The Big Ex, as promoters like to call it, is the first of fourteen such fairs held throughout the province each summer and one of the biggest.

I am but one of 70,000 who will pass through the gate by Saturday. On this, a Monday morning, I look happily to the week ahead and think of re-acquainting myself with the animals, the showmanship, the artistry and the conviviality of rural society. In particular, I am anticipating an opportunity to partake of the spectacle of strength and will which is ox-pulling. In Bridgewater as elsewhere in western Nova Scotia – in "ox country" – the ox pulls are the fair's most popular attraction.

I have loved ox pulling since childhood when I was introduced to this workingman's sport. In 1957, I sat in the exhibition building in Yarmouth, Nova Scotia, watching what was billed as the World Championship Ox Haul. As the pyramid of 200-pound weights grew higher on the drag so did the tension in the crowd. Each teamster, satisfied that enough weight had been added, settled into position between the heads of his team of patient oxen. Grasping a horn with one hand and twirling his whip in a circle above the team's back with the other, he let out with a resounding command – "Hauuuuul!" – and the oxen responded with a mighty thrust of their immense shoulders. The drag moved forward – grudgingly, inexorably, heroically.

That simple invocation, which melds man and animal to a common purpose, stirs my blood as much now as it did the first time I heard it. And I will hear it many times over the next few days. The variety of pulling contests will culminate in The Oland's International Ox Pull on Friday night, in which four Canadian teams will compete against four teams from the United States for the Oland's Cup.

But on Monday morning, the excitement and the crowds seem far away. There is time now to wander the grounds, to inspect the barns, to settle in and savour. I drink in the familiar sights and sounds and inhale the good smells – among which, as country-born, I count the earthiness of fresh dung. The best time of day at the Exhibition, in my opinion, is morning, when the exhibitors are about their business of watering and feeding, currying coats and braiding tails, or, like myself, simply admiring what the land and hard work have wrought. There is time now for casual talk before the crowds begin to pour in and the Ferris wheel begins to spin. Then, the Exhibition takes on a carnival spirit, with the frenzy, the bright lights, and the sounds of the city. Of course, that, too, is part of the fun and offers a welcome change for many of the country people who come here on a busman's holiday. For now, however, people's minds are on the show ring and the reward of ribbons, which by week's end will fly from one end of the barns to the other like flags on the halyards of a ship.

By mid-morning, a peaceful lull has fallen over the exhibition grounds. Sound travels cleanly and clearly through the air, and the most peaceful of those sounds is the nostalgic tok-tok-tok of the ox bells as the teams are taken out for their morning walk.

I follow the sound to the far corner of the fair grounds, where seventy teams are housed in the two barns. Nowhere – except perhaps in the heavy-horse barns – is so much care lavished upon the animals. A teamster takes great pride in the appearance of his team. To begin with, he tries to match a pair. Often he must travel throughout his district to find a match for a steer in his own herd – one of the same breed, build and, if possible, with similar markings.

Many teamsters prefer a crossbred ox. Hereford and Red Durham is a popular choice: the Hereford blood produces a good-looking, white-faced ox; Durham provides "the spark" for pulling as well as a "spreckle" of red colour. A yoke, painted red or blue, hangs above each pair of stalls, as does a name plaque. With few exceptions, the plaques read "Bright & Lion," the traditional South Shore names for oxen.

This morning, the teams are being yoked and paraded through the show ring to be judged in the categories Best Decorated and Best Pair. After judge Elzee Saulnier finishes his slow military perusal of the teams, like a sergeant major inspecting the troops, I join him in the shade of his ringside booth. I ask him what he looks for in a pair of oxen. "If I'm lookin' for a pair of oxen for myself I'd like to have a mated pair of oxen," Saulnier says in his French Shore accent. "Both look alike, both the same size, both travel the same in the yoke – we call that loose travellin'. They don't look like they're all humped up and their head down.

"And I like to see a nice set of horns on a pair of cattle. That's one of the main things because you meet people and you're always head on."

Those who meet a team of oxen head on see a pair of rather doleful and surprisingly pretty animals bound together by a wooden yoke. Yoke makers (a disappearing breed) prefer yellow birch for its toughness; with a saw, adze and drawknife, they shape the yoke to fit comfortably over the neck of the ox. To complete the fit, they gouge out grooves called horn boxes, into which the horns fit precisely. "Yoke's got to fit the ox like the shoe's got to fit your foot," one teamster told me. Each yoke is custom built and, when finished, looks something like a crude, heavy bow. Teamsters yoke the animals by winding about twenty feet of leather strapping around the horns and into grooves, called strap gains, at either end of the yoke. In the pulling ring, they attach the shaft of the drag to the yoke, making the connection between beast and burden.

As important as the functional paraphernalia are the decorative accoutrements. Each ox has a headpad. Traditionally, the headpads are "brassed up" with hearts, diamonds and shamrocks, and further embellished with rhinestones. Finally, each member of a team must have a neck strap for an oxbell, the source of the pastoral music of the ox barn.

THE OXEN, thus adorned, are the star performers at the Big Ex. On Tuesday, the day of the Grand Street Parade, many of the teams are yoked and teamed through the streets of downtown Bridgewater, re-creating a scene that might have been commonplace a century ago. I station myself on the last leg of the parade loop, which leads up a steep hill from the LaHave River to the fair grounds.

First to pass is the town crier, clanging his bell and looking uncomfortable in his heavy frock coat and fur-trimmed, three-cornered hat. Black Percherons, nostrils flaring, and Shriners on mini-bikes climb the torturously steep incline. Waves of marching bands roll up the street, now awash with boots, kilts and khaki. White furry hats, like tufts of cotton candy, appear above a rise. Soon, majorettes twirl and toss their batons while queens and princesses for a day wave greetings from convertibles. Floats, pulled by every conceivable conveyance from draft horses to Mack trucks, advertise the charity of local service clubs and the products of local entrepreneurs. The parade presents the community in cross-section, and no one, it seems, wants to be conspicuous by his or her absence. The town's major employer, Michelin Tire, flies the motto "Pulling Together," in clever deference to the region's symbol of progress and hard work. Last up the hill, in the position of honour, are the ox teams themselves, sure and steady of pace and unbothered by the heat or hoopla.

Oxen were a vital part of pioneer life in Nova Scotia and had some distinct advantages over the horse. First, they were cheap to feed, often grazing on marginal marshland that produced a wild crop of salt hay. The slow steady pace of the ox resulted in less damage to farm implements than occurred with draft horses, which tend to be quicker or, as teamsters say, "sharper." And when they became too old to work, oxen offered one final advantage over horses – they could be eaten by the farm family.

Horses eventually replaced oxen in most of Nova Scotia, but the ox held sway on the South Shore. Surefooted, they were better suited for the rocky coast, where they were put to work hauling seaweed for fertilizer, pulling fish catches from weirs, and winching boats ashore – all unsuitable tasks for the more temperamental horses. Of course, the ox cart was a popular form of personal transportation, and convoys of them often made the long haul from inland communities to the coast.

FOR THREE CENTURIES a dominant force in community life, oxen had all but disappeared from the rural landscape thirty years ago. It was then that a group of teamsters got together to form the Maritime Ox-pulling Association. It proved the salvation of the ox and, in the process, turned a pleasant pastime into a formal and popular sport.

One of those instrumental in reviving interest in the ox was Gordon Lohnes, a founding member of the association. A tall, lanky man with a mak'em cigarette stuck permanently on his lower lip, Lohnes is something of a father figure to the younger generation of teamsters. I have to arrive at the fairgrounds early in the morning to catch him before his daily work of supervising the show rings gets into full swing.

"Years ago they was pulling, but, at the time, they used to use the oxen. Now, most generally," Gordon says, softening his "r's" and speaking in the distinctive South Shore drawl, "we just keep them for the hobby of ox pulling, you see. So that's the reason the association was formed to keep the oxen going.

"You could see it coming up. If we didn't do something the oxen was going to go the other way. Now we got more people interested in the oxen that really don't need them any more than I do. But they just keep them because they like them."

Thanks to Lohnes and others like him, the ox has made a remarkable recovery. Today, the South Shore Exhibition is the only place in the province – or anywhere else, for that matter – where onlookers can see a hundred or more yoked cattle.

For me the patient strength of oxen symbolize the struggle to maintain rural traditions. Though the ox is no longer an essential component of a working farm, the people in ox country have been steadfast in their loyalty to the animal that built the country. They were not content, in a pragmatic gesture to modernity, merely to cast the ox aside as redundant. And they continue to show due respect for the ox with their painstaking attention to the look of the team.

Ox pulling honours the ox by giving it work. For those of us watching the ox pull, we see how man and animal can become a unit. Just as the oxen are yoked together, man and animal are bound in a heroic struggle when the teamster takes hold of a horn and asks them to "Haul!" It is good to be reminded of this relationship upon which rural society was founded.

TUESDAY NIGHT is reserved for the Canadian Qualifying Ox Pull, which will decide the four teams to compete against the Americans on Friday. The plodding teams enter the ring to the incongruous rhythm of "Bo Diddley," performed by Rompin' Ronnie Hawkins, who is just finishing his set in the adjacent outdoor arena. Ox pulling is a sport with a loyal following, and fans here are knowledgeable in the way hockey fans are at the Montreal Forum. I have the good fortune to sit beside an aspiring young teamster, who provides a running commentary on the herculean spectacle in the ring.

The teams pull in turns. Each has three tries to pull a 5,000-pound drag a distance of six feet, after which more weight is added. The four teams to pull the heaviest load will qualify. To begin with, the drag is on a cement slab. "It's a dead pull off concrete, there's no give," my interpreter tells me. "That drag seems to weld to the slab."

"Get up Lion, Gee, Gee. Step up Lion," shouts one unsuccessful contestant.

"They say teamin'," my friend confides, "but you're only teamin' the weak ox."

Of the thirty-nine teams, fewer than half move the drag the required six feet. There are heroic victories and failures. The crowd responds appropriately with cheers, applause or good-natured jibes. "He can't team. He couldn't ride a bicycle," a spectator comments, when one teamster slides in under the horns of his struggling team and lands ingloriously on his behind.

Teamsters display individual styles. Kendall Oickle, whose team moves the drag on the first try, is quiet and reassuringly unhurried. He never makes a quick or untoward movement or raises his voice above a whisper – and his team seems to respond in like style, quietly doing their job.

Others team with emotional fervour. Donnie Travis of Yarmouth County is one such high-pitched performer and, hence, a real crowd pleaser. Travis seems to be as much in communication with the bleachers as with his own team. "He should be a wrestler," says a voice behind me.

Travis wears his ball cap backwards and sports a tank top that shows his bronzed and muscled upper body to good effect. When the team fails to respond on its first try, he throws the cap into the dirt and kicks it like an irate baseball manager making a point with an impassive umpire. Regaining his composure, he stalks around the team, shortens the chain connecting the yoke to the drag, kicks away gravel in front of the drag, then ducks down, putting his head between the two oxen for a tête-à-tête, delivered in unctuous, audible tones.

"I said listen to me. Whoa, Lion, back haw. Now we got to haul. Now, Spark, haul!

"Come on, Spark, Lion. Bring it up heeeere!"

The team pulls the drag forward the mandatory six feet, Elzee Saulnier nods his head, and Travis throws his whip into the air to the wild applause of the crowd. To everyone's surprise, including Travis's, it seems, he has qualified.

Last up is Darrel Watkins. Of all the entrants, Watkins is my personal favourite. I grew up watching his father haul and then Watkins himself take over where his father left off – winning consistently and with style. Now, Watkins's own son, Darren, is capable of beating his father, keeping the winning tradition alive.

Win or lose, Watkins brings to ox pulling a riveting style. Other teamsters watch him to learn his secrets. "He's a smart cookie," one teamster tells me with grudging respect. "He knows just when to add on weight, and when to rest them to get a second wind. And he'll get three starts to your one. He'll be yelling 'Whoa,' but he'll be jiggin' that drag around – you gotta watch him." And watch him you do. The audience can't seem to take their eyes off him as he puts his team through their paces. He is a dervish of energy – circling, chiding, fidgeting – every action designed to concentrate the attention of the team on the task at hand, pulling the two-and-a-half tons of deadweight. Still, nothing distinguishes Watkins's style more than his voice. When he invokes his cattle to "Haul," he not only stirs the seemingly somnolent cattle into action; it is as if he disturbs the gods in their heaven.

I delight in his histrionics. He crouches with his hands on his knees and speaks to the cattle, eye to eye, in the teamster's equivalent of a mound conference. He "Whoas" the team back, flicking his whip at their knees; then, without warning, the Watkins's yell begins, rising up through his thin-legged, barrel-chested frame and issuing from a gaping mouth like a wind storm. His voice gains steadily in volume-- "Hauuuu . . . " – his whip twirls above the team's head like the cone of a twister, the oxen hoof the dirt, their heavy shoulders heave forward in unison; Watkins's voice reaches a hoarse crescendo – " . . . . uuul!" The drag slides forward but stops short of six feet.

Watkins clamps his mouth shut and cocks his head to one side in an attitude of dismay, as if to say, "Come on, guys, what do you think we're doing out here?" He then asks the drag attendant to unhitch the team, making me wonder if he is finished. I should know better. It is all part of the strategy. As he takes the team for a little promenade, he exhorts them quietly. Circling the team back between the rails, he backs them up, crowding them against the drag so that when they move forward they will have to lunge, uncoiling their power – and, in the process, will jerk the load into motion, overcoming the inertia of the drag against concrete. Again the yell from his heels, but this time Watkins backs up quickly, making the team come to him. And they do, bringing the drag forward the balance of six feet. To no one's surprise, Watkins qualifies for an unprecedented twelfth time and will join Donnie Travis, Kendall Oickle, and Leon Corkum in the ring on Friday night against the Americans.

The next day, I seek out Darrel Watkins to talk to him about the passion and skill he displays as a teamster. To me it is a privilege and, yes, to borrow the sportscaster's parlance, "a thrill" to talk to a man I have watched and admired for thirty years. He is a hero in the sense that he embodies what is best in his sport – a sport that has a cultural validity in this corner of the world as nowhere else.

"I fell through the ice when I was five years old," Watkins begins his story. "There was a little air hole behind me, and I remember my brother, with a friend, was ahead of me on the ice, and he said, 'Watch out for that hole.' I was just this little kid, but I can remember looking for that hole, and I was gradually slidin' backwards on my skates. First thing, I went into it.

"They hauled me out of there and I was soaking wet and cold. I went up to the house – up over the hill, across the railway track, over the field and into the house. The next thing I remember is asking my mother how many more exhibitions I was going to see. I thought I was going to die, eh, and that's all I was worried about. So I had this in me all my life I guess."

I want to know how Watkins does what he does so well.

"It's got to come natural," he says. "Probably some things I don't know I'm doin'. I've worked a lot in the woods and around the barn, and after a while, you pick up certain ways an animal responds to. Someone who just comes and buys a pair of oxen doesn't develop that kind of feeling."

Almost all teamsters speak of the rapport between animal and human. This finely-tuned relationship is a mysterious and fragile thing. Trying to make oxen haul a load when they are not ready or able is called "hanging the team," and it is the surest way to break a team's spirit. In the way that oxen in an ideal team should match each other in appearance and strength, the spirit of the animals and the temperament of the teamster must be a good match.

I spend hours observing this relationship in action, as there are pulls morning, evening and night for the various weight classes. One noon hour, with the temperature hovering around 30° Celsius, I sit in the bleachers with the wives of teamsters, the only other people in the sun.

"They're not true ox people," says Janet Sabean, gesturing dismissively toward the open door of the ox barns where the men have taken shelter from the heat. "They're in the shade, we're in the sun. We can see whether they made their three feet where they can't. They sit there and argue about it."

The women laugh with a conspiratorial glee.

"They get into arguments in the winter on how much they pulled and where they placed, and then we get out the books," says Barbara Hurlburt, indicating a little black book in her lap. Hurlburt records every pull: the weight pulled, the number of tries to do it, and the percentage of the team's weight versus the weight of the drag.

"When you sit here all day," she says, "it makes it more interesting to keep statistics."

Women are not just dedicated fans who sit in the mid-day sun and travel every weekend in the summer. Many of them have taken to teaming and have proven themselves more than a match for men in the ring.

"We hold our own," says Connie. "I've beat Donnie several times."

As Friday dawns the question on everybody's mind is whether the Canadians will be a match for the Americans. The Bridgewater pull is the first half of a home-and-home series. The same eight teams will meet again in New Cumberland, Maine, in September. In Bridgewater, they pull American style, a so-called distance pull. The winner is the team that pulls a pre-determined weight the furthest distance in five minutes. In Maine, the teams will pull Canadian style. There, each team will have three tries to pull a load a distance of three feet, at which time more weight is added. Under the Canadian system, the team that pulls the greatest weight wins. First held in 1957, these international contests have fanned a friendly rivalry. Usually the hometown crowds have little to cheer about, however, as the Americans usually beat the Canadians in Canada, and vice-versa.

One look at the American oxen reveals why they are better suited to the distance pull. They are, for the most part, Holstein steers, taller and longer in the legs, than the more compact, lower-to-the-ground beef cattle breeds that are preferred – primarily for their looks – by the Canadians. The American oxen dwarf the Canadian teams, so much so that they suggest the epic stature of Paul Bunyan's blue ox Babe.

There are other differences between American and Canadian oxen. Americans employ a neck yoke, a beam with a bow which passes under the neck of the ox, so that their teams are said to pull from the neck rather than from the head as Canadian teams do. As a rule, the yoke is unpainted and Americans dispense with head pads, collar and oxbells. To me the American oxen are pragmatic beasts in practical clothing.

However homely, the American ox is well chosen "to walk to victory" in the distance pull. But the stockier Canadian teams, with their lower centre of gravity, are better adapted to pull heavier loads in the Canadian-style pull. Watkins, for example, has won seven times in Maine, while victory in the international pull has eluded him.

Rain delays the pull until Saturday evening, when the bleachers begin to fill two hours before the pull. By 7:30, 6,000 people have assembled to greet the contestants. The Americans enter the ring first, flying the Stars and Stripes from their yokes, followed by the host teams, which answer with the Maple Leaf. The national anthems blare from the loud speakers and are absorbed by the sound of the midway.

A draw determines the sequence of teams to pull; the weight has been set at 6,400 pounds (12,909 kilograms), a load heavy enough to give the Canadians some hope of winning. That slim hope seems to vanish when Deane Anderson's team, a truly massive duo of Holstein-Chianina cross and the pre-pull favourites, quite literally walks away with the three-ton-plus drag. At the five-minute mark, the team has pulled the load a prodigious 331 feet 5 inches – nearly 100 feet farther than his Canadian predecessor, Kendall Oickle.

The last teamster to pull is Darrel Watkins. His team, breaking with Canadian tradition, is unmatched. Like the Americans, Watkins is primarily interested in how the animals pull, not how they look. And pull they do, at first, responding to Darrel's invocations like a team with real spark in them. They make the turn of the 200-foot course in two minutes, and it appears they have a chance of catching the Americans. But one ox begins to balk, and Watkins, try as he may, is unable to work his usual magic. He comes up well short, at 229 feet 3 inches, good enough for fifth place. Kendall Oickle, at 240 feet 9 inches, cops fourth place and saves face for the Canadian contingent by preventing a clean sweep of the top four spots by the Americans.

After the presentation ceremony, I seek out Watkins to ask how he feels about his performance. He shakes his head, flashes his bright smile and says, "There's always next year."

Like Watkins, I, too, find solace in the knowledge that there will be exhibitions, big and small, throughout rural Nova Scotia, this summer and for many summers to come – and that oxen will be there to delight the crowds.

Storming the Sand Castles
Greenwich, Prince Edward Island

AROUND ST. PETERS BAY, as almost everywhere on Prince Edward Island, the land eases gently into the water. In late May, seaside fields seem preternaturally green. Across the blue corrugations of the bay, red tillage ripples from farmhouses to the water's edge. Hard-edged strokes of unsullied colour: green, red, blue. Brakes of softwood border well-ordered fields that march off over rolling hills. Even to a casual tourist, this is a homey, knowable landscape. For me, a frequent visitor, the Island never fails to work its verdant mesmerism.

Every summer, 122,000 Islanders share this pastoral birthright with 600,000 tourists like myself who ferry across the Northumberland Strait to The Garden of the Gulf. Tourism ranks third behind farming and fishing in the Island economy. Even so, it is not so surprising that some Islanders who cherish peace and quiet view the tourist boon with mixed feelings. That has always been the case. As *The Garden Transformed*, a recent study of Island society, reveals: "Like the Anne [of Green Gables] novels, Island history has both a sense of ambivalence about bucolic isolation and a love/hate relationship with the outside world." Life on a small island has inured a simple truth: islanders value the land more than anything else.

One theory holds that such sentiment has its origins two centuries ago in the Island's unfortunate history of absentee landlordism. In the 1760s after the British had assumed control of Ile St. Jean, as the French called it, the entire landmass was divided into townships that became personal fiefdoms for friends of Whitehall. Some believe that the loathing ingrained in Island yeoman toward outside control of their land persists to this day, that it has become part of the collective unconscious of contemporary Islanders. Academic myth? Perhaps. But the Island's reaction to the persistent efforts of a group of West Coast developers to build a 1,500-acre (600-hectare) $40 million residential/recreational complex – modern-day leisure colony – on the shores of St. Peters Bay suggests that there is more than a little truth to the theory. Indeed, the proposal has sparked a controversy that has raged for three decades now.

In 1970, Robert Evans, president of H.W. Dickie Ltd. – a Duncan, British Columbia, real estate firm – flew over the north shore of Prince Edward Island. In place of a patch work of old farms on the Greenwich Peninsula bordering St. Peters Bay, he envisaged a 200-unit hotel/motel, 400 town houses, a championship golf course, an airstrip, and a marina. In 1971, he purchased the Cyril Sanderson place, a 500-acre (200-hecatre) farm at the tip of the peninsula that included a large sand-dune system jutting into the Gulf of St. Lawrence. The next year, he bought two more farms nearby.

In November 1972, however, the Liberal government of Alex Campbell cancelled one of these purchases – the Leith Sanderson property – and made a sweeping amendment to the Real Property Act that limited nonresident purchases to ten acres (four hectares) without cabinet approval. The measure was seen as a response to fears that speculators, encountering the new legislation protecting the Gulf Islands in British Columbia, had earmarked Prince Edward Island as their new haven. Evans' plans were further frustrated when the dune system was designated as an environmental protection area in 1975. Despite these setbacks, Evans and his partners – two businessmen from British Columbia and two from Seattle, Washington – have doggedly continued to pursue their plans.

For the Islanders, meanwhile, the Greenwich development has become a focal point for all that ails the Island psyche. To environmentalists, it poses a threat to a unique, pristine, sand dune system. Traditionalists see it as a symbol of the fraying of rural fabric on the Island. To others, it represents a hope for revitalizing an economic backwater and a progressive shift in attitude toward tourism. The issue has divided the cabinet, the community and even households. I first learned of the controversy in May 1984 and, as a longtime Island devotee, decided to visit St. Peters Bay to try to understand the passions that the land inspires in Island hearts.

St. Peters Bay is a 11.5 kilometre-long inlet on Prince Edward Island's north shore, eighteen miles from Charlottetown, the capital. The bay shelters three communities. At its head is the 19th-century shipbuilding centre of St. Peters, a hamlet composed of gabled and mansard-roof houses, a gas station, a general store, and two imposing wooden churches for 320 parishioners.

The community of Greenwich strings out along the peninsula that forms the north shore of the bay. Although it was once a thriving farming area, two decades of decline are now evidenced in its hay barns, their strong backs broken by disuse, and its houses, their grey faces masked by the saplings of the once proud homestead silver poplars gone to riot. The road ends at the Greenwich dune.

On the south side of the bay is the village of Morell (population 350) and the Red Head Wharf, its economic hub. By midday, the U-shaped wharf shelters the colourful lobster fleet: white, blue, lime-green and lavender long-liners returned from the day's fishing, which began at sunrise. Women in hair nets and men in white peaked caps come and go from the two fish packing plants. Morell is a vital, bustling community, the centre of the modern-day fishery, and St. Peters casts an envious eye toward the village, for it has usurped St. Peters' patriarchal position in the bay.

"In the coves of the land, all things are discussed," wrote Prince Edward Island poet Milton Acorn in "Island" and it was to the coves of the land that I went to hear what St. Peters Bay residents had to say about the development. At one of my early stops, at Cable Head West – north and east of Greenwich – I met Norbert Palmer and LeRoy MacKenzie, two fishermen who had spent the day netting gaspereaux, a herring-like fish used locally as lobster bait. Palmer's truck sat on a deserted beach that stretched to a vanishing point in the direction of the Greenwich dune: to the leisure-minded, a splendid vista; to the locals, a place of work.

I listened as Palmer and MacKenzie talked in the truck cab and wondered how many times such a conversation had been repeated at the general store, on the wharf and in farmhouse kitchens – wherever the question of the Greenwich development raised its head like some kind of exotic perennial plant. It was obvious that the two resented control of a common area by an outsider. It threatened their sense of freedom.

"Why do they want to put a tourist attraction in a place like that?" MacKenzie asked. "Why can't they leave it like it is? I don't want anybody telling me where I can and can't go."

"Mucky-mucks," Palmer snorted, using the local epithet for the well-heeled tourists whom the development has been designed to attract.

Others are less concerned with the common good than with the threat the development represents to the land itself. Although the Greenwich wetland and dune system has sustained traditional local use – hunting, trapping, fishing – for nearly two hundred years, it nevertheless remains one of the least altered natural environments on the largely agrarian and densely settled Island. That fact makes its cause dear to those like Daryl Guignion who feel a need to commune with uncultivated nature. Guignion, a wildlife biologist who agreed to guide me through the dune, lives near Morell and came to Prince Edward Island seventeen years ago [in 1967]. "We, as Islanders, deserve a few sites to enjoy and to be able to say to our children, 'This is what it was like,'" he said, as we drove along the Greenwich Road.

As we passed the Cyril Sanderson place, Guignion spotted a red fox, surprised by our downwind arrival, its bright back a giveaway in the green grass. "It's a tremendous area for foxes because of the small mammals," explained Guignion. Meadow voles and jumping mice inhabit the dune, and deer mice, shrews and redbacked voles find their niches in the adjacent woodland.

The leading edge of the dune rose up ahead of us, a solid white wave travelling inland at the dreamlike pace of three to six metres (ten to twenty feet) per year, now breaking silently on a summer field, inexorably drowning it. Dead tops of white birch stuck up through the sand like gothic candelabra gracing an immense white tablecloth.

THE GREENWICH SYSTEM IS A WANDERING DUNE, making it unique to Prince Edward Island and a rarity along the Eastern Seaboard, where most dune systems have been stabilized. It is this distinction that makes it so important to those who, like Guignion, are concerned with preserving the natural heritage of the province.

We ambled through the undulating landforms: a cat's cradle of hummocks, some bald, others tufted with marram grass. Climbing to the top of a 10-metre- (32-feet-) high crest at the centre of the mobile portion of the dune, Guignion said, "Try to think of this as a fresh meadow – that's what it was several years ago when we first came here to do bird surveys."

We had a full view of the Gulf of St. Lawrence, where the local lobster fleet was spread out between the beach and the horizon. Inland, a scrub zone of marram grass graded into distant bayberry bushes and wind-twisted white spruce, a natural plant succession that can occur in as few as thirty years in the process of dune stabilization.

Below us was Bog Pond, one of three large ponds interlaced with the dune. The combination of dune and wetland and the unusual productivity of St. Peters Bay led to a recommendation in 1974 that the area be declared an ecological reserve under the International Biological Program.

Black ducks and teal worked the reedy shallows of Bog Pond. "These ponds are full of life. There's an incredible array of animals here," Guignion informed me, listing mink, fox, muskrat and raccoon. The diversity of wildlife has made the area a favourite haunt for generations of local trappers and hunters.

Guignion, a past president of the Island Nature Trust – a provincial organization dedicated to preserving the natural heritage of Prince Edward Island – doesn't find such traditional use incompatible with site preservation: "Part of the Trust's plan would include use by people, but at a level that wouldn't be detrimental to the plant and animal communities that are there. We feel traditional use is quite compatible with preservation as long as it is monitored."

Even though the dune has been designated as an environmental protection area, there is little actual protection. It is, on paper at least, private property, but people come and go at will. This practise has led to depredation of the dune, especially from the increased use of all-terrain vehicles in recent years. I had seen two of the three-wheeled variety parked in a Greenwich Road yard.

After my firsthand inspection of the dune, I spoke with Dr. Ian MacQuarrie, a colleague of Guignion in the University of Prince Edward Island's biology department and the Island's foremost authority on dune biota. He compared the vulnerability of dunes to Arctic tundra, pointing to studies which have shown that just ten people following a single course can cause damage for a whole season. Vehicle traffic can leave scars that remain visible for years. Scarring results from damage to the marram grass root system which forms a dense underground net binding the dune together. Once exposed, the root bundles are easily undermined by the wind. In dune terminology, a blowout occurs.

MacQuarrie feels that massive development like the Evans plan, cheek by jowl with an important wilderness area, constitutes "classic land-use conflict." Inevitably, he said, there would be a spillover of people from the residential complex and a destabilization of the dune. MacQuarrie emphasized the importance of reconciling environmental concerns with the very real human needs in the area.

Born on a small Island farm himself, and still a hobby farmer, MacQuarrie described his love of the land as "genetic." He elicited a heartfelt sympathy – admirable and surprising in one identified with the environmental movement – for the fate of St. Peters and Greenwich. "At one time," he said, "this was a very fine farming area. But because of the major changes that have happened, its down to a handful of farmers. You've got a generation of people who have watched their children grow up and leave. They're quite bitter about it. To see a closely knit rural society falling apart like that is quite depressing. So I have trouble getting mad at people up there who support the development."

Despite its scenic attributes, St. Peters Bay has held to the old ways of Island life based on farming and fishing, eschewing the trappings of tourism that typify so much of the Island's north shore (notably at Stanhope and Cavendish). "It's frustrating for people at this end of the province," Aquinas Ryan, St. Peters' village chairman, told me. "They have been concerned with keeping the land in production, while other areas have opted for tourist development. Now they feel they've lost out."

There are still opportunities to make a working life in St. Peters Bay, but realizing them demands a versatile exploitation of all seasons and even the vicissitudes of weather. Norbert Palmer, who for me epitomizes the St. Peters Bay survivor, likened the local economy to a bag of jelly beans: "You like the black ones, the black ones are good; then perhaps you get sick of them, and you have to eat the red ones."

Lobsters are Palmer's mainstay. But he seines mackerel in late summer and fishes bluefin tuna that migrate into Gulf waters in the fall. He traps eels in the estuaries, and when a storm blows onshore, he collects Irish moss – a plant used in food and pharmaceutical manufacturing. North winds uproot the red seaweed from offshore rocks and bring it ashore at Cable Head, and then men, women and children flock to the beach in pickups for the harvest.

When "there's a fair shake of moss," as Palmer says, gatherers can earn a hundred dollars a day. "Some people might be at it for only one storm. The area is free, and if you have time you can go at it – if it suits you."

Palmer has recently added fox farming to his seasonal cycle, but his sanguine picture of personal freedom based on economic opportunism does not apply equally to all St. Peters Bay residents. For many, the bag of jelly beans is ten weeks work, followed by forty weeks of unemployment insurance. It is a pattern familiar to many Maritime rural communities.

THE ONE EXPANDING SECTOR of the local economy, and the only alternative to tourism development, is mussel culture. St. Peters Bay has been famous for its mussel productivity since the nineteenth century, when farmers cut holes in ice and dredged the harbour bottom for "mussel mud." The grey beds of mussel shells were then spread on the fields as a limestone substitute. Today, strings of white buoys mark the area where clusters of mussels are suspended on plastic socks as they mature for market. But the future of the mussel industry, like most everything else I looked at in St. Peters Bay, depends on the uncertain fate of the Greenwich development.

One of those caught between the development and the growing mussel industry is Russel Dockendorf, a proud seventh generation Islander, the descendant of a British Empire Loyalist of German extraction. All of the Dockendorfs farmed until Russel's generation. "It came to the point where you had to mechanize, which meant a large expenditure, or you had to get out," he told me. Dockendorf chose the latter course, following a route taken by many Maritimers economically expatriated by the demise of the family farm. He worked in construction in Goose Bay, Labrador, then in Ontario.

In the end, his heart led him back to his Island home ("Ontario? I don't know," he reflected, "it's all right if you're born there I guess"). He turned to the sea for his livelihood, and, today, he fishes for lobster and owns the St. Peters Bay mussel leases. Ironically, his business is now threatened by an influx of outsiders.

"If that went ahead and they got a marina and all that, it would be a real nuisance," he said. Dockendorf is a quiet man who gives the impression of wanting to avoid a controversy. A conflict is inevitable, however, if the development does proceed, because the mussels are most productive in the deepest portions of the bay, the same areas best suited to boating. Dockendorf stands to lose half of this mussel-growing area. For now, the potential territorial dispute has been laid at the doorstep of the federal Department of Fisheries and Oceans.

Banking on government support for his position, Dockendorf recently invested in a mussel-processing facility for Greenwich. The expansion will double his full-time employees to ten and will add an equal number of seasonal jobs. There is room for even more growth, but a 1981 environmental-impact assessment of the Greenwich development – the first ever commissioned by the provincial government – estimated that, at best, the mussel industry could generate only one hundred jobs; the dune development, on the other hand, might offer as many as 150. The service jobs would be seasonal and largely taken by women. They might provide a second income for families, summer jobs for local college students or a means for more young people to settle in St. Peters, rather than drift away to Charlottetown or off the

Island entirely. As one civic-minded supporter of the development noted ironically: "We'll lose our identity unless we get some new blood."

Others worry, however, that a seasonal population will disrupt community integrity. "What I don't like," said Russel Dockendorf's son, Russel Jr., as we stood on the Red Head Wharf below the Dockendorf packing plant, looking across to the spring fields of Greenwich, "is the absolute distinction between the rich and the poor. You may find there's a fence at the entrance to Greenwich, and beyond that, you don't go unless you're going in to clean rooms."

I tried to imagine sails spangling the bay, golf carts scooting over the green fields and condominiums peeking out through manicured woods: an affluent, daytime-television community transplanted to a landscape shaped by the hard labour and frugality of descendants of Highland Scots.

Already the Island has seen what would have been unimaginable a generation ago. Since 1950, two thirds of the working farms have disappeared, a trend accelerated in the last two decades by potato monomania and the currency of the bigger-is-better philosophy. These factors made the decline of Greenwich possible in the first place, according to David Weale, a University of Prince Edward Island history professor who is writing a history of Island farming.

"The philosophy of the time was the small farmer couldn't make it. So when hotshots like Evans came along, they naturally sold out."

Weale served as secretary to Premier Angus MacLean, a blueberry farmer who promised, but couldn't deliver, a "rural renaissance" during a two year tenure of power that ended in 1981. Still, Weale holds on to the slim hope that the small Island farm will make a comeback and with it, communities like Greenwich. "It might be a bit visionary," he admitted, "but I would like to think that the land can still provide a living for more, rather than fewer, people."

It does seem a vision born more of wishful thinking than of any pragmatic scrutiny of reality. There are now only two working farms on the Greenwich Road, where, two decades ago [in the 1960s], the local creamery truck made stops at twenty farm gates twice a week.

One of the extant farms belongs to Robert Rossiter. While not the typical century-farm, bed-and-breakfast type property, it is still pleasantly bucolic. Ayrshires grazed in the pasture beside the long farm lane leading to a new bungalow and a steel sided barn. I chatted with Mary Rossiter about the Greenwich development as she unpacked groceries from her weekly shopping trip to the Co-op, the last of the three general stores that St. Peters once supported.

"I think it would be nice," she said. "St. Peters will be a ghost town in a couple of years. Most of the people are already senior citizens, and I think, my God, we really need something. What is around for the young people unless you farm or fish or get a little job at the store? There's nothing for them here. And it's not like it's going to be a casino, like a lot of people have been claiming. If it's going to keep people in the community and add some jobs, I can't see a thing wrong with it."

Though some Greenwich households are divided on the issue, the Rossiters' is not. When Robert joined us in the kitchen, he was emphatic. "I look at it this way: You can't have your cake and eat it too. I've got four kids; you can't just think of yourself." He doesn't give credence to the idea that the development conflicts with farming. The bushes growing up on the Land Development Corporation fields along the Greenwich Road are there, he said, simply because local farmers no longer want to farm them.

I drove on toward Hubert Sanderson's farm, the unpurchased link in the chain of properties that Evans needs in order to proceed with the development.

"It used to be a great farming section," Sanderson declared, setting two steaming cups of tea on the kitchen table, "but since the neighbouring farms have been sold, you really got nobody to go to for a helping hand. There used to be three of us here who worked together. To me, it's changed here – quite a change." A heaviness settled in his throat.

Sanderson has always maintained that he wouldn't stand in the way of development, only that he wanted a fair price for the farm in which he has invested thrity-three years of labour. If Evans does not buy his farm, Sanderson doubts whether any other farmer would be interested in it now, because the character of the community has been so altered. "I was too late in selling the place, and I guess that's why I'm struck here yet," he said.

Our talk turned to the dune, and Sanderson warmed to the memories of his childhood. In those days, he said, the foredunes were a hundred feet high, and he and his brothers would dangle over the edge trying to catch cliff swallows. Catastrophic winter storms toppled them in the 1930s. He remembered the old Acadian burial ground at the mouth of the bay, the chapel cellar where he and his father rid the farm of fieldstone and two eight-hectare fields – long lost features of the landscape that were, as he said, "all sanded over now."

He also remembered an axe that Leith Sanderson had stuck in a stump when a winter storm drove him home from the wood grove that stood where the dune is now. It was not until thirty-five years later that the rusted axe head and the rotten stub of the handle were found. The inexorable movement of the sand exposed it, just as it had buried it more than three decades earlier.

Sanderson's story of the buried axe struck me as having a lot in common with the Greenwich development. Since the proposal first surfaced two decades ago, it has exhibited a capacity for going underground, then resurfacing unexpectedly.[1]

Greenwich has become a powerful and persistent symbol of the loving care that Islanders hold for the land – a care lyrically expressed by the late Island laureate Milton Acorn: Nowhere that plowcut worms heal themselves in red loam; spruces squat, skirts in sand or the stones of a river rattle its dark tunnel under the elms is there a spot not measured by hands.

Regardless of the outcome of the Greenwich controversy, its tortuous history will stand as a testament of the Islanders' deeply rooted attachment to the land – their tie that binds.

---

1. In 1995, the provincial government made a land swap with St. Peters Estates which had bought the land from Evans in 1985. The dune system has since been given protection as an adjunct of Prince Edward Island National Park.

III. To the Islands

The Last Lighthouse Keeper

St. Paul Island, Nova Scotia

"IT WAS ONE OF THE BEST STORMS I've seen. We had a really good blow, so it was a good farewell to St. Paul," recalls head lightkeeper Paul Cranford of his last tour of duty on St. Paul Island, N.S. – a jagged upthrust of rock twenty-five kilometres off the northern tip of Cape Breton Island. The storm revived memories of his sixteen years on this lonely Atlantic outpost: of the lightkeepers who, like himself, called St. Paul home, and of chance visitors to this wild place – snowy owls, storm petrels, eagles, and harp seals barking from the ice floes that hem in the island for three months every winter. He remembered with a shudder his first summer on the island when he tried to circumnavigate St. Paul in a sea kayak and was nearly swept away by the strong currents coiling about the rocks that have been the undoing of so many unfortunate ships.

Before its automation on November 6, 1991, St. Paul was one of only eight lightstations in the Maritime Provinces that still had resident lighthouse keepers. The Canadian Coast Guard decided in 1986 to automate most of the eighty-seven lightstations in the Maritimes, including those in the Bay of Fundy, the southern Gulf of St. Lawrence and along Nova Scotia's eastern coast. Wholesale automation of the Maritime lightstations contrasts sharply with policy on the West Coast, where most lightkeepers have been retained. In Newfoundland, the Coast Guard has opted to retain keepers in the more remote locations; eventually, however, twenty-five of Newfoundland's fifty-six lightstations will be automated. The Canada Shipping Act originally stated that St. Paul must be staffed, but the Minister of Transport approved the lightstation's automation in the summer of 1991 and the coast guard moved quickly to shut it down before the ice and winter storms made the task more difficult. As if in protest, the wind blew, making it impossible for the coast guard to get there safely. The boarding up of the lightstation's residences – sealing a 150-year tradition of people on the island – will have to wait until spring 1992.

I RESOLVED TO VISIT ST. PAUL in 1990, while it still had its keepers, but reaching this wind-strafed island proved daunting. It took six months of waiting and then, on the verge of reaching my destination, the weather again threatened to repel me. My first attempt to reach this desolate island was blown away by an icy March nor'easter. In July, my seat was taken by a member of the Coast Guard maintenance crew, making a routine quarterly check of the lightstation's electronics. Then, in October, a tempest grounded the helicopters. As I stood by, the winds blew the wind sock at a menacingly horizontal angle. "I hope you have a strong stomach," remarked Coast Guard helicopter pilot Arnie Lewis as he greeted me at the Sydney airport. "The winds up there are pretty strong."

Lewis usually depends on weather reports from Environment Canada, which receives its information – visibility, wind direction and speed – continuously from an automated weather station on St. Paul Island. That day, however, the computer was out of order, so Lewis asked the coast guard in Sydney to get an on-the-spot radio report from the keepers on St. Paul.

Weather permitting, the pilot must make two trips to St. Paul – the first to deliver supplies and, on that occasion, myself, and the second to transport two relief keepers. Lewis confirmed that we were going to give it a try, despite a 40-knot gale. The wind buffeted our four-seater helicopter as we veered over the water while breakers angrily pounded the black slate below. Squalls drove sheets of rain, which beaded on the cockpit bubble, further obscuring the mist-shrouded Cape Breton Highlands. Off Cape North, I looked down to see a Great Lakes freighter labouring toward the Gulf of St. Lawrence. Then St. Paul itself loomed, its high back seemingly hunched against the storm's lashings.

Lights at both ends alert mariners to the frequently fogbound, 5-kilometre-long island. We passed over the fibreglass tower of the Southwest Point lightstation, automated in the early 1960s and now served by a solar-powered flashing light. The helicopter dipped behind the cliffs of the eastern shore, which peak at two hundred metres above the swirling sea. Around a headland appeared the islet at Northeast Point, with its cluster of white, red-roofed houses and outbuildings connected by wooden walkways that thread their way through rocky outcroppings. On another day, it might appear a spartan, even barren setting, but that day it was a welcome sight.

The helicopter touched down gently on the wooden landing pad on the islet, and there was a flurry of activity as supplies and bags were unloaded and others stowed aboard. I ducked my head under the blades and braced myself against the cutting wind. It was only after the helicopter lifted off to retrieve the relief keepers from Neils Harbour, fifty kilometres south on Cape Breton Island, that I made introductions with Paul Cranford, the head lightkeeper. "Typical tropical day on St. Paul," cracked Cranford, whose lanky blond hair was battened down by a toque. "Today was a touch-and-go day. As a matter of fact, I didn't think the chopper was coming."

There was time only for a brief tour of the island station and its light before the helicopter was due back with the relief keepers. The wind, gusting ever stronger, nearly tore the red door from its hinges as we entered the lighthouse and climbed the flights of steel stairs to the top of the 10-metre white concrete tower. The beacon stands on a rise forty metres above sea level, making its light visible twenty-eight kilometres out to sea. A more powerful light-and-lens system was replaced five years ago by a revolving light capable of being converted to solar power, a changeover scheduled for the summer of 1992.

The sea was in an angry mood: two-storey waves frothed at the island's grey footings of needle-sharp rocks and sent spray and foam scudding halfway up St. Paul's spruce-clad flanks. "Just imagine your boat coming ashore on those rocks," Cranford mused, as we stood in the lamp room. "You wouldn't have a chance, and if somehow you did make it ashore you'd find little to sustain you."

INDEED, THIS WAS THE WRETCHED predicament and tragic end of many mariners before the erection of a light on this island, which sits in Cabot Strait astride the principal shipping lane through the Gulf of St. Lawrence. It is an area bedevilled by squalls, ice, fog, unpredictable currents, and the regular batterings of the stormy Atlantic. On Canada's East Coast, St. Paul is second only to Sable Island, the "Graveyard of the Atlantic," in the number of ships and lives that it has claimed, earning itself a similar epithet – "Graveyard of the Gulf."

In 1829, Capt. John Lambly, harbourmaster of Quebec, declared the island of St. Paul to be "probably the most dangerous to shipping that is to be found on the coast of British America." In justifying his claim, he noted: "It has been the scene of innumerable wrecks since the first settlement of the colonies, many, perhaps most of which, are only told by the relics strewed upon the rocks." The worst of the recorded disasters involved the *Sovereign*, a troop ship on its way to England in 1814 carrying British soldiers who had served in the War of 1812 and their families. The ship was blown steadily off course and inexorably onto the jagged shores of St. Paul. Of the 811 men, women and children aboard, only a dozen men survived.

Many of those lucky enough to survive the wreckage of their ship and the frigid waters eventually succumbed to starvation on the uninhabited island, which is devoid of mammals and home principally to sea birds in breeding season. Such was the fate of the crew of the barque *Jessie* of Prince Edward Island. The little ship grounded on the island's southwest coast during a January snowstorm in 1825. Their ship was a total loss but the crew managed to scramble ashore and salvage enough provisions to survive for ten weeks, as ice hemmed in the island and precluded chances for rescue. When a sealing ship's crew from Cheticamp finally called at the island that spring, they found the grisly remains, including those of Capt. MacKay who, near death, had wrapped himself in an expensive cloak. One of the sealers laid claim to MacKay's cloak and, a few months later, was wearing it on the streets of Charlottetown when he was stopped by MacKay's widow, who until then had no evidence of her husband's fate. The sealer told his story – not an uncommon one as sealers from the Iles de la Madeleine and Cape Breton Island regularly visited the island's shores in the spring expressly to recover the spoils of the previous winter's wrecks. Mrs. MacKay immediately had a ship dispatched to St. Paul to recover her loved one's remains.

The poignant story of the *Jessie* captured public sentiment and increased pres-sure on politicians to do what had first been recommended by Quebec's Trinity House in 1817 – erect a lighthouse on St. Paul. (Between 1805 and Confederation, the administration of lighthouses in the Gulf of St. Lawrence was under the authority of the Quebec Trinity House, the only independent naval authority in the British colonies.)

"Good God! Can nothing be done to erect a lighthouse on that fatal island?" raged an editorial in the Charlottetown *Royal Gazette* in 1834. But the carnage continued as Lower Canada and the three Maritime colonies bickered over who would foot the bill. On a single night in 1835, four ships were wrecked on St. Paul.

Finally, two lighthouses were completed in 1839 – one on the tiny islet of rock fifty metres from the north end of the island, and the other at the southern tip. This did not end the harrowing history of this "fatal island," however. Much of that history in the 19th century was interwoven with that of the Campbell family, who rendered seventy-two years of service on this outpost, as son and grandson followed in the footsteps of John Campbell, a native of Argyleshire, Scotland. The eldest Campbell supervised the first lifesaving station established at Atlantic Cove, midway between the two lights. His role was often as tedious as it was essential: "Upwards of seven months without any communication with any part of the world," lamented Campbell. "Revolutions and great changes may occur, without hearing about it until it be over."

Crisis punctuated the long periods of inactivity, as on the night of May 30, 1856: "Remarkably dense fog all day – firing the gun constantly at intervals of four hours. Fired an extra round at ten o'clock at night. About ten minutes after the gun went off we heard the ringing of a bell. A ship was on the rocks."

Campbell managed to get his lifeboat launched, despite his belief "no boat could live in such a sea," and by morning he had plucked, "with great difficulty," seventy survivors from the wreckage. Seventy-two of the Irish passengers perished.

Sometimes the lightkeepers themselves met with disaster. The first keeper of the Northeast Light, Donald Boone, went in search of two of his men who had ventured onto the sea ice in February after a seal. At dusk, a northeastern gale blew up; Boone, the two men, and a servant girl who had joined him in the search, were never heard from again. It was four days before John Campbell came by on a regular visit and rescued Mrs. Boone and her infant.

On December 20, 1955, George Gatza, keeper of the Southwest Light, went to pay a visit to the keepers at the other end of the island. At the time, a self-operated cable car provided the perilous transport across the narrow strait called The Tickle that separates the northern islet from the main part of St. Paul. As Gatza pulled himself across, the cable broke and he plunged to his death. Sixteen years earlier, New Brunswick author Carle Rigby had written this ominous description of the crossing in a book on St. Paul Island: "It is quite an experience, when half way across the chasm, to look down at the boiling sea and consider what would happen should the cable or truck ever let go!" Rigby also recorded that in the 1890s the island was crossed by a road and several paths joining a school, a telegraph and post office and a lobster canning factory at Trinity Bay that employed more than fifty workers.

A bridge was constructed across The Tickle in 1914, but was destroyed within a few years by wind and ice. After the cable-car tragedy, there was no physical connection to the northern islet outpost, and the keepers rarely rowed to the main island, which, in sharp contrast to the lightkeeper's barren perch, is covered with such a thick mat of wind-stunted vegetation that getting around is a difficult task. In Cranford's time, the keepers used only one of the former family houses as a residence; the second served as Cranford's music room and a woodworking shop for his fellow keepers.

UNTIL ITS CLOSURE, four men kept the lightstation on a rotational basis. Cranford, who first came to St. Paul in 1975 when there was still a light-keeping family living on the island year-round, believes the one-month-on, one-month-off system was better "in terms of morale and keeping the station maintained. It tended to keep you fresh." Though Cranford himself never suffered cabin-fever on the tiny islet, he once saw a fellow keeper "crack" under the strain of isolation when the helicopter failed to make a scheduled keeper change. That keeper subsequently transferred to a mainland station.

The two men on the island were on duty round the clock, each working a 12-hour shift. Cranford rose at 6:00 a.m., had breakfast, then went "up the hill" to check the equipment, including the three diesel engines that power the light. He called in the weather report at 9:15 a.m., and if there was no routine maintenance to be done that day, the rest of the time was his to use as he wished. Cranford, a musician and musicologist, immersed himself in the music of Cape Breton, Scotland and Ireland. He both collects and pub-lishes traditional music (using a desktop computer) and composes tunes on his 1870 fiddle. "I really liked the job," says Cranford. "I think it was the same with the other fellows. They enjoyed it and tried to make the most of their time. For me it was ideal for composing music. I'm a very fortunate man."

On occasion, the keepers have been called upon to respond to an emergency, such as when two Nova Scotia-based fishing boats foundered in the Gulf in De-cember 1989. They kept an all-night vigil in the light tower trying in vain to make visual contact with the vessels, which sank off Newfoundland's south coast. On other occasions, they have passed on radio messages for boats when the high-backed island prevented direct transmission to the mainland. "Once in a long while during lobster season a local fisherman got a hold of you by VHF or CB, and you gave him lube oil or diesel fuel to help him get home," says Cranford.

But the days of lightkeepers actually putting to sea to save the occupants of sinking boats, as the men at the life-saving station did, are long gone. In fact, officially, life-saving has never been a role of lightkeepers. In the case of St. Paul, it would have been difficult to put to sea, even if the keeper had chosen to. The skidway was destroyed by a storm in 1976, and the block and tackle used to haul up boats was removed the following year. During Cranford's last years on the island, there was no seaworthy craft other than a small skiff built by one of his fellow keepers.

After March 1992, the target date for full automation of the Maritime region, there will be only four staffed lightstations, attended by sixteen lightkeepers – at Cape Forchu, N.S., and Letete Passage, Gannet Rock and Machias Seal Island, N.B. Only two lightstations are likely to retain keepers, both in the Bay of Fundy. Lightkeepers on Machias Seal Island will lend support to Canada's claim of sovereignty in an area of disputed marine boundaries between Canada and the United States. After bidding farewell to St. Paul Island, Cranford became the assistant head keeper on Machias Seal Island and spent his first Christmas there in 1991. Fishermen from Grand Manan Island effectively lobbied for the retention of lightkeepers at Gannet Rock, the major sentinel over an area of intensive fishing. Eventually, however, all lightstations in the Maritimes may be automated, as was the once untouchable St. Paul.[1]

"Automation is a definite money-saver for us," says Dave Smith, regional superintendant of Marine Navigation Services, who estimates that the Coast Guard has saved more than $3 million in lightkeepers' salaries and maintenance and service costs since automation began. "We really don't feel that there was any reason to leave the lightkeepers on St. Paul," Smith says. "It's off the beaten track for pleasure boaters because they like to keep close to the Cape Breton coast. With today's navigational systems, there is no need for lightkeepers on the island anymore."

St. Paul, in fact, had been automated and monitored remotely by Coast Guard radio in Sydney for several years. Cranford and the other keepers performed only minor duties – painting the houses, checking fuel levels, phoning in weather reports – and kept watch on the operation of the light. There are now six central monitoring stations in the Maritime region keeping an electronic eye on the eighty-seven lightstations. The INTRAC computer keeps track of sixteen status points, including the operation of the

---

1. Machias Seal Island is the only remaining staffed lighstation in the Maritimes. Paul Cranford is one of the lightkeepers.

light and fog horn, checking the fuel levels of the diesel generators, and detecting if a break-in occurs at one of the lighthouses. An electronic eye even measures visibility in fog by calibrating the distance at which light is reflected back off the moisture in the air. "This system tells us right away if something is wrong," says Norman Porter, retired co-ordinator for the Coast Guard's lightstation monitoring program. He points out that this was not always the case even when the majority of lights were staffed, because the lightkeeper might be sleeping or away from the lighthouse for several hours. The system includes remote controls that let mainland personnel turn on the emergency light or standby generator. In short, the automated system appears to make lightkeepers redundant.

In the face of these arguments for technological progress, some sea-goers oppose the removal of lightkeepers from remote and dangerous locations such as St. Paul Island. The fishermen of Bay St. Lawrence, at the northern tip of Cape Breton Island, vociferously opposed automation of St. Paul when it was first suggested by the coast guard several years ago. "It's a shame they pulled the men off of there," says Freeman Morrison, a 49-year-old fisherman from Dingwall, whose father was the last lightkeeper at Southwest Point. "If you did run into trouble out there – and it's happened – the lightkeeper was always there." Morrison himself once received aid from the St. Paul lightkeepers when his battery failed and they lent him one to get home.

"There will probably be a disaster over the years, something will definitely take place if there's no one there to assist the fishermen," says Morrison, who describes staff on the islands as "a security blanket" for those who go to sea.

THE SOUND OF helicopter blades whipping the air reminded me that my brief visit to this lonely rock was nearly over. The keepers heard the noise and sprang into action. In his haste, Cranford dropped his fiddle case, but there was no time to check for damage. The relief keepers scrambled out and we took their places in the helicopter. "It wasn't so bad over the water," pilot Lewis informed us, "but it was a rough landing at Neils Harbour." We lifted off. Below, the seagirt rock where the Northeast Light perches was rimmed with tempestuous froth. As we approached the looming Cape Breton Highlands, I was acutely aware that the ritual of the changing of the lightkeepers is rapidly becoming another casualty of technological change, even here where the sea has exacted such a dreadful toll. For men like Cranford, the passage of such a tradition into history has become the stuff of lament, memorialized only by the mournful, elegiac sound of his fiddle. When Cranford's final shift neared completion last November, sad emotions found expression in two poignantly titled laments for fiddle: *Memories of St. Paul Island* and *Graveyard of the Gulf.*

Of Cabbages and Kings
Big Tancook Island, Nova Scotia

When the sauerkraut begins to smell,
    and it can't smell no smeller,
We take it from the barrel that's a-way
    down in the cellar,
We put him in the kettle, and it begins
    to boil,
So help me we can smell her round for
    40,000 mile.

           – "Sauerkraut Song,"
           from *Out of Old Nova Scotia Kitchens.*

"THERE USED TO BE A LOT OF CABBAGE here on this Island once," says Calvin Hutt, his husky voice and burly frame filling the low-ceilinged kitchen. "My God, man, don't you talk. We used to have nothing under five or six hundred dozen. Some fellows would have a thousand dozen, twelve hundred dozen, and they all went to Halifax. Now, you see, there was one time, most of them was shipped to the West Indies on them big boats – lady boats, they used to call them, those white ocean liners. Now, when that was given up, it was only down to Halifax to sell them to the wholesalers."

On Big Tancook Island, at one time considered the sauerkraut capital of Nova Scotia, Hutt was once known as The Sauerkraut King. Now in his early seventies, he is old enough to remember the days when cabbage was the economic cornerstone of island life. The biggest heads were shipped on two-masted schooners to Halifax, a four hour trip with a good breeze behind you. The smaller cabbage were cut into kraut and packed in hundred pound half barrels for export to the West Indies or for ready sale on mainland Nova Scotia. "Yes, we made lot of kraut," says Hutt. "One year we put in five hundred half-barrels – used to hold about ten gallons."

Hutt looks out the window at farm fields now gone back to alder and thistle, a grey scene made even bleaker by the low ceiling of grey Atlantic sky, and recalls a more pastoral season: "When we was making hay, we could hardly see each other, there was that much hay," he recalls. "We'd fill that barn up to where the swallows went in. Man dear, this used to be some place in the fall of the year, when the grass was taken off, and all the cattle was out on the land. Every fellow had his field fenced off, there was a lot of shareholders on this island, good croppers. In the fall of the year, pretty near everyplace you went past some fellow was cuttin' in sauerkraut. Yeah, pretty near everybody who had any land at all planted some cabbage."

In Nova Scotia, sauerkraut is generally associated with the South Shore, especially Lunenburg County, where German farmers were enticed in the early 1750s in order to feed the Cockney settlers and soldiers of the nearby garrison in Halifax. Among the staples the Germans supplied were cabbage, either fresh or in the fermented form of sauerkraut. Over the years, however, it became clear that the best sauerkraut did not come from the mainland but from a small island in Chester Basin – Big Tancook, one of 365 islands that stipple Mahone Bay. There are now fewer than a handful of cabbage growers and *Krautmeisters* on Big Tancook, but to sauer-kraut lovers in Blue-nose country, the Tancook name is still synonymous with quality. My purpose in coming to Tancook was to find out how Tancookers made their famous kraut.

BIG TANCOOK ISLAND, midway along the drowned coastline of Nova Scotia's South Shore, was first charted by the pioneer Atlantic cartographer,

Joseph Frederick Wallet Des Barres, in 1760. He christened it Royal George in honour of his patron, George III. The island's first settlers, perhaps owing to their German ancestry or to a simple lack of pomposity, rejected this British appellation in favour of the Mi'kmaq name, Tancook, which means "facing the sea" – even though, from earliest days, Tancook Islanders did not look to the sea for their livelihood. In 1829 Thomas Chandler Haliburton noted that the residents of "The Great Tancook . . . derive their subsistence wholly from tilling the land." During the Age of Sail, Tancook did gain a measure of maritime renown for the design of the schooner-rigged Tancook whaler, a speedy and sturdy craft as well suited to racing as to fishing. But it was still farming, not fishing, that provided the islands's principal occupation. It was not until the twentieth century that the sea began to dominate Tancook life. Today, fishing for lobster, cod, mackerel and herring has brought a new prosperity to many Tancook households and, in the process, decline to the island's traditional sauerkraut industry.

"The younger people on Tancook today are earning five times the money fishing that they can earn cuttin' in sauerkraut," says Arthur Stevens, the retired captain of the Tancook ferry, who still cuts in a few tonnes by hand every year for faithful mainland customers. "It's really not a money making thing, but it's an art that you hate to drop. I've got a feeling that it won't be many years when there'll be none at all on Tancook,"

Even the largest of the four remaining commercial Tancook *Krautmeisters*, John Cross, now considers kraut merely a sideline to his wage-earning job as a ferry deckhand. "There isn't money enough in it. I don't think if you counted your hours that you'd make $2 an hour at this."

In 1985, Cross netted $2,000 on his production of five to six thousand tonnes. Just a few years ago, Cross produced twice as much of his sought-after kraut, and twenty years ago, John's father used to keep a truck on the road peddling kraut under the E. & E. Cross label to the Halifax-Dartmouth area. Today, John's kraut is marketed by Hilchie Brothers in Chester, NS. Most of it sold in 5- to 30-pound buckets to general stores in eastern and northern Nova Scotia. "John makes real good kraut, his father did, too," says George Hilchie from his cramped waterfront office in Chester. "It comes up through the family." In the late 1940s, Hilchie's wholesale business moved more kraut than fish. Now the opposite is true. "It's a big dish but it's not as big as it used to be. Like you know, we used to sell a lot of salt herring and salt mackerel at one time. Now, the young people, two of them are working, got a microwave oven and they don't go into cooking herring or sauerkraut or stuff like that, and sales have dropped off from what they used to be years ago."

Despite changing tastes, Hilchie can sell all the kraut Cross makes and then some. Cross ships his kraut aboard the steel-hulled ferry that daily services Big Tancook and its diminutive neighbour, Little Tancook. It docks in picturesque Chester harbour and can carry freight and 150 passengers (nearly the entire population of the Islands).

Chester has none of the practical demeanour of the nearby famous fishing port of Lunenburg. It is the most New Englandish of Maritime towns. Boutiques outnumber the stores, and most of the Cape Island fishing boats anchored in the harbour have been converted to pleasure craft and are anchored in the harbour alongside a flotilla of expensive and colourful sailing yachts.

The fare for the two-hour round trip from Chester to Big Tancook is $1. After we steamed out of the harbour, flanked by peninsulas that provide a prospect of the sea for oversize Cape Cod houses, neatly shuttered and trimmed, manicured lawns rolling primly toward the shore like giant welcome mats, I turned my attention to the ferry bulletin board. Cod nets were advertised for $75. Bingo night promised a $100 jackpot. There were the cards of two competing satellite dish dealers posted alongside a notice about the dance to be held at the Tancook Recreation Centre, featuring a group named for a locally famous schooner, *Nyanza*.

We docked briefly at Little Tancook wharf, then shuttled over to Big Tancook, a collection of nearly flat topped, straight up-and-down houses I have always admired for their wonderful simplicity. Our first glimpse of the island was like a child's drawing; the houses seemed drawn with a penchant for bright colours and clean lines. There were aqua clapboard houses with aqua fences, there were mustard houses, even robin's-egg-blue houses, built into a hillside that sloped toward the harbour. As bright as the houses were, they were less garish than some of the boats. Nestled side by side within the protective L-shape of the wharf were lavender, lime green and pink fishing boats. Obviously, here was a community unfettered by mainland conservatism.

On the wharf to greet me was John Cross, a short, smiling man in his early forties, whose ancestors arrived on these shores more than a century before, bearing the surname Kraus and the Old World *Krautmeister's* secrets.

"What would you like to do?" he asked. "Maybe see the cabbage patch first."

In his black Ford pickup, we thundered over the pot-holed road toward the centre of the island. Three miles long and no more than a mile across at its widest point, Big Tancook is a comma-shaped islet that is perpetually sprinkled by Atlantic salt. Island vehicles hang onto their chassis by the thinnest of rusty threads. The corroded bodies flap like tattered rags as if they were going to lift into flight, and I guessed that there was not a muffler intact on the island nor a car that would pass a safety inspection. Like most islanders, John keeps a car on the mainland for highway driving and runs his truck on the five miles of island dirt road by whatever desperate means available.

We crested a hill and coasted to a stop at the bottom. John's half acre is the only sizeable cabbage patch on an island that a generation ago was boldly striped with fields of bulbous brassica. John's father also kept a dozen head of beef cattle; now there is not even a milk cow on the island and derelict trucks have replaced the oxcart. John has had to substitute commercial fertilizer for manure, although like his father, he still supplies organic content to his soil by collecting rock weed along the beach after winter storms. And despite islanders' abandonment of the land, many Tancook backyards boast at least a row of cabbage, enough to satisfy the undiminished island taste for freshly fermented kraut.

Although a late spring and too much rain in June, followed by an extremely dry summer, had conspired to stunt John's crop, there were some very handsome blue-green heads among his 5,000 plants. And Tancook cabbages have long been noted for their exceptional size. Judge DesBrisay, island hopper and amateur horticulturist, remarked on two Tancook Brobdingnagians in his *History of Lunenburg County*: "In November, 1894, Mr.

Sylvester Baker of the Island [Big Tancook] pulled two [cabbages] from his field, one of which weighted 25^1/$_2$ pounds and the another 23^1/$_2$ pounds."

On the mainland, "Danish Baldhead" and "April Green" are the favoured cabbage seed of commercial krautmeisters. On Tancook the the cabbages have a homegrown pedigree."You might as well say that this is the old type of Tancook cabbage," John says, as he selects the largest heads, lops off the outer whorl of leaves and tosses the squeaky, 5-pound missiles unceremoniously into the back of his pickup. "It's not like any kind you're going to find in those seed houses."

John's cabbage is a peculiar Tancook hybrid. When he took over the sauerkraut-making duties from his father a decade ago, most commercial growers on the island had already gone out of business. Wisely, John rescued a couple of cabbage from each of the island's best kraut makers' kitchen gardens, planted these together in the small seed plot behind his bungalow and has used their cross-pollinated stock as a seed source ever since. John doesn't know just how far back into the mists of time the lineage of this Tancook variety of cabbage reaches. But it probably pre-dates his grandfather and may have its origin in cabbage seed that his German ancestors brought across the Atlantic in the 1750s.

John stores his cabbage with the roots intact in two of the last cabbage houses on the island. They are derelict though still serviceable structures, with fieldstone basements and eaves that touch the ground. The roofs were once double-boarded and filled with an insulating layer of sawdust but now the inside boards hang loose, and the roof is covered with eelgrass for insulation. On the coldest days, John installs a kerosene heater to prevent the cabbage from freezing.

In the spring, he selects a half dozen of the previous season's best heads and replants them. He scores the head with a deeply cut X, out of which bolts a six-foot seed stock. In the fall, he harvests the seed pods, and the Tancook cultivar is perpetuated for another season.

The Tancook hybrid is a late cabbage – planted the first of June it is not ready for harvest until mid-October or later – and perhaps the fame of Tancook kraut has something to do with its hand-me-down horticultural pedigree. Calvin Hutt thinks so: "See, we raised all late cabbage, where on 'the main' [Tancook for mainland] they raise mostly all early cabbage. There's a lot of difference between late and early cabbage for sauerkraut. Early cabbage isn't as good: it doesn't keep like the late kraut, it gets softer. Late cabbage stays better, firmer. We stuck to the late."

The excellence of Tancook kraut may also have something to do with the sure hands of the Tancook *Krautmeisters*, who seem to have practised a kind of legerdemain. Kraut making is as much an art as it is a science. I tried in vain to acquire a written recipe for Tancook sauerkraut, but none exists on the island. The right way to make kraut has been passed on from generation to generation, like the rhymes of a ballad, with no apparent need for a more permanent record of proportions or method. When there were many commercial kraut operations on the island, each maker's formula was a jealously guarded secret. With only four *Krautmeisters* left, the Tancook method is in jeopardy of becoming a lost legacy.

THE INGREDIENTS COULD NOT BE SIMPLER: shredded cabbage, salt and water. There is no vinegar added to sauerkraut; the mixture makes its own "vinegar," actually lactic and ascorbic acid. This accounts for the sour tang and provides a good source of Vitamin C, which recommended it as a scurvy cure in the days of sail. Just how sour the kraut gets depends upon the relative proportions of these ingredients and the ageing of the kraut. Tancook kraut is not very sour at all.

In John's kraut-making room – a garage-like addition to the back of his house – preparation begins with trimming the cabbage head. Using a filleting knife, John cuts off about an inch of the stump, then peels back the outer whorls of green leaf with quick flicks of the blade. He removes the outer leaves to get rid of any impurities – dirt, blemishes – but also for aesthetic reasons. "You get clear of the green," he says, "it makes a whiter sauerkraut."

He then splits the stump three times, so that it will shred more easily. Some makers core the stump out completely, but John thinks that the stump has a better, milder flavour than the cabbage itself. "That's just my opinion," he says.

The kraut makers term for grating is "cutting-in." John cuts in between five hundred and a thousand pounds at a time. In the old days, all the cutting-in was done by hand using a "kraut knife," a simple device consisting of a wooden base with two blades set in it like the blades of a wood plane. (One blade will suffice but will only cut the cabbage half as fast.) Two small rails running along the edge of this base provide a trackway for a bottomless box frame big enough to hold a good size cabbage head. The cabbage is shredded by being placed in the box and drawn back and forth over the blades. John's kraut knife was three feet long, a foot wide, and made of pitch pine. Now little more than a curious bit of Nova Scotiana, in its working days it cut countless tons of cabbage. Vincent Stevens, not a day under seventy himself, told me that in his prime he could cut in a ton a day by hand, and only the day before, he had cut in several hundred pounds. "It's hard work, hard on your back and your arms. It's all right when you're a young fellow but when you get up in years like I am . . . . "

Today's large producers have opted for automatic cutters, albeit most of them homemade. John's father built the one John now uses. Powered by a small electric motor, the drive shaft is run off pulleys. The cutters are two scythe blades mounted on top of a vertical shaft like the blades of a propeller. A barrel top serves as a hopper, into which John feeds the cleaned heads, each head on its side to produce a longer, finer cut. "I try to get it as fine as possible," says John. The shredded cabbage falls into a bin, filling the garage with the clean smell of coleslaw. With his motorized cutter, John can cut in a ton in an hour.

Although the colour and shred of the cabbage may be important aesthetic qualities, the step that follows cutting-in is ultimately more important to the taste of the finished product. John packs and salts his cabbage in huge wooden puncheons, the largest of which holds a thousand pounds. John calls them "cherry barrels," but something more powerful than cherries may once have lined them, considering that Nova Scotia's South Shore was once as famed for rum running as for kraut making. He first applies melted paraffin wax to the inside of the barrel with a paintbrush – a sanitary measure, he says. Although the kraut is effectively sealed from contact with the wood, John maintains that "it gets a better flavour out of wooden barrels than say plastic or fibreglass." This has less to do with the kraut picking up flavour from the barrel than with the fact that wooden barrels maintain a more constant temperature, an important factor in the making of kraut—too much heat can cause spoilage, too little can retard fermentation.

John packs the cabbage in layers of four to six inches in depth, then compresses each layer by tapping it with a large maul. Some still use a wooden stamper that resembles the old fashioned butter churn. At one time, the cabbage was compressed by being stomped on with bare feet, like grapes. This may be more lore than historical fact but Tancook children, who still travel by ferry to high school in Chester, have to endure the mainlanders' sobriquet "Sauerkraut Stompers."

John sprinkles only a shallow handful of coarse salt on each layer of cabbage. "The more salt you put in it the more sour it'll get," he says. "You don't want to get it too sour." In search of the elusive recipe, I note that he uses about a handful of salt to every fifty pounds of cabbage. But this is not a hard-and-fast ratio either, as John points out. Depending on the time of the year, he uses more or less salt. For instance, he uses more in the fall when the weather is warmer, to retard the speed of fermentation, and less if it has been a particularly wet season and he wants to control the amount of brine the cabbage will make.

In John's opinion, the best type of salt was Turk's Island salt, but he can no longer get it. He now uses the same fishery coarse salt that island fishermen use to salt cod. He tried fine salt, but found it had a tendency to soften the cabbage because it dissolved more quickly. Salt keeps the kraut crisp by drawing juices from the cabbage – which is 90 percent water.

Left for twenty-four hours, salted cabbage will make its own brine. However, John prefers to add a little water after he has packed the barrel to the top in alternate layers of cabbage and salt. "I might use a little more water than some," says John. The more salt you put on the cabbage, the less water you will have to add, but also, the sourer the kraut: a delicate trade-off. John's goal is to avoid making the kraut either too salty or too sour. "I like something that you can take a bowl out and take a fork and sit down and just eat it raw," which is not the type of astringent kraut one remembers reluctantly eating as child. For cooking, John says, most people prefer a more sour kraut. As with maple syrup, it is a matter of taste: some people like strong-tasting, vinegary kraut, others prefer a lighter tasting kraut. John adds five three-and-a-half-gallon pails of water to a 500-pound batch of salt-ed cabbage.

The last step is to cover the kraut and weigh it down to ensure that the cabbage is always immersed in the brine. John stretches clean plastic over the top of the puncheon, fits over it a piece of plywood cut to the inside di-mension of the barrel, then weighs the cover down with a chest-sized, smooth beachstone – or "popple stone," as it is called on the island. The word (one of many in a rich local dialect) probably derives from the verb meaning "to heave – as in choppy sea." The sea washes the stone smooth as a plate, which is why John prefers it to rough granite that collects dirt. Main-landers might not be able to duplicate his recipe without the popple stone, John jokes, but he adds that weighting the cabbage by some means is essen-tial. The weight forces from the cabbage juices containing natural sugars that are the fuel of the fermentation process. Also, the weight ensures that the cabbage remains immersed under the brine. If the cabbage were allowed to float to the top of the brine, it would probably become contaminated with yeast mould and turn an unappetizing "black and all the colours of the rain-bow."

After salting and weighting, there is little to do until the cabbage is fin-ished fermenting, usually in two to three weeks. John does check to see that his barrels aren't leaking, or that the powerful, gas-producing fermentation hasn't blown off one of the barrel hoops – not an uncommon an occurrence, it seems. "That's why I've always got spare hooping around," he says.

Two weeks after my first visit, I returned to Tancook to sample John's kraut. The clean smell of coleslaw that had perfumed John's garage on my last visit had been replaced by a slightly illicit whiff of fermentation. I dipped out a handful of the finished sauerkraut, noting that its colour was the same as the freshly cut cabbage – a delicate white with a hint of pale yellow. Its taste had just the right tartness for my liking. This was the real thing, I thought: Tancook kraut, kraut without the "sauer."

"Good," I said. "It's not sour at all."

John smiled: "I think it's got a good flavour to it. It's not real strong. You could eat it whichever way you wanted to. You could cook it, you could eat it raw, some people fry it. You could use it much the same as a salad, like a coleslaw if you wanted to, whereas if it was real strong the only way you could eat it is if you cooked it."

Most islanders will tell you they prefer to eat their sauerkraut "ror" – raw, that is. If they do subject their delicate kraut to cooking, they simply boil it with corned beef. However they choose to eat it, it must be kraut made by Tancook *Krautmeisters* from cabbage grown on Tancook. They will brook no substitute.

When I went to the wharf to catch the ferry on Sunday, John was dressed for duty in his navy blue deckhand's uniform, transformed from *Krautmeister* to mariner as were so many Tancook Islanders before him. But as a newly-made mainland convert, I carried his secret in my right hand – a 30-pound bucket of Big Tancook Sauerkraut.

The Glory and the Grit
Grand Manan, New Brunswick

GRAND MANAN REVEALS ITSELF SLOWLY. I did not so much as catch a glimpse of the island before the ferry *Lady Menane* nestled against the pylons of the berth at North Head, after our two hour fog-bound passage from Black's Harbour, New Brunswick. Then the Bay of Fundy fog hung over the island in stubborn billows for the next week, enhancing the elusive character of this island which for most mainlanders is a place permanently shrouded in mystery.

For those better acquainted with the island's virtues, it is a well-guarded secret. Year after year, for decades, painters and photographers have been drawn to the vistas of spruce-crowned capes receding into sea mist, the becalmed harbours bustling with boats, the wooden manors of 19th-century sea captains and the smokehouses poised on stilts above the Fundy tides. Generations of birders have found Grand Manan a place of wonder: even John James Audubon was impressed with the 275 species found there and did some of his sketches on the island. Latter-day naturalists come to see what may be the world's rarest whale, the North Atlantic right whale, which summers in the Bay of Fundy. Willa Cather, the great American novelist of the early twentieth century, was so taken with the island's charm and quietude that she chose it as a spot to write many of her books. For all, it has been and remains a place to jettison the concerns of the mainstream, to be alone with nature and oneself, a true island of the spirit.

For some the qualities that set Grand Manan apart from "the main" are enough to qualify the island as a country of its own – and reason enough to make preserving the island way of life a common cause among Grand Mananers, born or naturalized. One of these proud island patriots is fisherman David Outhouse who grew up on the other side of the Bay of Fundy at Tiverton, on Long Island. Owner of a herring seiner, he is often away fishing at night, but I caught him home relaxing during the day. In the driveway was a vintage, canary yellow Cadillac and in the yard was a flagpole flying an unfamiliar ensign: boat, lighthouse and maple leaf set off against a field of sea-blue.

"I had an idea always about wanting a Grand Manan flag," he explained. "I always figured Grand Manan was a special place, set off by itself. It's sort of a unique place."

He paused to reflect on his own meaning: "Well, it kind of rolls you back in time, maybe, when you come here. And I like it the way it is. I hate to see any changes in it. So I thought it would be nice if Grand Manan had its own flag."

Wedge-shaped in profile, the island kingdom of Grand Manan is twenty-five kilometres long and twelve kilometres wide. It is the largest of an archipelago of twenty islands straddling the Bay of Fundy and Gulf of Maine boundary. Passamaquoddy Indians from Maine simply called it Mun-a-nook or "island in the sea." Twelve kilometres from West Quoddy Head, the easternmost point of the United States, and thirty-seven kilometres from mainland New Brunswick, it is far enough from either shore for the people to have developed their own distinctive character and independence of political spirit. Descendants of United Empire Loyalists who settled the island in 1784, Grand Mananers do not think of themselves as just New Brunswickers. They are Islanders first. They are Canadians, to be sure and proud of it, but with enough close family and business ties to Maine to render their speech most reminiscent of that of New Englanders. As one woman explained in the mellow tones one hears throughout the island: "Gen'ly, we ah a bit soft on the ahs."

But whatever else the alliance, to be an Islander is first and foremost to be allied to the sea. Disembarking from the ferry at North Head, visitors inevitably saunter down to the wharf to look over the fleet of seiners and longliners, trawlers and draggers, instinctively drawn close to that which makes the island tick. It was there, on my first trip to Grand Manan, that I met Floyd Brown, now eighty-four, a retired lobster fisherman and weir owner. He is on the wharf most days, keeping track of the comings and goings, and he is generally willing to discuss Grand Manan's privileged place in the fisherman's universe.

"Around here, there's always something different." he said. "They go netting fish and line fishing – for cod, pollack, hake and haddock – and they got seiners and weirs, of course. Then there's lobster and scallops. And if you get right up against it, you can go clamming. There's lots of places they only got one thing. When it goes down, you're out of luck. Here, there's always something to go to."

The diversity of sea resources, fuelled by tidal upwellings at the mouth of the Bay of Fundy, makes Grand Manan a prosperous place by Maritime standards; there are few "poor-mouthing" fishermen to be found. Grand Manan is the only Maritime offshore island that has been able to maintain the population base it established in the 1880s when herring stocks boomed.

Like their ancestors before them, many Grand Mananers still fish with a primitive device called a weir, or "ware," as it is pronounced on Grand Manan. These heart-shaped pens, which at a distance look like gossamer colosseums, are connected to the shore by a long line of twine-strung poles called the fence. When the herring follow the flood tide inshore at night, they strike the weir fence and follow it offshore in an effort to go around the obstruction. Instead, the fence leads the school in through an infinite figure eight, the hooks of the enclosure constantly leading them back into its centre. The Islanders are proud of the weirs and name them as they might a boat: Sea Wall, The Dream, North Air.

FISHING BY WEIR, explained Brown, "is the worst damn gamble you ever seen." Some years he said, a weir may not "fish" at all; other years, the same weir may be full nearly every tide. It is then that the island's debts are paid off, new cars and boats are purchased and the kids get a holiday in Disneyland.

I once witnessed a big payday at one of the island's largest and most whimsically named weirs, The Mumps. Struggling against the racing tide, fishermen worked from dories to set a purse seine around the inside perimeter of the weir. That task completed, a rope strung through rings around the bottom of the net was drawn in, or pursed, thus enclosing the fish inside a giant bag. As the net was raised to the surface, the water under the boat turned a cloudy green. Millions of iridescent herring scales floated in the water like a galaxy of rhinestones. Six fishermen clutched the net's cotton mesh with white-knuckled determination and leaned their collective weight into raising the bounty of fish. As the tide and teeming fish slowly yielded to man and machine, the scene before me – viewed from the seine skiff's cabin roof – was magically transformed: the sea was drying up. Instead of water, there were fish, a seething, electrifying mass of herring. Those on the surface, suddenly finding themselves out of their element, flapped desperately against one another, beating the scales from their silver bodies in a death throe that created a milky plume which steadily expanded toward the perimeter of the weir. One of the fishermen, pausing in his labours, glanced up at me and said, "Isn't it a pretty sight when they dance like that? It makes them scale better when they dance too."

Before the day was over, I had watched 115,000 kilos of herring pumped from The Mumps – a haul worth $23,000 to the weir's five partners.

The small herring were destined for a sardine factory in Maine. In the nineteenth century, before the canning process was developed, small fish were either discarded or used as fertilizer or a source of oil. Large herring were preferred for the burgeoning smoked herring trade in Europe and West Indies. In 1884, 8 million kilos of smoked herring were shipped from Grand Manan, making it the world's largest producer. While the market for smoked herring lasted, the half dozen small villages that hug the low-lying eastern shore of the island enjoyed unusual prosperity.

A century later, many of the weathered smokehouses perched above the water in Woodwards Cove serve only as billboards for adolescent graffiti. But puffs of pungent smoke have been issuing from under the roof caps of more and more smokehouses in recent years, promising a partial revival, if not a full-fledged return, of the industry that was once the cornerstone of the island's economy.

Hovey Russell, one of those anticipating a turn in the fortunes of smoked herring, has reopened some of the smokehouses in which he learned the arcane art from his father. An alchemical essence – earth, air, fire and water – emanates from the dark doors of Russell's buildings. A hundred years old, their very timbers are preserved in herring oil.

"Smells good, doesn't it?" a worker remarked as he went about his morning routine of laying fires. Half-cured herring hung above him, tier upon tier, in amber legions that seemed to glow with their own light, like the smoky chimneys of thousands of low-burning lamps.

The fire builder made small piles of kindling, slab wood and sawdust on the gravel floor. With a shot of oil and the touch of a torch, the fires blazed up momentarily, then died down to begin their daylong smouldering.

Russell – now in his sixties – learned how to smoke herring at the age of thirteen. "The fire has to burn low, no blaze to it whatsoever. You can burn them too. You have to watch what you're doing, all right," he said, indicating the brine tanks where the herring are salted before being strung on pointed sticks for hanging in the smokehouse.

"If all goes right, the finished product is ready for eating in a month. You take them home and boil them with some new potatoes, you got something good to eat."

Not everyone agrees with Russell. The taste for smoked herring, as for all salted foods, has declined in recent decades in North America. Inflation has ravaged the traditional Caribbean markets. Last year, 340,000 kilos were produced, a paltry amount compared with that of a century ago but reason enough for Russell's optimism about the prospects for a resurgence of the grand old industry.

"I think it's really picking up because we've had people from New York and different places, and they want to know when the herring's going to be done. The same people was here last year."

People return to Grand Manan with the alacrity of pilgrims. To most, life on the island seems governed by a less insistent clock than that of the hurly-burly world left behind. However, according to Eric Allaby, local historian and harbour master, the belief is simply not true: "One of the illusions of the place, of course, is that the life of the fisherman is pretty laissez-faire and easygoing. But, in actual fact, what seems like a very easy going kind of timetable is ordered by the tides or the wind or the weather – it's just a different set of rules than what the more artificial parts of society live by." Allaby's remark itself reveals a common Grand Manan conceit: life on the island is the real thing, while mainland existence is, at best, a pale imitation.

My own initiation into the strictness of the tide as alarm clock came my first morning on Grand Manan. It was 4 a.m. and still dark when I rolled from the comfort of my bed, intent on catching the early tide at Dark Harbour. Surrounded on three sides by cliffs and bounded at its mouth by a great seawall of beach stone and driftwood, the salt lagoon is the only safe anchorage on the west side of the island. In sharp contrast to the sheltered coves and gentle marshes of the eastern shore, the west coast, with vertical cliffs of basalt rising one hundred metres from the sea, is an ironbound nightmare to mariners. Dramatic as its name, Dark Harbour is a seasonal home to dulse pickers and cottagers, and its sole connection to the sea is a narrow channel that was dug during the nineteenth century and is negotiable only at high tide.

I WAS GOING DULSING. Grand Manan is particularly noted for its dulse, a red seaweed that grows luxuriantly on the island's rocky coast. In 1984, the island exported 125 tonnes. Rich in vitamins and minerals, much of the dulse goes to health-food stores. It is used to flavour soups and stews. But many people – Islanders especially – like to eat the seaweed as a salty snack, fresh from the sea, sun-dried or cooked on the stovetop. Dulse grows all around Grand Manan, but to Leroy Flagg, one of my companions that morning and the island's best-known dulse buyer, there is only one dulse worth picking – Dark Harbour dulse. The high cliffs, he says, shade the dulse grounds at their base, preventing the rockweed from getting sunburned. Also, the strong tidal currents on the west side of the island seem to favour the growth of the dulse while keeping it clean of mussels and mud.

It was a Sunday morning, and the highest tides of the month, the so-called dulse tides, were past. Perhaps that was why only a handful of drowsy dulsers had shown up, rather than the dozens that set out regularly to pick between the tides. Perhaps, too, the poor turnout had something to do with the dance at the curling club the night before.

After cautiously winching Flagg's Lunenburg-built dory up and over the protective seawall's crest, we launched ourselves into the pearl-grey waters of the outer Bay of Fundy. We cut a clean wake through a mysterious void of dense fog and grey sea. Only the ephemeral weirs – ghostly houses for air and water – gave relief to the seascape.

We put ashore in the shadow of the cliffs to the north of Dark Harbour, where we found a dense patch of luxuriant dulse. I marvelled at Flagg's knack of knowing where to bring us despite the fog that was almost thick enough to obscure the towering coastline. "You can't fool me on the dulse," said Flagg. "I know every rock and curve on the coast. I suppose I've picked over every rock five thousand times. I can always find good dulse because I can keep it in my mind. I know where we picked six or eight weeks ago."

Flagg's right arm was in a cast and sling, but he set about picking with his good hand, displaying the same unharnessed enthusiasm he has had for the task since he was twelve years old. "I like the sound of dulse; I like that snap." Clutching a mittful of ruddy, glistening Dark Harbour dulse, he held it up proudly: "This here is the only dulse in the world."

Handful after handful pulled away with ease. A good picker can gather enough dulse to yield fifty kilograms (100 pounds) after it is sun-dried on a field of beach stone. Flagg pays pickers 80 cents per pound for the finished product. We had two hours between the tide's uncovering the dulse rocks and covering them again, and the rhythm of the picking made the time pass quickly. We loaded our half-dozen 25-kilo (50-pound) burlap bags into the dory and sliced our way home through the fog.

Ironically, it was the fog, a most unlikely quarry, that the first summer people came in search of. Before the advent of air conditioning, fog was considered just the palliative for hot sticky nights. Droves of the well-to-do flocked to the seaside hotels that lent an air of Old World gentility to the Eastern Seaboard.

Today, most of these resorts are in shambles. One survivor of the bygone era of steamer trunks and straw boaters is the Marathon Inn which rises above the tiny fishing community of North Head like a haughty dowager. In 1977 it was a hundred years old and in a sorry state of disrepair. It was then that Jim and Judy Leslie of Toronto answered an ad for the sale of the Marathon. The Leslies eagerly took possession and set out to restore the down-at-the-heels inn to its former glory. They hoped to capitalize on what Jim describes as the island's "escape aspect," a perennial attraction to urbanites. In creating an ambience to match their renovations, the Leslies decided to offer beer, wine and spirits with their meals, and they took the seemingly innocuous step of applying for a liquor licence. In doing so, the Leslies ran afoul of the Islanders' deeply held conviction that Grand Manan should stay the way it has been or once was.

It was the surprise beginning of a long, hard battle for the Leslies and a resounding introduction to the gritty determination of their new neighbours. Grand Mananers, it seemed, had done without a drinking establishment in the past, and they were not about to have one now. Many residents were still bitter about the opening of Grand Manan's single liquor store, which they felt was not only contributing to the deterioration of island morality but also creating a safety hazard along the island's single stretch of road.

Clutching Bibles and babies, the teetotalling congregations of Grand Manan's Ministerial Association, counting among themselves more than 800 of Grand Manan's 2,600 souls, made a pilgrimage of protest to the provincial legislature in Fredericton each time the Leslies submitted a new application. Until 1984, when the license was finally granted, the Leslies' application, and concomitant mass exodus to Fredericton, was an annual event. While most of the arguments posed by the Islanders were both moralistic and pragmatic, many also contained a sentiment that perhaps lay even closer to the heart of the matter. "I'm not against tourists," one Islander grumbled, "but I'm against changing things around to suit them." Another, ruddy with anger, was even more succinct: "We don't like change on the island."

Such resistance runs deep in Grand Manan. No sooner had Grand Mananers lost their battle with the Marathon Inn than the island's citizens mounted a campaign against another threat to the Island's status quo. Panic rippled through the community when it was learned that Moonies – followers of the Reverend Sun Myung Moon's Unification Church – had purchased two of the island's lobster pounds to supply church retail outlets in the eastern United States. The Grand Manan Ministerial Association, representing the island's seventeen churches, was harshly critical of the Moonies' avowed motives. "The Moonies are so two-faced at times that it put fear into me," said Reverend Wayne Robertson of the Central Wesleyan Church. "They're not here just to buy and sell lobsters. They must have come to Grand Manan to further the Unification Church."

To an outsider, it might seem that one more church would make little difference – already there is one church for every mile of road. One explanation for the God-fearing nature of the people is offered by Daniel McGee, pastor of the Emmanuel Pentecostal Assembly: "I guess fishermen see how humble they are in the scheme of things because of the elements. Every day on the water, they see the awesomeness of creation."

Apparently, awe and humility have yet to breed religious tolerance. Ronald Benson, a lobster-pound owner and fish processor, echoed the island sentiment: "Most of the concern is the Unification Church as such, not the business aspect of it. This is the main concern of the citizens of the island – that we not lose any of our young people, or anyone, to that cult."

Although the Moonies have not yet proved to be a threat to local fish buyers, most Islanders remain vigilant. One Mananer who seems nonplussed by the commotion is Buddy McLaughlin, who sold the lobster pounds to the Moon-ies. McLaughlin does not appear to be worried about being censured by his fellow Islanders. "I've got broad shoulders," he says offhandedly. Neither does he share the view that island-owned fish operations would not be able to compete with Moonie-run enterprises. He puts his faith in his own shrewd business sense – another island trait, judging by local prosperity. "We've bought and sold these particular pounds three times now," he says, then adds wryly, "each time at a profit."

Though the wider world sometimes impinges on this sea-girt kingdom, for the most part irksome mainland issues can be ignored or regarded at a comfortable, even smug, distance. After being on the island for a while, a visitor begins to believe what everyone has been saying: Grand Manan is a place apart, not only in setting but also in spirit. Islanders enjoy the independence that isolation breeds. "They don't have no bosses to Grand Manan," said Gleason Greene, an 87-year-old raconteur and former boat designer. "Grand Manan is an easy place to live. You can make a living easy, as far as that goes. You got no bosses; you don't have to run by the tick of the clock. You can go where you want to go. Of course, you go on the tide when you're fishing. You go just the same, but nobody drives you. You go on your own."

For many, the ease that Grand Manan engenders is something they grow into and come back to renew. Some enquire about real estate; others are so hard-bitten by Grand Manan's version of "islomania" that they stay – despite themselves. Robin and Mary Wall, for example, knew the first time they set foot on the island that they wanted to make Grand Manan their home.

In his mid-fifties, Wall left his longtime post as art teacher at a community college in Cornwall, Ontario, where, he admits, he and his wife had been perfectly content. On Grand Manan, they cleared away alders, designed and built a printmaking studio and joined the church and historical society – all within a year. They are now firmly rooted.

"What the hell is it about this island that attracts so much?" Wall puzzled as he showed me his prints of weirs, smokehouses and rocky shores that reflect his artistic conversion to the island's iconography.

Mary, who now works as the island's first school psychologist, immediately began to answer his question, making an extemporaneous list of island virtues. It evokes childhood – not one's own, she pointed out, but the state of mind. There is also the neighbourliness of the people: the Walls have opened their door to find anonymous gifts of illicit gulls' eggs – "Delicious," they confess – or a string of stream-caught trout. And when they were building, neighbours dropped by to ask if they needed anything and to pitch in.

Wall listened, nodding. "You know, it just doesn't feel like Canada here. It's as if I'm in my own country. I like that . . . " He paused, looking at the print in his hand, and I silently finished the thought for him, the thought that would complete his transformation from mainlander to Islander: "And I'll work to keep it that way."

Island Pastoral

McNutts Island, Nova Scotia

TASHA, A SEVEN-YEAR-OLD BORDER COLLIE, is balanced with her front paws on the gunnels of the *Bar-Tender*, a Cape Islander fishing boat, as we approach the rocky shore of McNutts Island at the mouth of Shelburne Harbour. Though we are still too far from shore for me to distinguish sheep from the bulks of grey granite boulders, Tasha obviously can smell them as she thrusts her nose eagerly upward, sniffing the sea air. Ranger, an older sheep dog with a black spot around one eye that looks like a pirate's eye patch, joins Tasha at her lookout. These two "salty dogs" are all anticipation, eager to get ashore and on with the task at hand – to round up the sheep which roam wild on McNutts Island off Nova Scotia's southwestern shore.

Islands are scattered like pieces of a jigsaw puzzle along the deeply indented coastline. Sheep have been kept on many of them for more than a century. Romantic theories abound as to how they got there. It is said that sheep were placed on some islands to provision shipwrecked sailors; on others the first sheep may have been survivors of shipwrecks. A more plausible version of events is offered by a Dr. J.F. Ellis in his turn-of-the-century report, *The Sheep Industry on the Atlantic Coast of Nova Scotia:*

> "In the early days when the horse was a novelty in
> this region and public highways were little used,

the fisherman's only means of travel was his boat," he wrote. "Consequently a great many of them lived on these islands. But of late years they have nearly all moved to the mainland, and at present only a very few of the islands have any inhabitants. However, the sheep, left on these islands by the old inhabitants, thrive and do well... "

In this century, the practice of keeping sheep on islands was carried on by fishermen-farmers who occupied the islands seasonally for lobster fishing or the gathering of Irish moss, a commercial seaweed. As late as 1960 there were 8,000 sheep on islands from Canso on Nova Scotia's eastern Atlantic shore to Brier Island in the outer Bay of Fundy. Often several owners – in some cases, descendants of the original island inhabitants – managed the sheep co-operatively, and shearing time became an occasion for a big picnic, a kind of island reunion.

The number of island sheep has since dwindled to 2,000 (following a general downturn in the sheep industry), and flocks are restricted to thirty islands in southwestern Nova Scotia. A handful of island sheep owners persist in the time-honoured practise there, because sheep seem to thrive despite the harsh offshore environment, and often it proves more profitable than intensive management on the mainland.

Walter Perry of Central Chebogue, Yarmouth County, runs the largest island sheep-farming operation in the province. As I drove into the farm yard, three border collies circled about the car to greet me, and soon their master emerged from the white farmhouse with a welcoming hand extended. At seventy-seven Perry is a vigorous man with bushy black eyebrows, a shock of white hair and ruddy complexion. He showed me into his kitchen where he had spread out on the table maps of the coast showing *his* islands – Mud, Seal, McNutts and Emerald Islands, among others.

Perry bought his first purebred flock of sheep in 1932. "I guess I was born to have sheep," he said with a smile, "because I like them, and I always seemed to have pretty good luck with them." As a boy he had helped a local farmer raise lambs on Crawley's Island at the mouth of the Chebogue

River, but Perry did not get into island sheep for himself until the 1950s, when a Cape Negro Island sheep owner offered him his flock at a price he could not refuse. He now has seven hundred ewes on eight islands, in addition to 125 at his mainland farm which borders the tidal Chebogue River.

Traditionally, island sheep were raised primarily for their wool. "I think the women used to be more interested in the sheep years ago," said Perry. "They did their own spinning and knitting mittens. Quite often you'd find the women were doing more shearing than the men, who were probably out fishing when women were doing the farmwork."

In the past, the transportation of lambs to market was a practical constraint, whereas wool could be processed locally or stored and shipped in any season. As barren ewes, rams or wethers (castrated males) will give double the wool clip of a pregnant or lactating ewe, they were often retained to the detriment of the lamb crop, which today is the key to success in the sheep business.

Like most contemporary sheep producers, Perry was more interested in maximizing the lamb crop than the wool harvest. To increase lamb production, he saw that the island flocks had to be managed more carefully. It was therefore vital to remove rams in the summer months and return them in early winter so that ewes would lamb in late spring, thereby increasing chances of survival for the lambs. This meant more trips to the islands rather than the once-a-year shearing frolic.

That was fine by Perry. "There's a challenge and a pleasure there that's hard to describe," he said. "A walk around any island is a pleasure, I think. There's always something different to be seen. I guess there's some beachcomber in me, too." Sadly for Perry, a heart attack two years ago has kept him ashore, and he now leaves the beachcombing and the round-ups to his two sons, Tom and Ron.

When Tom and Ron Perry arrived at the wharf in Gunning Cove on a balmy evening in mid-July, the captain of the *Bar-Tender*, Clifford Van Buskirk, quipped, "Time to leave off fishing and go sheeping." Van Buskirk was accompanied by his brother, Dwight, their 13-year-old nephew, Randy, and Randy's friend. Clifford, one of eleven children of the former McNutts Island lightkeeper, is now a full-time fishermen but continues to keep sheep, a hobby that began when the Perrys gave him a pet lamb.

After the hour-long run out Shelburne harbour, Van Buskirk steered his boat around the north end of the 20-square-kilometre island where we put over a punt into the water. Heads of curious harbour seals poked above the swells as we rowed ashore, leaped onto the slippery rocks and scrambled to higher ground. McNutts was named after a notorious 18th-century character, Colonel Alexander McNutt, who settled on the island in the 1760s after an attempt to found a Utopian colony, New Jerusalem, at what is now Shelburne. In her book, *Offshore Islands of Nova Scotia and New Brunswick*, author Allison Mitcham, notes: "Islands such as McNutts were not . . . so easily tamed as their early inhabitants hoped. McNutt's has always defied the incursions of civilization." And so it is today.

We followed a narrow sheep path through the thick tangle of underbrush which grows to the edge of the island's splash zone. Telltale wisps of wool clung here and there, but it was not until we arrived at the lighthouse grounds that sheep came into view. This so-called lighthouse flock moved off warily and we split into three groups to encircle them and drive them to the beach. We would later be joined by another sheep farmer, Elizabeth Hyde, and helpers to gather the three flocks on the island.

"This is the most fun for us," Ron Perry said as we picked our way through boggy ground to the rocky shore. "Just to see if you can do it. It's a challenge. It gets in your blood after a while."

Part of the challenge for us on this evening was to get the job done before nightfall. On a wooded island such as McNutts it is best to drive sheep in the evening, Ronnie explained, for it is only then that the sheep come to the shore from the woods where they seek shade during the heat of the day. In the woods, they are nearly impossible to find or retrieve.

The sheep threaded between the deserted lighthouse outbuildings in obedient file. I was surprised by the orderly progress of the flock, and asked whether island sheep were in fact "wild" when compared to mainland flocks. "They're not so much wild," Ron said, "I'd say they're foxy, they're cautious."

As if to affirm his observation, a small group of ewes and lambs suddenly bolted. "They're going for the woods, better send the dog out," Ron shouted, and the "king dog," Ranger, followed in hot pursuit. It was a quarter of an hour before he reemerged at the heels of the errant sheep. One panicky ewe headed for the water where Dwight Van Buskirk had to administer a football tackle to keep the animal from plunging into the waves.

"If sheep get pressured too much, they get suicidal, and they'll even drown themselves," Tom Perry explained. "I've had to go for a swim more than once.

"Let her rest," he urged. This proved the most dramatic episode in the four-hour hike which took us halfway around the Island. The sun set in a vivid display on the western shore, and the evening star rose through a salmon-coloured sky. Soon we had only our flashlights to show us the way as we stumbled on behind the sheep lulled by the anxious bleating of the lambs and the deeper maternal calls of the ewes.

I overheard two boys holding counsel in the dark. "It's like in an old Western movie," one said. I took his meaning, as one reinforced by the terms *roundup* and *drive*. However, what we were doing is formally called a *gather*, which, I thought to myself, would find its closest analogy in the outer islands of Scotland. By the time we reached our shearing corral, the tide was high, forcing us to ford a shallow creek. With a little encouragement, the flock passively crossed over into the makeshift corral.

After six hours sleep, we were up again to do another sweep of the island in an attempt to gather the sheep we had let pass through our human net, or others that had fallen by the wayside. Among the latter were the "swaybacks." It was easy to pick out these lambs from the flock – their hind quarters sway back and forth uncontrollably, making it next to impossible for them to walk without stumbling. The partial paralysis is caused by a demylenization of the spinal chord and is attributable to copper deficiency in the diet.

Swayback is endemic to some islands and not others. McNutts has a high incidence – up to 20 percent of lambs may be affected – but even on McNutts there is a variation between the "lighthouse flock" and the "pen flock" at the other end of the island, which is almost free of swayback. According to Mac Fuller, Agriculture Representative for Shelburne and Yarmouth counties in southwestern Nova Scotia, swayback on the island may be related to a gull colony at the lighthouse and its influence on the vegetation. Fertilized by a steady application of bird droppings, the rich vegetation in the area may be depleting the soil of copper. Longtime sheep farmers have commonly associated swayback with the presence of seagulls, much to the scepticism of professionals at the Nova Scotia Department of Agriculture. But farmers may have a valid point, said Fuller. Another factor may be sandy soil types which are often copper deficient. Acid rain, a major problem in the region, may also be affecting what little copper there is present in island soils.

For the past several years, the department has funded a program to prevent swayback; it encourages farmers and veterinarians to inject liquid copper into ewes in the last trimester of pregnancy. However, success of the program depends on the ability to land on the wind-battered islands in March – a risky business at best.

WINTERING ON THE ISLANDS – some of which are bald and lack shelter – is perhaps the greatest threat to the flocks. Elizabeth Hyde, who owns the largest flock on McNutts and is its only year-round resident, knows well the perils sheep face in winter. The cold winter affects them more than a heavy snowfall, she said. "They seem to know where the hay is and they'll dig away at the snow with their hooves." Inevitably, however, there are losses.

As we talked, we spelled each other in carrying a swayback lamb to reunite it with its mother at the shearing corral. We came across evidence of last winter's severity in the carcasses of ewes and lambs; there were also old orange lichen-encrusted bones of the generations of island sheep that had lived and died there. Up ahead were the survivors, wending along the shoreline and reminding us that life goes on.

Until fifty years ago, little new stock was introduced to the islands. The sheep were described as having distinctive deer-like faces and probably were descendants of sheep from the British Isles. Common breeds such as Scottish Blackface, Suffolk and Cheviot have since been mixed in, but island flocks remain characteristically robust. "Mother Nature does the culling," says Yarmouth veterinarian Tommy O'Brien. "As a result they tend to develop a hardier breed than on shore,"

O'Brien has treated island sheep since 1978. "Production of island sheep is good, and in some cases higher than on shore," he noted. "It's amazing the body condition these animals will have. Even after lambing they will have high body fat." He attributes the good conditioning of ewes to the virtues of kelp, their primary winter forage. Kelp has a high protein content, essential amino acids, and a salt balance close to that of the body. Because it is naturally salted, the inherent food value is preserved. "It is as good a wintering feed as you can find," said O'Brien. "Provided there is enough kelp being brought ashore by good winds, they'll do well."

Several years ago, the population of common green sea urchin, which feed upon kelp, exploded along the Atlantic seaboard and, as a result, greater sheep mortalities were experienced on some offshore islands. It underlined how sheep depend on land and sea for nourishment, and how these two ecosystems are intimately connected in this offshore world. Sheep feed primarily on kelp from October to May, then switch to forage inland. "They eat bay berry bushes, it flavours them; wild roses, it flavours them; wild mint," Elizabeth Hyde observed. "They're the best tasting lamb in the world."

Ann Priest, an actor and part-time sheep farmer helping Elizabeth Hyde that day, guided her dog, Tess, with whistles, hand signals and soft-spoken words. Tess, in turn, did an admirable job of bringing the stray sheep to the corral where the shearing began mid-morning and proceeded all day. I watched with amazement as professional shearer Bill Oulton cut the fleece from a sheep in ninety seconds flat. I tried my hand, upending a ewe and clamping her between my knees. She showed remarkable patience with my novice effort, but half way through decided she had had enough and made her escape. Tom Perry, who could not contain his amusement, finished my ragged job.

The sheep were treated for parasites and vaccinated against tetanus. The tagged ewes were checked to see if they were lactating, and the lamb crop divided up among the three flock owners.

By the end of the day we had sheared 120 sheep, and everybody, weary from the two roundups and hot work, found a soft bag of wool to rest on as sandwiches were eaten. "To me it's more like a picnic, though after the twentieth sheep I start wondering how many more there are," Tom Perry remarked. "I always enjoy the community aspect of it." I asked Randy Van Buskirk, who was nursing a sore knee that had been butted by a rambunctious ram, what he thought of his first island sheep shearing. "It's fun," he replied, adding with enthusiasm. "And tomorrow they dock the tails!"

On this trip, all lambs would have their tails clipped, male lambs would be castrated, and mature rams removed to a nearby island. (Several South Shore islands bear the name Ram Island, probably because they were used to segregate the rams from the flock during the summer.) In September and October, island sheep owners will return to pick up their market lambs, leaving 10 percent of the ewes to maintain flock numbers. Again in December, they brave high seas and bad weather to return the rams to the islands. "You take your life into your hands to make a landing in a small boat," Walter Perry had said before we set out on our trip. "You've got to have a good man on the oars and another man with the ram in the stern of the boat. And before she touches the ground, that ram's got to get out of there and up over the beach, and you've got to be ready to get rowing out before the next roller hits you. I've done that a good many times."

The risks inherent to island sheep farming are balanced by greater profitability. On islands there are no fencing or feed costs as the sea acts as fence and forage provider. There are fewer predators on islands than on the mainland, although last year two island flocks were decimated by coyotes that swam from the mainland. Raising island sheep requires less work because the animals do not have to be tended everyday. However, the cost of transportation to and from the islands offsets some of the gains.

I concluded that to undertake this offshore adventure one must not only love sheep but islands too. It was well past dark before the *Bar-Tender* pointed its bow toward Gunning Cove. Clifford Van Buskirk was going home to the mainland, and then to sea again to fish. "It gives me an excuse to go out around the lighthouse twice a year," he said, reflecting upon his island sheep enterprise.

His statement struck a responsive chord. I realized that in Nova Scotia island sheep rearing is not simply a business but a carry-over of a vanishing maritime culture. Now that nearly all lighthouses have become automated and the communities that sustained island families are no more than cellar holes and memories, island sheep help keep that historical offshore connection alive, for Van Buskirk and other Nova Scotians too.

Bottom Line

Georges Bank

CAPTAIN GARY FROST STANDS AT the centre of the shiney varnished wheelhouse, pondering an impressive array of marine gadgetry: four Lorans, two radar and an old fashioned brass magnetic compass mounted in front of the wheel. The scene beyond the nine bridge windows – a green-grey, undulating expanse of moody ocean flecked with dainty storm petrels – could be anywhere in the non-descript North Atlantic, but as Frost's checkings and cross-checkings confirmed, we were on Georges Bank, 160 kilometres southwest of Yarmouth, Nova Scotia, and a scant five kilometres from the newly drawn, and uneasily maintained, boundary line that defines the limits of Canada's jurisdiction over the richest fishing bank in the northern hemisphere.

Our position was critical, for Frost's 36-metre wooden scallop dragger, *Adventurer II*, was steaming full throttle toward the line, towing two 4-metre-wide scallop drags along the sea bottom, as we have been almost constantly since our depth sounder signaled our arrival on the shallows of Georges twenty-four hours before. Frost was keen to work as close to the line as possible, yet to cross it would mean the loss of his boat and the end of his career – at the age of thirty-five. The same fate awaited the captain's counterparts from the United States but as Frost was quick to point out, the threat has not always proved a deterrent: "This is where a lot of the activity has been. Now it's all shells." By "activity" Frost meant Amercian scallop boats running the boundary line to scoop up Canadian scallops.

Frost is a confident man who loves his boat and the Bank, and he likes to talk about both. I shipped aboard the *Adventurer II* primarily to learn about scallop fishing but soon discovered that one does not fish on Georges Bank these days without also learning about politics and confrontation. "Couple months ago," Frost recalled, "there were three or four Americans across the line in the nighttime, and then one guy got brazen around 9 o'clock in the morning and came across."

This illegal activity continues two years after the International Court of Justice in The Hague handed down its binding decision on the marine boundary dispute in the Gulf of Maine. Canada had claimed less than half of Georges Bank, while the United States had petitioned for complete control of Georges based on what it argued was historical dominance of the region. After hearing 9,600 pages of testimony, the International Court of Justice made the predictable politic decision, splitting the claims down the middle. Canada was granted one-sixth of the bank, a 60- by 120-kilometre section known as the Northeast Peak. Reaction in Canada varied from "disastrous" to ecstatic," but no one denied that the decision gave to Canada the best part of the scallop ground and important groundfish spawning areas. Historically, the Northeast Peak has yielded 60 percent of the total Canadian and American scallop catch, and hence American skippers are tempted to cross into Canadian territory despite the risk of heavy fines and the threat of confiscation of their million-dollar vessels.

An independent breed, accustomed to roaming the Bank at will, fishermen of both nationalities must now exercise restraint, and many are finding it difficult. Traditionally, Canadian fishermen exploited Georges side by side with Americans, and many regarded each other as friends. One Canadian scalloper I spoke with considered the Americans as "almost like family." There is truth in his sentiment, for the eastern United States and Nova Scotia have exchanged goods, services and personalities, as well as fishing grounds, for two centuries.

Georges Bank sticks out like an upturned thumb between Massachusett's Cape Cod and Nova Scotia's Cape Sable. For more than a century it has been a favoured fishing hole of people from both sides of the Gulf of Maine, and prior to the 1977 claims by Canada and the United States to a 200-mile (320-kilometre) limit, it was the haunt of foreign fleets as well. One Russsian trawler captain remarked that Georges Bank was nothing less than "an oceanic miracle."

All the oceanographic criteria are met to nurture marine organisms. The Bank is shallow – as recently as the last Ice Age it was an emergent island – thus, well shot with the sunlight necessary for photosynthetic production. Furthermore, as part of the Gulf of Maine–Bay of Fundy system, Georges is subject to strong tidal action, which results in vertical mixing of seafloor nutrients. The presence of nutrients tumbling through light translates as biological productivity; at Georges Bank, however, the combination has resulted in a productivity estimated to be four times that of the legendary Grand Banks. Its nurturing capacity is obvious even to the casual observer. In my few days on the Bank, at any given time I might see whales feeding or shark fins knifing the waves and, always, hundreds of seabirds skimming the waters – all signs of the fishy riches lurking below the bleak surface, which billows and falls like the roof of an enormous big top.

In the northern hemisphere Georges is an unmatched fish producer. In 1985, Canadian landings of all species from Georges were worth $52.7 million at the wharf. Of that total, the scallop fishery was by far the most valuable, bringing in $39.5 million. Lobsters added $1.6 million, and groundfish such as cod and haddock made up the balance of $11.6. Georges Bank alone accounted for more than one third of the total Nova Scotia fishery and generated an estimated 3,600 jobs.

Obviously, the high stakes scallop fishery is not taken lightly by men like Frost. He reminded me that there are fifteen wives and maybe seventy-five or eighty kids counting on him and his boat. For that reason Frost is attentive not only to his own approach to the line, but to any transgressions by Americans. Squinting into the radar screen Frost saw six amber blips, a mile and a half into the American side. Although we cannot yet see them through the fog, Frost knew that they were American scallop draggers, and in his mind, there was no doubt that they were simply biding their time, waiting for the right conditions to cross the line and plunder *his* scallops. "They just stay on their side of the line, and when the weather gets right for them to take a jump, maybe the six of them will come at once."

THE RIGHT WEATHER would be southwest winds and more fog, exactly what the marine forecast had been calling for all day. At the moment, however, the fog was lifting ever so slightly, and to starboard we could just begin to make out the silhouettes of two big stern trawlers, National Sea Products' boats out of Lunenburg, dragging the Banks for groundfish. Frost trained his binoculars to the "no'rd," where he picked up a third vessel on the horizon.

"That's our coast guard. I know it, I know it, I know it." He handed over the binoculars just in time for me to see the long grey vessel swing round and begin plowing water in our direction. Frost whooped with laughter, exhilirated by the mock chase. "He thinks we're Americans trying to sneak back across the line, or if we're Canadians, he wants to tell us we're getting too handy to the line." Frost swivelled and grabbed the radio behind him: "Fisheries Patrol Boat, *Cygnus*, Fisheries Patrol Boat, *Cygnus*, this is the *Adventurer II.* O'er." Then turning to me Frost said, "If they're playing cat and mouse with the American boats he might not come back."

The game of cat-and-mouse has been played almost non-stop since the line was drawn. There have been forty-four reported incursions into Canadian territory in the intervening two years. Eighteen of the offending boats have been brought into Nova Scotian ports and given fines from $25,000 to $45,000 plus the loss of their catch. In the opinion of many Canadian skippers, Gary Frost among them, the only measure that will eventually put a stop to the violations is for the department to seize a boat.

"That's what you gotta do, you got to make the fine so steep, that it won't even enter your mind to cross the line. See, now when you catch them, seize the boat, and put a couple hundred thousand dollar fine – that would stop it, in my opinion. But when you're given a $30,000 fine, and there's fifteen guys chippin' in on it, it doesn't do much, you see. If you get 4,000 pounds of scallops a day, they're gettin' five bucks a pound, that's

$20,000 right there. And it's amongst fifteen guys, like I said, that's the way they're doing it. Now these six guys we seen might be all buddies, right? And they might have it all lined up. They left the dock, and they said, 'Look, we're goin' close to the line, and if we get caught, whoever gets caught, whatever the fine, we'll split it.' You see, now, that's the way they usually do it."

In January 1987, Frost and others got a portion of what they have been pressing for, when Canada announced a substantial increase in the maximum fine – from $100,000 to $750,000. In the past the Department of Fisheries and Oceans has requested from the court confiscation of the offending vessels – albeit unsuccessfully – and it will continue to do so whenever it thinks the abuse warrants it.

Ultimately, the stakes are so high that perhaps there can be no certain deterrent. Some American captains feel that they have to take the chance of running the line to keep a crew and make payments on their vessel. Even the possibility of losing their vessel may not dissuade them in the end. According to one DFO official, "A lot of them say, "Take my boat, the bank owns it anyway.' "

Access to Georges Bank has been equally critical for Canadians. Many believe a line drawn more favourably for the United States would have meant not only financial ruin for a few fishermen but economic ruin for the whole region of southwestern Nova Scotia. Since the mid-1800s, fishermen from more than thirty small ports along a 320-kilometre stretch of Nova Scotia coastline have been sailing what was originally called St. Georges Bank. First, they put to sea in saltbank schooners searching for cod, and then later in modern steam trawlers in pursuit of halibut, haddock and swordfish.

The scallop fishery did not begin until 1945, but it quickly assumed prominence after Captain John Beck returned from an exploratory trip to Georges with 8,000 pounds (3,630 kilos) of "deep sea scallops," the Georges Bank mollusk that many seafood connoiseurs consider a delicacy second to none. Word spread along the coast, and the next year, boats began gearing up for Georges. By the mid-1960s Canada dominated the scallop fishery on the Bank, with fifty offshore draggers working the Northeast Peak and

Northern Edge – the tip of the thumb to which they were pretty much limited by distance from port.

It is a 12-hour trip from Yarmouth, home port of the *Adventurer II*, to Georges Bank, and as I was to learn during my days on board, those in transit hours are the only ones in stints of up to a week when the crew of fourteen, the captain and mate are not frantically working to "make their trip" of 26,000 pounds (11,800 kilos).

"You can't lose time in this," explains Frost. "It ain't like any other fishing. It's average, the fishing's got to go on a solid average, you don't get a big day. If I get 3,500 to 4,000 pounds [1,600 to 1,800 kilos] a day, I'm well satisfied."

WE RODE A FOG SWELL all the way out, Frost vehemently and alliteratively cursing the fog for the entire distance. The depth sounder indicated our arrival on the Bank. "She comes up pretty quick," said Frost, referring to the shallowing water. At dusk the veil of fog lifted long enough for us to see that three other scallopers were on the Bank – "Lady boats," belonging to Comeau Seafoods of Meteghan, northeast of Yarmouth.

Turning on the radio as we wallowed in grey hills of water, Frost tuned in to hear someone's thoughts about their lawn back home: "I think I'll try some Kentucky bluegrass – it's nice and green." Frost cut in to ask what the scallops were like, and the voice came back with barely a change of tone: "Meats gone out of them – o'er." Frost, though, was anxious to get a few scallops in the hold, after checking the depth – ninety fathoms – he gave a blast of the horn, the signal for the crew to "shoot away."

"We'll take some here," he said, "then we'll look around for better bottom." The book on Frost is that he's a real dog for new bottom: "He'll find scallops where nobody else can find them," I was told. The winch cable sang through gallows' blocks. Frost let out a length of "wire" equal to three times the depth plus ten fathoms for good measure. This ratio (the same as that used by fish trawlers) usually settles the two-tonne rake on the seabed. Frost went slowly until the rake was in position, then he gave the boat throttle. Each tow is three and a half to four kilometers and takes about twenty minutes.

The rake looks and functions like a giant dustpan. As it is towed along the bottom, scallops and other bottom dwelling creatures, rocks and trash, are swept into the net of chain-mail and rope. It is an unsubtle device, and for every scallop caught, another is probably crushed by the rake's rambunctious passage.

The horn sounded again, and the deckhands and winchmen moved into the waist of the boat to receive the rake. They did so with an unsettling nonchalance, considering what they were grappling with. Three men worked each side. Two deckhands attached boom hooks to the rake, turned it and then cleared the deck while the winchman, who operates the boom cable from a safer position, below the wheelhouse, brought the rake crashing nose first onto the deck. Scurrying across the tossing deck once again, the deckhands detached and repositioned hooks so that the winchman could upend the rake, spilling its contents onto the dump tables.

The emptying of the rake is a continual fascination, for one can never be sure what will appear from the nets. Scallops, of course – pink, white or brown, plain or patterned, large and small – but also, if the beds being dragged are old ones, as many half shells as live scallops. And with the scallops comes the rest of the benthic marine ecosystem, as well as a portion of the sea bottom itself in the form of sizable boulders.

I soon become familiar with a rogue's gallery of sea-bottom monsters: yellow and orange spotted deep sea skates, conger eels that are half-fish, half pouting look-alikes for Mick Jagger, and, without exception, monkfish – perhaps the ugliest members of this menagerie. They vary in size from a half meter to more than a meter in length, most of which is head – a spiny, abhorrent visage, wide as it is long, bisected by an enormous mouthful of tiny razor sharp teeth. The relatively insignificant tails, called "monkey-tails" by the fishermen, are delicious, I was told, and much sought after by Japanese buyers. If there are few scallops to be had, the monkey-tails are iced away. As well, there are non-descript creatures like "sea-pumpkins," which I at first mistook for blobs of oil. One day, there was the rare catch of a manta ray, a creature that must be lovely in the water gliding on its sea wings but on deck looked like a collapsed mass of grape jelly. One of the deckhands posed with it and then unceremoniously kicked it through the scuppers.

For their part, the fishermen ignore the zoological curiosities, with which they are all too familiar and which make their task of picking scallops more difficult. Legs spread, head between their knees, my shipmates bent to their task of sorting through the trash, flipping scallops into plastic baskets with lightning speed as they sorted through the marine trash. Once I got my sea legs, I picked for a few hours each day. "Good job for a strong back and weak mind," said one of my fellow pickers. It's also hard on the hands: it's common to go through a pair of heavy rubber gloves every two days.

Once the tow had been sorted through, Frost again sounded the horn. The dump tables were lifted, depositing the trash back into the sea, and then gently returned to the deck. A crewman appeared and as the boat listed to his side, he cracked the handcuff holding the rake with a maul, and it plunged once again toward the riches of Georges Bank.

SHOOT AWAY, DRAG FOR TWENTY MINUTES, haul up, dump the contents of the drag on deck, and shoot away again, a never ending frantic cycle in the quest to return to port with 11,800 kilograms (26,000 pounds) of fresh deep-sea scallops.

Frost is a driver. In 1985 he caught more scallops than any other captain in southwestern Nova Scotia's Sweeney Fisheries fleet. He went to sea at age eleven and had his Captain's ticket by twenty-one and the command of a scallop boat at twenty-four. He is anything but a fairweather captain: when the other boats have headed for home, Frost is still fishing.

"I wish you could be here when its blowing fifty or sixty," said a longtime crew member. "I tell everyone to clear the deck until the gear stops flying,"

While there might be occassion for grumbling in the forecastle, the crew of the *Adventuer II* fares better than most of their counterparts, and that is compensation enough. In 1985, the *Adventurer II*'s crew share was twice as much as that for many boats. As well, the crew respects Frost's willingness to shed the trappings of rank. "He won't ask you to do anything he won't do. He doesn't stay in the wheelhouse and yell at you, he gets down on the deck and picks just like you. You don't see that in too many boats."

Frost has steel rods in both legs, the result of his putting a car up a tree at age nineteen, and the rods seem to inspire respect from those who work with him. By the time he's fifty, doctors have told him, he will be in a wheelchair. Now, though, several times a day, he leaves the therapeutic comfort of his $1,100 captain's chair, shouts an obscene salutation from the bridge, then bolts for the deck to start picking.

The scallops are whisked to the shucking room. In fact, it is not a room at all but a cramped corridor on either side of the galley and the aft cabins. There, every scallop – by my reckoning 750,000 on our trip – must be handled once again. The men stand at a long steel trough, rocking heel to tow in a kinetic trance. Each has his own customized kitchen knife, ground, curved, tapered and taped to his liking, that allows him to work at top speed. The knife is inserted between the two halves of the scallop, and one flip of the wrist ejects the bottom shell and viscera out a facing open bay – to the delight of the greater and sooty shearwaters ("hags" to fishermen) who follow the boat faithfully. Another flip of the wrist scrapes the remaining shell clean, and the scallop meat – the muscle – falls into a stainless steel pail. A fast worker can fill a bucket an hour. On the first trip of the year, the men frequently get "shucker's wrist," an inflammation that swells their forearms to twice their normal size. I could keep at it for an hour at a time before my wrist began to give out – not to mention my back and legs.

I ADMIRED MY SHIPMATES' STAMINA. There was a constant clacking of knife against shell like the sound of castanets or musical spoons. In my bunk, with a porthole that looked into the shucking room, I went to sleep and woke up listening to the cacophony. When they are into scallops, as they were then, the men work double shifts, knowing that the sooner they made quota, the sooner they will go home. That means eight-hour watches, with just four hours to sleep and eat before starting again. "We'll go right out for a week now, no stops, sixteen hours a day," said crewman Dave Reid.

A retired scallop captain once defined the fishery as "slavery without a whip." All of the *Adventurer*'s crew agreed that almost any other kind of fishing is easier but scalloping is where the money is right now. Most of the crew started fishing one thing or another when they were in their teens and have known little else. Most, including the captain, have only an elementary school education and, therefore, have few options to make comparable wages ashore. In a good year, such as 1986, Frost can make $60,000 to $80,000, and the crew around $30,000 for a hundred days at sea. These are deceptive figures, quoted on level ground, far from a deck that on a good day rocks in a 20-degree arc, and is buffeted by a 30-knot breeze which dumps water down your neck when you are picking and shoots spray into your face when you are shucking. At the end of the day, you fall into a narrow bunk in the ship's forecastle.

To a man the crew believe that they earn every penny. "People ashore think we got an easy job, lots of money. But they would be shocked at what we do," one of them said. "Sure, we're six months on the water but you do twelve months' work. And you're away from you're wife and children. It's hard, hard on everyone."

"In most jobs there is a rising and falling rhythm, times when you work at top speed and times when you coast," another observed. "Not so in scalloping. Everything's a mad rush. It takes its toll. The money is good but by the time you're thirty-five, you're through. Look around, they're all young fellows."

The frantic business of icing away scallops continued around the clock. After the *Cygnus* had passed our stern, heading south along the line to show the Maple Leaf to the American boats, Frost ordered the drags pulled as he didn't want to be caught fishing over the line. It was the only time during the days that I was to spend on *Adventurer II* when the drags were deliberately idle. But not for long: the *Cygnus* passed, Frost took one last look at the Americans, and then wheeled to starboard. As he did, he shouted through the open wheelhouse window to the deck crew who had been enjoying the brief and rare respite, "Okay, boys, let's make some money." The horn sounded, a maul was swung, and the drags shot away.

North of Nain
Cut Throat Island, Labrador

IN THE HIGH RIDING BOW of the 6-metre speed boat, feet planted resolutely apart and holding hard to the painter, is Abraham "Aba" Kojak, a 50-year old Labrador Inuit fisherman. At the back of the boat is Aba's son, Jacko, gunning the outboard motor as you might expect any 19-year old would do – for all its worth – so that the boat rides off the ramp of each wave crest, then slams into its deep trough, shooting sharp slivers of pain through my back and neck muscles. I sit huddled in the middle, watching as father and son pass finely tuned signals between one another. Without trying to shout instructions over the sounds of the motor and the boat's pounding, or resorting to hand signals, Aba directs Jacko where to steer and when to alter course. He accomplishes these commands, with a slight, almost imperceptible, nod of his head, to port or starboard.

Jacko responds by cutting around the end of Blow Hard Island. As he does a flock of black guillemots splutters into flight, exposing their bright coral-red feet. As the bracing air whips my face, I take in the unfamiliar sights of the northern waters. Several hundred yards to starboard, there are two grounded icebergs. One looks remarkably like a country church, with its single spire at one end and an oval window eroded by wind and water through the other. The bergs shine as if lit from inside, brightening an otherwise melancholy seascape. Suddenly, directly ahead of us, a minke whale surges to the surface, spouts and disappears. "Grumpus," notes Aba, applying the local name for the small rorqual. Overtop the barren mound of Blow Hard Island, which is grey and cracked as an elephant's hide, loom the snow-capped, serrated peaks of the Kiglapait Mountains, reflecting the pinkish light of the sun rising from the pewter-coloured Labrador Sea.

Jacko eases off on the throttle – to my relief – and we ride on the chop to check the nets anchored to the lee shore. As the landwash pitches and tosses our small boat, a deep sound reverberates across the water, disturbing the profound quietude of this subarctic wilderness and seeming to vibrate my very ear bones. My first thought is, 'Sonic boom from a NATO low level flying exercise.' Aba looks up from his net, cocks his head to one side and says, in his perfunctory way: "Iceberg breaking up." Sure enough, on our return to Cut Throat Harbour, I note that my "country church" iceberg, warmed by the mid-summer sun, has split into two pieces. This event provided the first of many occassions for me to marvel at how intimately Inuit like Aba know or, perhaps it is no exageration to say, communicate with the land.

During the week I am to spend on this remote island, I will often pause to contemplate the coastal landscape of glacial peaks and low granite islands capped with tundra – at once exhilirating and intimidating in their austere grandeur – and to reflect on how the Inuit have survived here for centuries, so effectively that archaeologist William Fitzhugh of the Smithsonian Institution wrote: "It seems impossible to find a spot which has not been modified in some tangible way by Inuit hands."

Though Jacques Cartier never ventured as far as northern Labrador, ironically, his notorious epithet, "the land God gave to Cain," has often been invoked to describe the coast. It is useful, if only to invoke the emotional impact of the landscape, which can inspire a shudder in someone from more equable climes. In many places, wind has stripped the white granite to the bone; elsewhere a few patches of yellowish green turf have been able to establish themselves in the interstices of stone. And even in August acres of snow cling to the north facing slopes. To a Euro-Canadian such a land might appear so utterly worthless it deserved a rebuke from God.

This transparently ethnocentric view does not take into account either the diverse resources of this outwardly inhospitable environment or the skills that the Inuit have devised to exploit them. For the Labrador Inuit the ocean has always been the prime source of sustenance here – whales, seals, fish and seabirds abound in the icy waters of the Labrador Sea. But the land, too, has been a good provider, for herds of caribou migrate to and from the coast, and other animals and plants contribute to the Inuit diet in season.

The barren islands and deep fiords of the northern Labrador coast, a remote region stretching nearly five hundred kilometres from Nain to the Arctic Circle, have been the Inuit homeland for much of their long occupation of Labrador. Glowered over by the highest mountain ranges east of the Rockies, the Kiglapaits and the Torngats, which rise precipitously from the sea, it is one of the last wild frontiers in North America and is unpopulated for most of the year. However, as soon as the ice leaves the coast in late June or early July, Inuit families – grandparents to infants – return to the land of their forebears to engage in the fishery for arctic char and Atlantic salmon. The fishery is the mainstay of the Inuit economy but life in summer fishing camps is also a matter of cultural survival. It is in the camps that the children learn by watching their mothers and fathers how to survive on the land as their ancestors have done for millenia.

As fall announces itself, often with a blustery September gale off the Labrador Sea, Inuit like Aba Kojak move south again to Nain, which is Labrador's most northerly permanent settlement. For many, it is a reluctant transition from a world in which traditional skills suffice to a world dominated by southern values. "I like it here better than in Nain," Andrew Kojak, Aba's 23-year-old-son, told me at Cut Throat. "Too much money problems in Nain. Around here we can just live off the land." Another Cut Throat fisherman, Alec Dicker, echoed Andrew's sentiments: "I'd rather be here than in Nain," he told me. "Hard on money, hard on yourself. Lot of trouble in them big old communities."

Canada's north has undergone drastic change in the twentieth century, and northern Labrador has been no exception. At the turn of the century, there were five permanent settlements north of Nain – Killinek, Ramah, Hebron, Okak and Nutak – reaching to the very tip of northern Labrador.

However, in the late 1950s, the triumvirate of power in northern Labrador, namely the Moravian Mission, the International Grenfell Association and the Government of Newfoundland, decided to resettle residents of the two remaining northern communities, Hebron and Nutak, to Nain and Hopedale. Nain, once situated midway in an unbroken string of coastal communities, thus became the most northerly, and the biggest, permanent settlement in Labrador.

NAIN IS TUCKED INTO the head of a deep bay four hundred kilometres by air from Goose Bay. Flanked by imposing grey hills, it enjoys a pleasingly dramatic setting. But its reputation as a place afflicted by poverty, social violence and poor sanitary conditions preceeds it. Happy kids playing in the sandy streets, where a stranger is sure to receive a friendly greeting, help to to distract attention from, but cannot mask, such third world problems as communal water supplies, open sewers and makeshift housing. At the centre of town is the fishplant, Nain's economic hub, and across the way is Nain Church. On top of the quaint steeple is a vane stamped with the date 1771 – the year the Moravians (Unitas Fratrum), a German Protestant Missionary sect, succeeded in extending its work from Greenland to the coast of Labrador by establishing their first mission-cum-trading post here.

The Moravians exerted powerful control on the economic life of Labrador for two hundred years, but today, even though in Nain you can hear an Inuit brass band, replete with horns, violins and cellos, play baroque music at Christmas and Easter, their influence on day-to-day life has diminished considerably.

As one external influence waned, others swept over northern Labrador. World War II and the Cold War that followed saw the construction of a U.S. Airbase in Goose Bay and radar stations elsewhere along the coast, which lured Inuit off the land into a wage-earning economy – a trend abetted by resettlement in the 1950s. However, the Labrador Inuit now face the greatest challenge that they have yet encountered to their way of life. The deterioration of the fishery in the 1980s, coincident with the loss of the seal pelt market, has resulted in "a level of social and cultural disruption not previously known [on the coast] and unmatched in other areas of the province or nation," according to a 1986 Royal Commission Report on Renewable Resource Use and Wage Employment in the Economy of Northern Labrador.

The social statistics bear out this grim assessment. Infant mortality rates are one-and-a-half to three times higher in Labrador than in Newfoundland; Inuit children suffer a high incidence of skin diseases and ear infections; half of all school children have a bout of tuberculosis; and alcohol abuse is rampant among the adult population.

Perhaps no statistic is more disturbing than that related to suicide. The rate of Inuit suicide in northern Labrador is three times that for native populations nationally, and five times the average rate for the Canadian population as a whole. Particularly discouraging is the fact that most victims are young, fifteen to twenty-four; in this age group the suicide rate is seventeen times the national average. "They are screams of desperation," says Commission Report author Carol Brice-Bennett, who relates these numbing statistics to the breakdown of traditional cultural values and, at the same time, an absence of economic opportunties in the northern communities.

I understood that the social problems, so pervasive in Nain, virtually disappeared when people returned to their summer fishing camps. In order to see the more traditional, and happier, side of Inuit life on the land, with the permission of the provincial Department of Fisheries, I booked passage aboard the collector boat, *The Setting Sun*, which ferries fish, families and supplies back and forth between the camps and Nain.

IT IS A 10-HOUR, 150-KILOMETRE PASSAGE, along some of the most spectacularly scenic coastline anywhere. On the Labrador coast the Canadian Shield meets the North Atlantic – two titanic forces seemingly in conflict. The jagged prominences of the Kiglapait Mountains (Kiglapait means "saw-toothed" in Inuktitut) rise magnificently, 1000 metres from the waterline, like great sea fortresses erected against the sea's batterings. After a mercifully calm run (on my first trip to the Labrador coast, seven years before, I had been caught in a frightful gale off Cape Kiglapait), we arrived at Cut Throat (Sillutalik) at dusk. Aba came aboard for a chat with captain Chesley Webb and to pick up his expected visitor. Recognizing that I must be him, he offered his hand: "Don't be lonely, boy. Don't be lonely," he said by way of introduction, his deeply-lined face cracking open with a wide grin.

Once onshore Jacko and two younger boys, Joshua and Gus, eagerly helped me set up my tent. Dispensing with tent pegs, which would have found little soil over the ungiving rock anyway, they anchored my tent as the Inuit have always done, with the generous granite rocks scattered over the island tundra.

"How do you like living in camp?" I asked in the manner of a southerner on a sojourn at a public camping ground.

"This isn't a camp," Jacko corrected me. "This is my home."

Jacko was right. Northern Labrador has been "home" to his people for a very long time. Paleo-Eskimoes of the Pre-Dorset culture were in northern Labrador four thousand years ago. Ancestors of the present day Inuit belonged to the Thule culture, a highly sophisticated people with origins in the western arctic. They spread into northern Labrador, seven hundred years ago, from eastern Baffin Island by way of Resolution Island and the Button Islands, appropriately called Tutjat, or "stepping stones." The Thule quickly moved southward into the rich whale hunting regions between Killinek and Saglek, in the process replacing the resident Dorset culture, which did not have the technology to capture whales or to fully exploit other marine resources. By the late eighteenth century, these adroit and spirited maritime people had occupied the coast of Labrador from its tip at Cape Chidley to Hamilton Inlet.

Travelling the coast today, it quickly becomes apparent that northern Labradoreans are a mixed race. There are pure-blooded Inuks, the Inuit; the Kablunangajuit, or "not quite whites" in Inuktitut; and the "Kabalanks" or whites, sometimes called Settlers. (There are also the Innu of Montagnais-Nascapi origin who live in the coastal community of Davis Inlet.) Sandra Gwyn used the apt analogy "Pitcairn Islanders," to describe northern Labradoreans. Ninety percent of northern Labradoreans claim some Inuit heritage and, admirably, Inuit and Kablananjuit see themselves as one people bound as much by lifestyle as bloodline. A single organization, the Labrador Inuit Association (LIA), reflects this mutual respect, by representing all four thousand native Labradoreans of Inuit extraction. Success in Labrador has always depended, and still does, on a high degree of co-operation among people. That they share their resources and help each other out – unquestioningly, it seems – are the lessons that a harsh land has taught its inhabitants.

The Labrador Inuit have always concentrated their activities on the coastal islands and at the mouths of bays, where they could intercept the arctic char as they migrated toward their spawning rivers, and Atlantic salmon as they moved north along the coast in late summer.

Aba has been coming to Cut Throat Island since 1971. Like most Inuit fisherman Aba brings his family with him when he comes north to fish. Aba's youngest son Jacko mans the boat with him; two older boys, Kelly and Andrew, have their own boat; another son, the eldest, fishes independently in Okak Bay. Two younger boys, grandson Joshua and adopted son Gus, help out onshore, washing the fish and packing them in ice. Andrew has brought his own family, wife Dora and their 5-month-old daughter, Eva – so that three generations live together under one roof, the rule rather than the exception in northern Labrador where the extended family still holds sway. Aba's wife Louisa looks after the household, happily leaving behind the modern conveniences of Nain for the more traditional lifestyle of Cut Throat, where she washes clothes by hand and cooks on a stove fashioned from an oil barrel: "I'd live here all year round if it was up to me. I hope we can always live this way," Louisa says.

The nine-member Kojak family comfortably shares the cramped quarters of a one-room shanty, spartanly appointed with crude bunks cushioned by caribou skin mattresses, a table where the family eats and wiles away evenings playing Scrabble and Yatzee under a single lightbulb powered by a gasoline generator. "It's so peaceful here, except for that generator," Louisa says.

Aba stays in touch with Nain by means of a battery-operated shortwave radio. Through the Nain Fish Plant he can place orders for sugar, flour, salt, tobacco – the northern staples; as well, the Fish Plant calls him regularly to check on the weather, the amount of fish they can expect and to see if he needs more ice.

I quickly acquired the moniker "Harry Kablanak" on Cut Throat Island. This alliterative pun (note the "K" in "Kablanak" is pronounced like "H") poked fun both at my appearance, bearded and bushy-haired, and my own obvious roots. I took the ribbing as a sign of Aba's acceptance, and soon found myself welcomed into family life on Cut Throat.

Daily routines revolved around checking the nets, first thing in the morning and again in the late afternoon. Aba always carried a rusted shotgun in the bottom of the boat, for every excursion on the water is also an opportunity to put meat on the table. "We have to hunt. We have to have something to eat. No refrigerators in Cut Throat, boy," Aba explained one day, after he had taken an unsuccessful crack at a flock of overflying geese. One morning when the sea was taut as silk, on returning to shore he observed: "Lots of seals this morning."

"Did you get one?" I asked.

"No, can't eat old seal meat all the time."

The Kojak men often spent the afternoons mending nets that had been torn up by grounded icebergs or, as happened this spring, by roving polar bears which had drifted south on the ice. The children wiled away time by fishing barehanded for "baby sculpins" in the tidepools, or roving the tundra in search of lemmings to provision a pair of pet, unfledged rough-legged hawks. The women, meanwhile, tried to keep up with the round of washes and meals. "Always something to do in Cut Throat," observed Louisa, who professes not to miss the amenities of her Nain home.

Perhaps the hardest thing for a Kablanak like myself to learn is patience in conversation. While Aba mended nets, I punctuated the silence with questions. Answers were often slow in coming and, I discovered, might arrive, out-of-the-blue, the next day. So I learned about the effect of the sealskin ban on Inuit life in Labrador: "No price on sealskins," Aba offered. "Not worth nothing. Greenpeace is a hard crowd. They want us to live on potatoes."

I was impressed by the calmness displayed by Aba, a kind of measured response to life, which perhaps had something to do with the harsh realities of survival on the coast. "It's hard to live on the Labrador," he told me. "Always living off the land. That's our life – we eat seal meat, deer meat, birds, partridges, pigeon eggs. . . . "

One evening Aba showed unusual animation, when, from his cabin window, he watched a hunting party arrive back from a trip to Hebron. "Lots of deers," he said, excitedly, when he saw the caribou lashed to the bow of the boat. The next morning I arrived at the cabin to find the family gathered around a leg of fresh caribou.

Dora was chopping a roast into pieces for the stew pot, but each of the men, including young Gus and Joshua, had his own knife and was helping himself to a portion of the burgundy-coloured meat. Aba seemed to relish the fat in particular. When he noticed my interest, he said with characteristic humour: "You can tell people Aba eats everything raw in Cut Throat, even sculpins."

He handed me his knife to try a piece for myself. "Small piece," he cautioned. "Don't make yourself sick."

Everyone in the family contributed to the supply of "country food," as wild game is called. Even young Gus caught two unfledged ptarmigan one day for the stew pot. With every meal, there was *baniksiak*, an unleavened bread that Louisa whipped up by the dozen in a frying pan.

Summer is a busy time as everyone is putting food by for the long winter ahead. Aba's neighbours – after sharing fresh meat with everyone – began drying what was left. I watched as a woman cut the meat into thin strips with sure strokes of her moon-chaped *ulu*. She then hung up the meat to dry on squares of fishing net suspended on poles. This curing method, similar to the traditional sun-curing of cod, will yield a product, called *kikkuk*, that will keep for two to three months. Also hanging nearby like brightly coloured socks were arctic char. Each fish had been split, then scored crosswise every few inches. After smoking for twenty-four hours it is dried for two more days to make *piksik*, a chewy, earthy-tasting delicacy. On a nearby beach rock, a hunter had unceremoniously perched a caribou head, sporting a magnificent set of velvety phase antlers. Jacko cut off the tip of one of the antler prongs, peeled back the velvety covering, and, with the point of his knife, fished out a piece of pale yellow marrow, which he offered to me. At first I politely refused this local delicacy, but, in the end, I relented to his peristence and nibbled on a corner. It was salty and chewy like a toffee; however, I ate only half and surreptitiously let the rest drop to the beach.

"We'll make an Inuk of you yet, before you go back to Kablanak land," joked Jacko.

Coming from Kablanak land, I was surprised by the extent to which the Inuit of northern Labrador did subsist off the land. So-called "country food" contributes significantly to the regional economy; in fact, it is the single most important source of income along the coast. As well, country food is an important factor in the health and social well-being of Labradoreans, according to a study by Memorial University of Newfoundland's Faculty of Medicine.

THE LABRADOR INUIT Association was formed in 1973 with the clear objective of maintaining a way of life in which hunting, fishing and trapping continued to be of prime importance. Life in the communities still centres around these traditional pursuits, even though people only relocate to camps during summer. Snowmobiles and speed boats have made it possible for hunters to use the traditional, family-based hunting areas but to continue to live in communities like Nain. Exploitation of species changes from season to season. In summer people primarily pursue char and salmon; in fall they hunt seals and migratory waterfowl; in winter, caribou; and in spring, seals, fish, migratory birds and caribou all contribute to the subsistence economy. Black bears, rabbits, hares and porcupines are hunted as well, and fur-bearing animals are trapped.

As important as subsistence hunting and the food fishery are, the Inuit of northern Labrador have long been engaged in a cash economy as commercial fishermen. In fact, the Labrador Inuit are unique among northern aboriginal groups in Canada, for they have been actively engaged in a commercial fishery of one kind or another for more than two hundred years – first for seals, then cod, and since the 1960s char and salmon.

In the last decade the cash economy – and the family life that depends upon it – has been undermined by loss of the seal pelt market, but even more significantly, by declining arctic char stocks in the Nain and Okak Bay areas.

The latter problem can be traced to resettlement, which irrevocably changed northern Labrador, displacing families, disrupting harvest practices, in effect, upsetting the whole economy based on the commercial fishery and subsistence hunting. In the thirty years since resettlement, Nain's population more than doubled to 1,100, putting intense pressure on the thinly distributed subarctic resource base, in particular the fish stocks in Nain Bay and nearby Okak Bay.

One day as Aba and Jacko and I were setting out a new net on the back of Cut Throat Island, Aba said: "Used to be a lot of char around here until the end of August. Not any more. Ten years there's not going to be nothing around here, maybe in five years time. No char, no nothing."

He paused and breathed out heavily: "If we lose the fishing people will go on welfare – nothing else we can do."

Inuit fishermen in northern Labrador face a number of problems peculiar to Labrador, Aba explained. First the season is shortened due to ice, which makes it practically impossible for Inuit fishermen to get the minimum of ten weeks necessary to qualify for unemployment insurance. The federal government has so far refused to adjust the Unemployment Insurance regulations to take the harsh weather conditions of northern Labrador into account. As a result, Inuit fishermen find themselves without an income in the spring when they most need it. "You can't get no ten weeks fishing in the Labrador," says Aba. "UIC cuts off May 15 and fishing starts June 15. It's really hard when we got to get ready for fishin', no money in the pocket. And we can't get credit for to go fishing. You can hardly make a living these days." As well the provincial Fisheries Loan Board has been reluctant to finance Inuit fishermen in the purchase of bigger boats, which would allow them to diversify into the offshore ground fishery. So the Inuit of Labrador find themselves caught in a bureacratic Catch-22: no money and no credit without money.

We secured the net to a rocky point and pushed off. Aba pointed behind me to the great mauve eminence of Cape Mugford rising in dramatic steps to its glacier-capped peak: "When I was eleven, I lost my uncle through the ice, seal hunting near that big high peak."

"What did you do?" I asked naively.

"I walked back home to Nutak, fifteen miles." he said matter-of-factly.

There was a moral in this story – at least for me. I realized that survival for Aba's people now depends as much on their ability to win battles with government to secure access to and management of the resources of the coast as on the skills passed from one generation to another. Aba reluctantly recognizes this fact, and for this reason when he leaves Cut Throat, he will return to the LIA office in Nain. Aba is chairman of the local Fisheries and Wildlife Committee (Omajunik kamajet) and also a land claims negotiator for LIA. It means travelling to Ottawa and St. John's. "It's hard to leave home when you got to look out for a large family," he says. And, he admits, for a man who grew up in a community (Nutak) where there was no school, no wildlife officer, no RCMP, and everyone spoke Inuktitut, it is hard to deal with bureaucrats. But it is work that he feels compelled to do, if his sons are to have a chance to live off the land as he has done.

"It is hard to go back into the office," he told me, "I don't want to but I have to."

It has taken ten years just for the LIA to get to the negotiating table with the federal and provincial governments (which they finally did in 1988). During this time their economic position has deteriorated markedly, so that they are entering negotiations in an atmosphere of urgency. "People here can't afford any delays," Judy Rowell, Environmental Advisor to the LIA told me. "The erosion of the economy and of the lifestyle is the most serious threat they've got right now."

Recently, the LIA and both levels of government signed an agreement, committing all parties to a resolution of the claim by 1994.[1] Central to the Labrador Inuit claim is their attempt to secure priority rights to the fishery adjacent to the coast. LIA claims that the fishery has been and still is the backbone not only of their economy but of their culture. "Cash income is essential for an Inuk," an LIA brief to the Senate Standing Committee on Fisheries states unequivocally. "Without cash an Inuk has no rifle, no ammunition, no fishing gear, no transport, no fuel and no meaningful occupation."

The Labrador Inuit claim that their aboriginal "right to fish" applies not only to coastal waters but to landfast ice (which may extend twenty kilometres offshore) where Inuit hunt seals in winter and spring.

---

1. The Labrador Inuit Land Claims Agreement-in-Principle was signed in Nain, June 25, 2001. The Labrador Inuit settlement area consists of 75,520 square kilometres of land, as well as some 44,030 square kilometres of tidal waters within Canada's 12-mile (20-kilometre) limit.

The Inuit now enjoy exclusive access to salmon and char in waters adjacent to their coast, but they also want priority rights to northern cod stocks, for which they currently have no quota. LIA maintains that they do not want to exclude fishermen from the Island of Newfoundland, who have been coming to Labrador to engage in the summer fishery for generations; they simply want first crack at the groundfish stocks. It is sure to prove a contentious issue in the land claims debate.

For now, Aba and his fellow fishermen want a faster and bigger collector boat that would allow them to return to the northern fiords of Nachvak and Saglek, where char stocks are healthier. Their requests have been met with silence, however. "Government is hard, especially the province," says Aba. "They don't want to give you nothing."

Pushing the summer fishery north is essential, if the traditional Inuit lifestyle is to survive. LIA has stated its ultimate goal is to re-establish a permanent presence in the far north, probably at Saglek where there is a DND airstrip from which fresh char could be flown to markets in Montreal and New England.

I wondered whether this would ever happen, whether the people themselves – young people especially – wanted to return to the far north to live year round. My brief time on Cut Throat Island had convinced me of one thing: Labrador Inuit need to maintain their way of life in the summer fishing camps, where people work together for the welfare of the family and neighbours, without the interference of institutions ensconced in Nain. On the land – harsh, lonely and challenging as it may seem to someone like me – people have a sense of belonging and of being in control of their own destiny. Contemplating this, I flashed on the image of Aba Kojak in the bow of his boat – resolute and unshakeable – guiding his son through the familiar, home waters of the Labrador Sea.

The Devil's Work is an Ark of Sand

Sable Island

"THERE SHE IS, THERE'S YOUR ISLAND." Thus did my cabinmate, Russ Miller greet me on a June morning. For twelve hours, the Canadian Coast Guard vessel, *William Alexander*, had beat across the riled sea; now she lay uneasily at anchor. I peered sleepily through the porthole. The sky was grey; the Atlantic, the colour of a heavier metal. In between was an incongruous slip of white land, Sable Island. My island? I suppose it is, technically. I am a Nova Scotian, and this place – to me, until that moment, more fabled Avalon than real domain – has been Nova Scotia's easternmost territory since the province first established life-saving stations there in 1803. Whoever may claim it, Sable still belongs to the North Atlantic first, and to Maritime history, because it has been so voracious in its appetite for men and ships, rising from the waters where no land should be.

What was it doing here, two hundred kilometres from the nearest landfall of peninsular Nova Scotia? "The devil's work," wrote onetime Sable wireless operator Thomas Raddall, in his novel *The Nymph and the Lamp*. Perversely, Sable sits in the middle of the North Atlantic's busiest shipping lanes, where until the invention of radar it regularly renewed its right to the notorious epithet "Graveyard of the Atlantic." Geologically, it is a relict of the Ice Age, 1,000 metres of sand deposited by the retreating glacier 10,000

156

years ago. Most of that thick blanket of sand is now a submerged fishing bank, which made fortunes for some sons of Gloucester and Lunenburg but cruelly harvested others.

Sable, the island, is an emergent promontory. Its unlikely latitude-longitude (44 degrees N, 60 degrees W) is near the convergence of the Gulf Stream and the Labrador Current. However, this seems to be mere coincidence. It is a local and tidally-generated current, spiralling around the island, that actually holds it in place against the tireless battering of the waves. Its rhythmic dunes are the work of the wind, blowing at 25 knots from the northeast when I arrived. A beach craft, which looked like war surplus from D-Day, was being used to ferry 3,000-gallon tanks of gasoline to the weather station, an outpost of Canada's Atmospheric Environment Service. Taking into account the surf, I opted for a dry-footed landing by helicopter.

One must have an express purpose for setting foot on Sable and the blessing of the Canadian Coast Guard, the island's jealous guardian. Sable is seasonal home to those who do research on fisheries, oceans and wildlife and to various provincial and federal officials, all charged with overseeing this sandbar's flora, fauna and residents. In recent years oil drillers have plumbed the sands, and oc-casionally writers like myself have come to plumb Sable's less tangible treasures. I was the guest of the Canadian Wildlife Service and stayed with seabird bio-logist Tony Lock at his small hut near the east end of the 36-kilometre-long crescent.

SABLE HAS AN ABRUPT WAY OF IMPRESSING certain verities upon its transients. The cycle of decay from birth to death seems foreshortened here, perhaps only because it is so glaringly obvious. Evidence is everywhere on the ground, as I discovered on my first walk. I kept to the better worn wild horse paths to avoid the nesting ground of terns. They seemed unimpressed by my care. Wisely mistrustful of any intruder, however well-intentioned, they swooped overhead and raised a screed of protest at my approach. Gulls, an ever-present threat to the terns, nest here too. I found four spotted gull's eggs in a nest constructed of dried marram grass and horse dung, the two most available building materials – one, after all, is the other in different form.

A little further on, I nearly stumbled upon a dishevelled horse carcass, flaps of reddish hide draped over the skeleton as over the wire frame of a mannequin. The nose and eyes were gone. Soft-parts of animals disappear quickly on Sable but in the absence of large predators all else is achingly persistent. In the days ahead I become accustomed to the remains of seabirds, seals, whales and horses. Sable had begun to wrap a cowl of sand around this victim. It is constantly covering, then disinterring its prey, a fact which was distressing to its inhabitants in the nineteenth century, when the dead were often sailors thrown ashore by the sea's violence.

The East Light blinked its warning over the top of a high dune. I headed in the direction of this landmark, again unprepared for what I found over the rise. There was a weathered house, three-quarters buried. I slid down the slope of the dune, and, stooping, entered by an upstairs window. The bedroom closet was nearly full of sand, the door casually ajar. I crawled to avoid bumping my head on the lintel. As I entered the upstairs hall, the damp, chilling breath of the house rose up the open back staircase. It was suddenly dark and unsettling. For a moment, I considered easing myself into the bowels of this entombed house. However, I had no light, and my courage abandoned me completely when a bird suddenly burst from a back bedroom and bucked out a window. I retreated, leaving the spirits of the house to rest, and wended my way back to camp, eager to share my discoveries. Dick Brown, pelagic seabird biologist, informed me that he had slept in the same house in 1970. On Sable, sand as the measure of time has a poignant everyday relevance.

Tony Lock was fond of saying, "On Sable you live the slimmed down life." Long walks become my daily regimen. I wandered the landscape (aimlessly as the horses, it seemed) foraging for flotsam, which is everywhere. All glass is exquisitely sandblasted. Even the most mundane item, such as a Pepsi bottle, has a misty charm after Sable's sands, driven by North Atlantic winds, have had a few weeks to work on it. The dunes are difficult terrain, not the least because the dry sand gives way at each step. I soon came to prefer the more compacted sand of the beach, even though this more dynamic environment was not as rich in artifacts. However, every several hundred yards, there were herds of twenty or more harbour seals and their pups. (Sable is Atlantic Canada's largest harbour seal breeding ground.) Their dish-shaped faces with inscrutable coal-black eyes would bob up from the surf, and I was always accompanied by one or more of these curious creatures. On my second day, one hauled out for a closer look before bustling back into the sea. This almost human, beckoning behaviour made me feel that it was expecting me to follow, to assume its likeness, become a sleek form with flippers.

EACH DAY, MY COMPANIONS – Lock and Brown and Canadian Wildlife Service biologist Colleen Hyslop – used a rocket net to catch immature Common and Arctic terns which seemed content to spend most of their time loafing on the beach. The adult males, on the other hand, frantically foraged out to sea, returning with silver sandlances in their bright coral beaks for prospective mates.

Late in the afternoon of the third day, we too decided to make a foray away from camp. We hopped on our bikes and headed for the East Bar, the five-kilometre spit of barren sand that is one end of Sable. The green sea was driven ashore on a southeast wind, the breakers advancing over the bars which run parallel to the island and were the nemesis of so many ships. The further we went east, the darker, colder and more melancholy the day became. Seemingly in sympathy with the worsening weather, the bar itself became utterly barren, except for the tiny disasters which had converged there.

When I visited, Sable's shores were littered with all sizes of new lumber. The wood, I learned, had been carried on the Gulf of St. Lawrence current as it swept around the edge of Cape Breton. Like hay in a haystack, the boards stuck out of the sand at every angle. Old tree trunks, worn smooth, and oil rig refuse added clutter. And there was the usual carnage: a seal fatally wounded by a shark bite. Among this unremarkable refuse was a 12-metre section of a 19th-century top-gallant mast. Cracked and weathered, it nevertheless bespoke the grandeur of the ship which like five hundred others had met its end on Sable's shores.

We maneuvered through the rubble to the tip of the bar, where we were greeted by a great herd of grey seals. Three thousand grey, white and buff lozenges of fat lumbered into the crashing sea as we bore down on them. The fleeing seals left the air rancid in their wake. In January and February, the scene must be even more impressive – as must be the stench. Then, herds of 20,000 and more frequent Sable's bars: 12,000 breeders, 6,000 pups and as many as 4,000 non-breeders.

If reminders of death are everywhere on Sable, one realizes that one is also in the midst of great fecundity. Anytime I cast my eye around, seals were feeding in the waters or sunning on the beach; horses were feeding in the marram or galloping beside the surf; seabirds were filling the air with shrill sound. Sable is sanctuary as well as graveyard. Oppressive in light of human history, it is nevertheless a majestic natural place.

As we turned for home, the sun broke through the cobalt sky. The whole complexion of the bar was suddenly transformed. Minutes before it had been a dreary expanse; now it seemed to shine with inner light. We came across a grey seal pup with a piece of green fishing net tangled tightly round its neck. Using a flexible piece of one-by-three lumber as a teeter-totter and the seal as a fulcrum, Colleen and I pinned the frightened animal. It hissed like a cat and showed its formidable row of curved teeth as Lock cautiously cut the net free. We continued on, our spirits lifted by our own act of samaritanism and the ever strengthening light that now bathed the whole island – a green and white moon shape curving into a sea rich with life.

Like the weather, one's mood changes suddenly on Sable, moment to moment, from one day to another. The next day I found myself, unaccountably, restless and anxious. I mentioned this to Dick Brown, who has undergone many long voyages. He recognized the syndrome. Three days afloat, the exhilaration wears off. It begins to set in that you're trapped, there's no where to go.

SABLE, AN ARK OF SAND, has its unique fauna. Perhaps the best known is the Sable Island horse. Horses were probably first introduced by Andrew LeMercier, a Boston clergyman, who tried to colonize the island in the early eighteenth century. Today the Sable Island horse is considered a breed apart and is one of only a few wild populations on the planet. But wild seems too strong a word to describe these creatures, which have reversed the usual trend toward domesticity. They are stoic, doleful, and to a degree, sociable – perhaps the less inflammatory term "feral" suits them better. After several days it occurred to me that I had not heard so much as a whinny out of them. They roam the island in small, discrete herds of families or bachelors. We had our resident group, which was somewhat non-conformist: three scraggly stallions and an unusually sleek chestnut mare. Occasionally they stopped by to scratch their ragged hides against our thin- walled shack or to crop the marram. I responded to a commotion outside one day, to find Lock muttering: "Eating my grass. They cause all these blow-outs."

Marram, with its tessellation of deep roots, holds the island together. Men and horses have disturbed this finely knit fabric, however, making the island more vulnerable to the force of storms which regularly sweep over it. Barrier dunes are breached, the bars shift, the island's interior is gouged out. In fact, the shape and dimensions of Sable have altered significantly as can be seen from a comparison of early and contemporary surveys of the island. A reliable map by Joseph Des Barres in 1776 shows a major lagoon in the interior of the island. Wallace Lake, as it was called, remained navigable from the sea until late in the nineteenth century. Now it is much diminished in size and entirely landlocked.

Fortunately, the island has its own underground lens of fresh water, and the wind, however fierce, can only remove the sand to the water table. Our well was located at the bottom of a blow-out behind Tony Lock's shack. The hand pump was mounted on a platform out of reach of the horses, which also used the blow-out as their water source. One day when I went for water, I found them digging their own well with their front hooves, pawing away the sand to make a shallow depression that quickly filled with water. I returned minutes later to find the horses gone. In their place were two Ipswich sparrows using the horses' well as a bird bath. These pale-grey sparrows, which overwinter on coastal sand dunes in the Central Atlantic States, breed only on Sable.

The well that became a birdbath struck me as an example of domestic co-operation between creatures sharing a small island. As one might expect, cramped co-habitation is not always this compatible. For the terns, which nest in the marram, the relationship with the ever-foraging horses is fundamentally antagonistic. Horses leave broken eggs and trampled chicks behind them.

Lock believes that there has been a drastic decline in the number of Sable terns. Described as immense at the turn of the century, the colony may then have numbered one million individuals and acted as a refugium for the species on the east coast. For at least two hundred years the terns have shared Sable with horses, so it appears their decline to contemporary estimates of 2,500 cannot be attributed primarily to them. More recent immigrants have caused the most havoc. Terns are being heavily depredated by herring gulls and great black-backed gulls, whose population explosion along the entire East Coast has spread even to this most offshore of islands. In Lock's opinion their proliferation at the tern's expense begs some kind of control. The horses, meanwhile, will remain unmanaged and inviolate. They are protected by law, public opinion on the mainland, and the sentiment of any lucky enough to share their island.

Lock pointed out, "Man can't live on an island without wanting to introduce something." The island's earliest colonists introduced cattle, sheep, hogs and, of course, horses. Horses are all that remain of man's attempts to domesticate this Atlantic landscape.

SABLE-BEFORE-HORSE must have been a more verdant place. In exclosures around the fisheries research station cabins, the marram grew to luxuriant heights compared to the close cropped grasses elsewhere. Other flora flourishes, however. One of the tern nesting areas is named the Strawberry Colony. When I was there, the ground was awash in the pale blossoms. Parts of the island's interior are generously vegetated while others – such as Bald Dune, at twenty-three metres the island's highest point – are utterly denuded. From its prominence one day, I counted forty-seven of the island's estimated population of 350 horses. This number represents a peak in a cycle which Lock has shown is dictated by the weather. Every seven or eight years, there is an unusually high snowfall on Sable and as many as one hundred horses starve to death. The population cycle begins anew.

On the morning of day six, I returned as I had come, holding hard to Lock's all terrain vehicle as we scooted along the south beach and Wallace Flats (once the site of Wallace Lake). A fixed-wing aircraft was due to land on the beach, but fog, which can wrap the island for days and weeks, descended in earnest. The flight was grounded in Halifax. It was for the best. A mechanical check revealed the tail section was seriously rusted. I was on Sable until another plane could be mustered or a Mobil Oil helicopter came our way. I settled in to see how the other half lived, those for whom Sable was home for months on end.

The manning of Sable is no longer important to ships, which can steer well clear of the island's treacherous shoals. The heart of the island's practical purpose is the Atmospheric Environment Service Station. Sable is one of thirty-three so-called upper air stations in Canada. At each one, theoretically at the same moment, technicians release a hydrogen weather balloon into the atmosphere. This probe of the world's changing weather – nowhere more changeable than on Sable, it seems – is repeated twice daily, at precisely 8:15 a.m. and p.m., Sable time. It is one of two atmospheric events that mark the daily lives of Sable denizens. The other is the overpass of the transatlantic Concorde. Its sonic boom rattles the station windows, jolts you into the day. Paul Workman, the island's handyman, perhaps best summed up life on Sable: "In a way, it's like a space station here: the work is routine but highly technical, the number of people is limited [six], and each person has a specific purpose for being here."

FOR EACH PERSON THE ISLAND also comes to have a different meaning, which, I was beginning to appreciate, was what my cabinmate had implied the morning I first caught sight of Sable. *Your island, my island* — Sable enters each individual's mythology in a highly personal way.

Near the end of my sojourn I met Sherod Crowell, another highly skilled technician, who helps locate the giant jack-up rigs precisely over their drilling sites, work he had done for a decade. It hadn't taken long for Crowell to fall in love with Sable. "It was August, all the wild roses were in bloom," he recalled. "I've been passing through for a long time. It's like home now." Throughout the 1970s, Sable offshore oil and gas production seemed imminent; now, with cheap oil flowing once again, there were just two rigs still drilling on Sable Bank, and the bank's prospects as an oil producer were dim. For Crowell, this meant a reluctant cutting of ties.

After lunch at Nova Scotia Government House, a modular hut of fibreglass whose entrance is an overarching gate of a whale rib and a ship's rib, Crowell led me to the Rose Bowl, a natural depression rimmed by a profusion of wild rose bushes. It is said the roses were planted by keepers of the old Main Life- Saving Station as a memorial to a French ship that went ashore here with great loss of life. We observed an impromptu moment of silence.

Sable provides a welcome opportunity for a person to do some mental beachcombing, collecting memories like flotsam and jetsam. Said Crowell: "I look inside myself a lot, which is not a bad thing. It's a good place to think."

But for Crowell the island was not only a good place to get, and stay, in touch with himself. He had gone beyond mere introspection, confessing that he had come to feel a kinship "with all the lives that have been lived here." Or, for that matter, lost here. Sometimes he had felt something, or someone, as he worked alone at night. There was nothing occult about these encounters with Sable's past spirit. It was an expression of respect for the place, which takes many forms for those willing to open themselves to it.

Now that the oil boom is over, there will be less reason for people to visit the island, to disturb, or commune with, its spirits. Sable can return more to its natural order.[1]

My last afternoon on Sable I gained a glimpse into what that order might be. I checked my impulse to roam and took up a station on a high dune, with a view inland and a prospect of the sea. Shafts of light muscled through the marram grass. A very young foal dozed several yards away, nestled in the long grass, as a herd of seven shaggy, thick-legged Sable horses grazed mindful of but uninhibited by my presence. The water's shadows were aqua and mauve. Fat harbour seals loafed on the north beach while in the shallows mothers passed on to their pups the aquatic acumen of their

---

1. Cancelled in 1986, the Sable Project was revived in the early 1990s and began to produce gas in 1999.

race. One mother propelled herself on her back, supporting her pup, who swam above her. Rolling, they dived, their heads reappearing in unison. The mother's flipper dunked the pup, and they were off again. All around older pups exploded out of the water, splashing down with adolescent exuberance and showmanship. Further offshore the slow shadows of grey seals feeding: a ponderous ballet. Sable's much maligned land and sea were nurturers that day. I walked back to the Staff House, which was as peaceful as an Edward Hopper painting, remembering what a young weather technician had told me: "When it starts to feel like home here, it is time to leave."

IV. Close to the Ground

Mining A Thin Seam
Wasn't God's Idea
River Hebert, Nova Scotia

THE BANKHEAD REARS UP LIKE A COLOSSAL, black-boned skeleton exhumed from the tidal mud. It looks so rickety, I question last night's decision to defer a life-insurance option. Even Ron Beaton, owner of the coal mine in River Hebert, Nova Scotia, says, "It's a relic." It's the last unmechanized thin-seam mine in the province and, in it, one hundred men daily hack out coal, as their grandfathers did. River Hebert has mined coal for 130 years and, in the 1930s, nineteen men died here in explosions. Successive provincial governments have subsidized Beaton's mine to protect jobs. But last spring, dangerous gas levels revived old rumours that the mine would shut down forever, and mine officials give it two years at best. Meanwhile, the men keep going down. Most are under thirty; some have no skills to sell, just their youth and strength.

Underground manager Ralph Henwood accompanies me on the tour and, as we board an empty coal car, a light mist billows from the slope's black mouth. I lie propped on an elbow, heeding Ralph's warning to keep my head down. The spring sun vanishes behind us. Ralph shouts above the rumbling track: "This mine takes you back to the turn of the century. In

Springhill, the slope was arched with concrete." My lamp scans the hardwood pit props. Water spits on us from sagging, cobweb-festooned roof supports. It takes only a couple of minutes to travel through the millennia of geological years to the first level: 2,500 feet (762 metres) underground. Disembarking from the coal car, I stoop to avoid striking my head on the slant roof, and a rat scurries down the dark tunnel ahead of me.

A few hundred feet in from the slope, Ralph stops to check for methane with his meter. Water and poor roof conditions have also plagued the miners, and the word is that the men are into "bad ground." Now a concussion recoils from deep in the mine's bowels. The rock walls, roof and floor shudder, and "BUMP" whiplashes into my mind. Smoke sucks past me, as adrenalin flushes my veins. But Ralph reads my look of alarm and gently advises, "They're blasting at the coal face."

Pandemonium greets us at the face: Curses and barked instructions compete with the deafening rhythm of the shaker pan. Miners' lamps cut through the dust and smoke. My mind and gut tighten to accommodate the claustrophobic dimension that is the men's working space. Miners kneel, or lie on their sides and backs, to shovel their bed of coal into the pan. They have no choice. The wall is only thirty-three inches deep and pitches at a sharp angle. An older miner snarls about the position in which someone on the night shift has left the cutter (a big chain that undercuts the seam). Irritably, he prods the roof with his pick. "And this roof isn't too goddamned good either."

"The roof is slate," Ralph tells me. "That's what makes it dangerous. A sandstone roof is much more stable."

Squirming under the roof, I flip onto my back and, to ease myself down the grade, dig in heels and elbows. In places, there's barely room to fit myself between the "packs" of hardwood timber that buttress the roof. Rows of packs recede into the dim distance where the coal has been extracted. The weight between the face and the main slope has squashed some to a fraction of their original height. Where the roof takes on weight near the wall, men keep wedging in more timber. Still, it is as if each miner were an Atlas, bearing his slate-skied heaven on his own shoulders and knees. Every eight or nine days lately, the roof has been "taking a set"; with a thunderous warning, the stone above squeezes your crawl-space closer to extinction.

When we reach the lower level, I regain my feet. "That's a weight off your shoulders" has never had more meaning. And at the top of the slope the light of spring has never been more welcome. At noon the men stretch out on the narrow benches in the lunch room. Ribbing soon gives way to stoic talk: of the Glace Bay miner who died last night in hospital; of the first anniversary of Hector McKeigan's death at River Hebert. "Carelessness causes most mining accidents," one miner says. "It's always the good roof that kills people." I reflect that there may never be another pit like the one these men know, and perhaps that's just as well. As one man who spent fifty-two years in River Hebert-Joggins mines told me: "I don't think God ever intended Man to mine a thin seam."[1]

---

1. The River Hebert mine flooded and was closed in 1980.

After the Bump

Springhill, Nova Scotia

THE DIGNITARIES ARE STANDING with military attentiveness against the sun-blasted stucco of the Miners' Hall, an elongated structure crowned with a cupola. Wooden racks that will soon be filled with memorial wreaths have been propped up on either side of the monuments. A loose crowd has assembled on the street. Women and children are perched on a retaining wall; a clutch of old men rally around a telephone pole.

"Great day to be going down No. 2," one offers.

"I've been down better," the other replies, dismissively.

The hushed conversations are abruptly curtailed by the dropping of a needle onto a well-used recording of *O Canada.*

It is the kind of ceremony that is repeated in towns and cities across Canada. But this act of remembrance is not taking place under the leaden ceiling of a November sky. It's June, and the cenotaph is across the street. The memorial that commands attention is a white sandstone figure, a mustachioed miner who has overlooked Main Street in Springhill, Nova Scotia, for nearly a century. His pedestal bears 125 names. At the base, thirty-nine names are engraved on a footstone, and a few feet to his right is a headstone with yet another seventy-five names chiselled into its granite face. Each name represents a man or boy who was lowered into the coal-rich depths

172

under this town of 5,225 citizens only to be hoisted to the surface crushed, battered or burned by the explosions of 1891 and 1956 and, finally, by the 1958 Bump that put an end to big-time mining in this hilltop town.

The town's courageous struggle for survival in the late 1950s engaged the sympathy of the world. This day, a hundred Springhillers are quietly remembering their own – spared the fickle attention of the media's interlopers. They are honouring not only the men who died in the headline-making disasters but all 424 men who have lost their lives in Springhill mines, the majority in the day-to-day accidents that are a grim fact of life in any mining town.

In *Blood on the Coal: The Story of the Springhill Mining Disasters*, Roger David Brown writes that Springhill was first settled in 1790 by three Empire Loyalists. Originally, coal was mined from outcrops – surface deposits – and sold to blacksmiths. Commercial mining began in 1849. By 1891, when the first and most tragic of the disasters struck, there were 1,350 males working in three Springhill mines. Many were boys, who performed the menial, but back-breaking, tasks.

At 12:43 p.m., February 21, 1891, a massive explosion ripped through the mine, the result of a slippage of stone that allowed flame from a routine blasting operation to escape into the gassy, dust-filled workings. "The explosion at Springhill was different from the two other major mine disasters the town was to endure," Brown writes. "After 2 o'clock, a little over an hour after the explosion, no survivors came out of the mine. There was no miracle."

On November 1, 1956, another explosion rocked Springhill. A seven-car train loaded with coal had become unhooked and gone on a wild careering rampage through the haulage slope of the No. 4 mine. At the 4,400-foot (1,340-metre) level (the depth of a mine is measured on the slope, not in vertical feet), it jumped the track and crushed a 2,200-volt cable. A wall of flame roared to the surface and shot two hundred feet (61 metres) into the cold November sky. Three walls of the bankhead collapsed, and people came running to the foot of Main Street, many to help in the rescue effort, others to stand helplessly by, waiting. For some, the wait was not in vain. Although thirty-nine men died, eighty-eight others emerged from the mine's depths. One group of forty-seven survived for three-and-a-half days in the gas-filled mine by notching a compressed air hose that remained intact, then breathing its life-giving oxygen.

Although two of Springhill's major disasters were caused by explosions, the most ominous characteristic of the Springhill mines was their tendency to "bump." In the forty years prior to 1958, more than five hundred bumps had been recorded in the No. 2 mine.

SIMPLY DEFINED, A BUMP IS A ROCK BURST, a sudden failure of the coal seam brought on by excessive stress. The coal itself is violently expelled into the working area, and in major bumps, the floor heaves, crushing everything in its wake.

Restricted to relatively few mining areas in the world, bumping always occurs in association with a strong roof stratum, such as the hard sandstone that overlies the Springhill coal seams. In long-wall mining, as practised in Springhill, the miners' safety – strange as it may sound – depended upon the roof collapsing behind them, in the waste area, as the seam of coal was extracted, thus allowing for a gradual release of pressure. The strong sandstone roof resisted caving in, however, and as more coal was extracted, this solid beam of rock acted as a cantilever, putting more and more pressure on the coal face, until it burst, or bumped, in colliers' terms.

In 1958, the No. 2 mine, which had been worked continuously since 1873, was the only mine left in Springhill. It was also the deepest coal mine in the world, having been mined to a vertical depth of 4,340 feet (1,320 metres). Bumping had begun to occur at the 2,000-foot (610-metre) level, and the frequency had increased with depth. Most were mild pressure bumps that nevertheless accounted for more than one hundred fatalities. Every Springhill miner knew that a major shock bump was coming; he just hoped that it wasn't on his shift.

The tremor was registered at 8:06 p.m., October 23, 1958, on seismographs in Sept Iles, Quebec, and in Ottawa. Seventy-five men lost their lives. But after six-and- a-half days, and the near abandonment of hope by rescue workers, a group of twelve men were found alive. Two days later, another group of six were disinterred from their living grave. They had been eating coal and bark, and in the final days, they were forced to drink their own urine in order to survive.

The relatively new medium of television kept a constant vigil over the unfolding drama, and reporters dispatched their stories to newspapers across the continent. The miners' ordeal became a parable of human endurance, and Springhill itself entered the lexicon of the North American collective unconscious. Springhill still seems to occupy a paranoiac dark pocket of the mind, a place where a fear of the earth suddenly collapsing under you is palpable.

The durability of the town's hard-luck image naturally displeases many Springhillers. Except for the ritualistic observance of the town's tragic history, many would just as soon forget the three dates commemorated on Monument Hill. That is particularly true for the men who actually survived the disasters.

Hugh Guthro was trapped in both modern disasters: for two-and-a-half days at the 4,400-foot (1,340-metre) level in 1956 and for six days at the 13,000-foot (3,960-metre) level in 1958. I almost expect someone of heroic stature, but Guthro is a small, wiry man – an advantage in low-roofed mines. He sits at the kitchen table, cupping the knee of his drawn-up right leg in both hands, a compact posture that he no doubt often assumed in the mines.

He talks freely: "I know one night, I nearly choked the daylights out of the wife." He demonstrates, crooking his arm like a wrestler applying a headlock. "You know, something happened in the mine that night, and I pretty near choked her to death. I was saying, 'Get down, get down, the roof's coming in.' Christ, she would tell me about it in the morning, and I wouldn't remember doing it. But this was after the Bump and that . . . but that was twenty-five years ago. I don't think too much about what really did happen, now."

In the aftermath of the 1958 Bump, Guthro, like many Springhill miners, was forced to leave his hometown to find work. He went to Labrador to work for the Iron Ore Company of Canada. But in 1960, when the Syndicate Mine opened, he was back digging coal in Springhill. When it closed in 1970, he moved to the River Hebert Mine, twenty miles (35 kilometres) away.

175

He thought nothing of returning to the mines, despite being buried alive twice. Like most miners, he is philosophical about the dangers. "This was a way of life, and this is the way everybody worked here." And he was proud: He preferred mining to unemployment. Today, however, he is happy with his job at the Surrette Battery factory. A mine is the furthest thing from his mind. "I'm fifty-five years old. You start thinking. Well, when you get this far in life, you don't want to go back into a mine."

TODAY, IF YOU DRIVE INTO SPRINGHILL from the New Brunswick border, the first intersection brings you hard up against the town's mining past. The Miners' Hall and monuments stand at the top of Main Street. Facing the hall are two rather large wooden churches; opposite, there is a Lucky Dollar store. It has seen better days. The asphalt-grey siding covers a false western storefront; attached is a boarded-up warehouse. Proprietor Fraser Mills produces a bottle of pop from the walk-in meat cooler, claiming that it is the coldest in town – an honest boast. I learn that it is a family business, and I ask what effect the mine closing had on merchants.

"Since the war, really," he offers, "we all knew something violent was going to happen, and of course, it did. But that pretty much was the low point. After that, it had to get better."

Fires have left a visible mark on Springhill – even more than the mines have. Driving down the steep serpentine incline of Main Street, I was struck first by its incompleteness, then by a lack of architectural continuity. A fire in 1957 levelled much of the upper half of Main Street; another in 1975 took up where the first left off, destroying eighteen buildings in the lower half – leaving the town without a commercial district to speak of.

The rebuilding process has been painfully slow. There is a new Stedman's, a modern split-level municipal building and a Bank of Commerce, which probably had something to do with the benevolence of the bank's prime-time attraction, singer Anne Murray. A large blow-up poster of Springhill's most famous daughter, framed in a Nova Scotian tartan border, hangs on the municipal building's brick facade. "Welcome to Our County" captions a girl-next-door image of Murray.

Springhillers are proud of the international acclaim accorded the smoky-voiced daughter of a local doctor. They are also grateful for the face of success that Murray has helped put on the "hard-luck town" – the media's cliche of convenience since the 1950s. For many, that epithet has been a matter of personal shame. A Springhill resident describes her first trip as a teenager away from her hometown: "When you told people you were from Springhill, they looked at you as if you had some kind of disease – that was before Anne Murray made it."

A few wooden stores that remained intact at the lower end of Main Street emanate a kind of fusty charm. Lorne Smith, thirty-seven, runs a lunch counter at the front of one of the town's oldest businesses, the Springhill Candy Kitchens. A vinyl stool at the black arborite counter was as good a place as any to get an inkling of the town's feisty spirit.

Smith does not so much serve his customers as taunt them into good-humoured acceptance of what he's handing out: fries, burgers and a good ribbing to boot.

"Since you're hanging around doing nothing, you want to pick up that waste? And try not to limp."

It is the type of repartee that one almost expects to find in a mining town where poking fun was developed to a high degree. Smith was obviously a good student. He is one of many Springhillers who came back to his hometown after a decade away. Pressed for his personal reasons, he replies, "I had a young family then, and I wanted them to grow up seeing the same things I did."

Things have changed considerably, however, since Smith was a kid in the 1950s. There are no longer two hotels and six menswear shops. Now, there isn't even a theatre for a children's Saturday matinee.

Smith attempted to revive his father's clothing business, but the venture ended in bankruptcy. He accepts most of the blame, but he also discovered that after the fires, customers had gotten into the habit of shopping in the shire town of Amherst, twenty-five kilometres northwest of Springhill.

"You can't think with your heart. You got to think with your head," Smith says, unconvincingly. He is a bit like the town itself – heart-strong, proud, tenacious and more than a little philosophical; tragedy teaches you that if you're going to survive. "The trauma people went through, you won't find that any place else. In that sense, this town is great," he concludes emphatically, just to be sure that I don't go away with the wrong impression.

The spirit that prevailed over the succession of disasters in the 1950s has had to carry on in the face of chronic economic ills. Mayor William Mont contends, with justification, that, economically, Springhill is only twenty-five years old. There was no phase-out period: One day, 1,400 men went to work; the mine bumped; and that night, it was all over.

The town has converted the old mine grounds at the base of Main Street into an industrial park. The mine buildings are now occupied by small manufacturers of plastics, batteries and furnaces. They have proved themselves reliable employers – even during the recent recession. But the mainstay of Springhill is the federal medium-security institution located on the outskirts of town. Over a beer at the Lamp Cabin Tavern, a guard tells me: "It used to be the pit, now it's the joint."

The prison provides far fewer jobs (350) than the mines did at their peak. But the $20,000-plus institutional salaries have given Springhill a surer economic base than the mines were able to in their last days, plagued as they were by frequent shutdowns.

Economically inconstant, the mines were, nevertheless, a unifying force for the community – something the prison will never be. If for that reason only, many Springhillers lament their passing. "Any coal-mining town has a very strong esprit de corps among the population," Mont explains. (Mont worked in the mine's machine shop but is now a prison employee.)

"It just made for a family type of attitude, or feeling, with the townspeople – but that's slowly disappearing. As you get people who never worked in the mines, and their fathers are dying off, and they don't know anything about the coal-mining era, it'll be like any other town."

To understand the character of a coal-mining town, it is necessary to know something about what takes place in the cramped workings that spread under it like a subterranean maze. It is there that loyalties and interdependencies which bind the community into a hermetic whole are forged.

In a one-industry town like Springhill, mining was an economic imperative. "You see, that's the way it was when we was growing up," a former miner savs. "We just followed down in the footsteps." But given the choice, most miners would take the pit over any other workplace. The explanation most often given for this mystifying attachment is "Mining gets into the blood."

HARRY MUNROE IS A DIRECT DESCENDANT of Henry Swift, the underground manager at the time of the 1891 explosion. All of his people were miners. It was the romance of the miners' oral tradition that first attracted him to the mines as a boy: "I used to be fascinated to hear them talking about the mines. I couldn't wait to get down into a mine and see what it was like – they never pictured it as a place you wouldn't like."

Now fifty-five, Munroe, like many other Springhill boys, went into the mines as soon as he could, at the age of sixteen. The realities of life underground didn't disillusion him: "There was never two days the same in the mine. It was like every day was a challenge.

"And of course," Munroe continues, taking visible pleasure in his subject, "the thing, too, was that the miners themselves were like a breed of people who are separate. I don't know where you'd ever find people like them. They made their own entertainment. Maybe this was one of the ways of shedding fear . . . it was the sense of humour that took away the drab of the job."

Men actually went to work hours early to pick up on a yarn that had been spun out the day before. The company provided a place, known as the Pest House, for just that purpose. Today, old miners carry on the tradition in the basement of the Miners' Hall, on the steps of the federal building or on several sidewalk "liars' benches."

This camaraderie found its practical expression in the buddy system. For reasons of safety, miners always worked in pairs. Ultimately, their interdependence was couched in the sacred miners'code: in case of disaster, miners on the surface would work without rest until the last living man, or the last body, was found. Munroe actually ended his mining career as a Draegerman, carrying out that grim charge after the Bump.

Dominion Steel and Coal Corporation (DOSCO) sealed off the entrance to the No. 2 mine in July 1959. Although DOSCO had operated the Springhill mines since 1913, no provision had been made for the fate that awaits all mining towns – someday, the mines shut down for good. "I know fellows that worked forty-seven years who didn't get a cent," recalls the United Mine Workers' last local secretary, Cecil Colwell. "When No. 2 bumped and didn't reopen, all these men were never offered a pension. At the time, there were no pension funds at all."

Money poured into the Springhill Disaster Relief Fund from all over the world, eventually swelling it to $2 million. But that only compensated the widows and the very needy men who were either disabled by the disaster or too old to find alternative employment. They received $40 a week. Many men, who had known nothing but the mines, simply had to pack their bags and leave. Springhill's population shrank from more than 7,000 to less than 5,000.

THE COROLLARY OF "Mining gets into the blood" is "Mining towns die hard." Although large-scale mining was brought to an abrupt halt by the Bump, mining has never entirely stopped in Springhill. Immediately after the closing of No. 2, illegal bootleg mines sprang up wherever there was an outcrop of a few accessible tons of coal in old workings. The last bootleg mine was closed in 1981, causing a furore in the local press.

Currently [1984], there is a controversial strip mine on the outskirts of town, the planned first phase of an underground mine. A political decision is pending on whether to press ahead with the second phase.[1] The surface (or strip) method of mining flies in the face of a century of mining tradition in Springhill. To Springhillers, a mine must go underground to be considered a mine. If you broach the subject of the strip mine with the former miners who meet everyday "overtown," on the steps of the federal building (a sort of open-air Pest House), you may get a shrug and a guttural dismissal of your loose use of language. If they discuss it at all, it is as a conundrum and an irritation. "I don't see what kind of mine they're supposed to be startin' out there."

---

1. The underground mine was never developed. Today several industries use thermal water from old mine workings to heat their plants.

Mary Raper was attending night school when her class was interrupted by a dreadful bang. As she ran from the school, she asked the janitor if a car had hit the building. "No," he answered. She knew better than to ask, for her husband had been telling her for months that there was going.to be one big bump and that nobody would come out alive. Some did, but not John Raper.

"It was six days before they got my husband. It was just pure hell," Mary recalls from the living room of the two-storey home that her husband built. On this quiet, well-kept side street, whose entire length is visible from Mary's living-room window, eleven other families lost a father, a husband or a brother. There wasn't a Springhill home unmarked by the 1958 disaster.

For Mary, it was not the first bitter encounter with the tragedy that so often envelops mining towns. Her father, who was a miner in Durham, England, was killed when she was sixteen. "It just seems to go right through," she says, sadness clinging to her broad accent. "Thank God, my children won't be killed in the mine." It is a sentiment that many Springhill widows share.

It is unlikely that there will ever be another major tragedy in a Springhill mine, as provincial regulations now prevent mining at a depth below 2,000 feet (610 metres), where serious bumping began to occur. But a question that gets its due in the sidewalk congresses is whether one hundred or two hundred men will be found to work the new mine – especially young men.

Guy Brown, the local Liberal Member of the Legislative Assembly, supports a small mine, but only for the men put out of work by the closing of the Syndicate and River Hebert Mines. He is adamant that a mine is not a long-term solution for the town's young people: "Let's not take our young people who are nineteen and twenty and put them into the ground if they know the thing will close in fifteen or twenty years."

Old miners seem loath to accept that ineluctable fact. The rhythm of the mines – the mechanical underground cacophony and the esprit de corps which manifested itself in the human ebb and flow between shifts – is the pulse that still controls their passions. It runs deeply and richly through their beings. They cling tenaciously to the notion that the only thing which will ever do Springhill any good is another coal mine.

Even if the new mine gets the green light, the way of life in Springhill will never again be dictated by the advance of a 400-foot-long wall of coal. Those days are gone forever. But remembering Springhill the way it was remains important – not just to those who lived it. It is more than a nostalgic exercise or old men clinging stubbornly to the romanticism of mining.

In *The Road to Wigan Pier*, published in the 1930s, George Orwell wrote: "Our civilization is founded on coal. . . . In the metabolism of the western world, the coal miner is second in importance only to the man who ploughs the soil. He is sort of a grimy caryatid upon whose shoulders everything *not* grimy is supported." On the eve of 1984, Orwell's observation about civilization's dependency on coal is no longer true. But as a description of a way station in civilization's advance, it remains valid. And for the world of the mining town, that utter dependency on coal is always valid until there is no more or until the price paid for extracting it is too great in either economic or human terms. This was Springhill's fate.

IN SPRINGHILL, MEN FOLLOWED THE SEAMS OF COAL deeper and deeper into the earth, beyond the point where the coal could be hoisted to the surface at a profit and, tragically, beyond the point where the coal could support the mass of earth above it. It was as if society had forgotten why these men went into the underworld every day, following rhythms we no longer understood or even cared about, until the world caved in under their little town. Then we focused our attention on every detail of their dark lives, with a blinding and sometimes cruel intensity. We witnessed their courage and endurance and extracted what moral lesson we could from the heartrending drama. It is a lesson worth remembering, especially as the consumer society scrambles to satisfy its materialism and as coal once again becomes an acceptable energy source.

I stood in the June sun, trying to pay respect to the men who climbed into the man-rake, never to see the light of day again. But I got closer to them at the Springhill Miners' Museum.

Retired miners lead you through the washhouse, where clothes are hung from the ceiling (like effigies) by ropes and pulleys, as if the shift were going to return, don them and head for home. Finally, they guide you to the black mouth of a mine tunnel. You awkwardly descend the 30-degree slope. Ninety metres down, you strike coal. Children and adults can try their hands at picking some – it is harder than you imagine.

Then without notice, the electric lights are momentarily doused. Your breath catches in a fleeting second of remembrance in the absolute darkness – blacker than coal or night.

Prest's Last Stand
Mooseland, Nova Scotia

THE TAIL OF HIS L.L. BEAN SHIRT FLYING, Murray Prest strides through the woods with the fierce energy of a man charged with an urgent mission. Occasionally, he stops to cast a wary eye over the carpet of spruce needles. He points out the stumps of yellow birch that are now reduced to rich reddish mounds of mulch camouflaged with a moss cap – fertilizer for the forest floor. At the base of a tall, straight red spruce, he kneels to note that the squirrels have been scattering the seed, a sign of the tree's reproductive maturity. He spies and clutches a mat of moss that is the pedestal for a red spruce seedling no larger than the size of his thumb, gently overturns the clod to determine whether the young tree has established a secondary root system. Satisfied that it has, he replaces it, then moves on up the hill, contemptuously brushing past a dead balsam fir pole that has been choked out by the faster growing overstory of red spruce. "Nature's way of spacing red spruce" is all Prest can muster by way of a compliment for the undistinguished fir.

It has been thirty years since Prest selectively cut over this ground, working the hardwood hills for the yellow birch – "Then, you could go to hell and back for a good hardwood tree, it was worth something" – and taking the mature red spruce for sawlogs. But he took care to leave the young spruce to mature, thinking that he would be back to harvest them when they had produced a seed crop for a future generation.

This time-proven forest practice was typical in Nova Scotia when Prest began working in the woods in the 1950s. Even as a boy, he learned the practical and moral principles of good forestry by watching the Eastern Shore woodsmen.

"I remember them working a crosscut saw in between trees, and if there was a little tree standing there, they would say, 'Don't cut that one down, that's one for the young fellas! I mean, there's no such thing as that kind of care or concern for the forest today.

"We're destroying our forest, we're mining it, and we're destroying it as fast as we can," he says, bracing himself against a sturdy spruce. "Now, if I could just see that level off . . . . I'd be happy if I could see that indication."

Murray Prest has lived all of his fifty-eight years in the tiny village of Mooseland. It is tucked into the forested interior of Nova Scotia, midway between the pastoral elm-lined Musquodoboit River Valley and the Eastern Shore, a rocky, sparsely populated stretch of coast between Halifax and Cape Breton Island. Surrounded by rivers, lakes and bogs and underlaid with granite and the merest dusting of topsoil where the glacier left any at all, it took a gold strike to put it on the map in 1858. That's when the first Prest came to Mooseland seeking his fortune, one hundred years after his ancestor had been given a land grant on the Eastern Shore as separation pay from the British Army.

Mooseland's gold rush days lasted until the early 1900s. Then people turned to the rich resources of the woods. There were virgin stands of the unusually diverse and productive mix that characterizes the Acadian Forest: red spruce, yellow birch, hemlock, white pine and rock maple. Mooseland's water-powered mills turned out everything from molasses puncheons (80-gallon casks) for the West Indies to hardwood tongue depressors. Log drives down the Tangier River fed Canada's first sulphite pulp mill at nearby Sheet Harbour. Even during the depths of the Great Depression, there was no lack of work in Mooseland.

In 1946, when Murray Prest returned home from active duty as an Air Force gunner, there were five mills. Everyone expected the war to be followed by another depression, so timberland was going dirt cheap. The young entrepreneur, only twenty-one, saw his opportunity, bought up land and opened his own mill. He quickly established markets for his quality hardwood and softwood in New England, the Caribbean and overseas. Eventually, his five younger brothers joined the booming family business.

Today, an unnatural calm hangs over Mooseland and the Prest Brothers Mill. A "No Trespassing" sign warns visitors off the empty lumberyard. Across the way, the schoolyard, too, is empty. The mill sports a new coat of grey paint, but its serviceable exterior is deceptive. Inside, there is only a hollow silence. The saws and planers long ago went to the auction block. It has been nearly a decade since the resinous smell of newly sawn lumber or the high-pitched wail of a saw charged the Mooseland air.

Mooseland, which survived so long because of the woods, is now caught where it is – for a while longer, anyway – in spite of the woods. It is an intriguing and supreme irony that is certainly not lost on Murray Prest: "We're right in the middle of the woods. We should have been able to carry on forever," he notes in his disarmingly unguarded way.

Premature retirement does not suit Murray Prest. His brisk movements belie the kind of physical energy that abhors being penned up in the house. His face has the ruddy hue of the outdoorsman; in fact, he spends a good deal of his time in the woods, cruising his lands, hunting and fishing. But he has also dedicated long hours to the study of the evolution – or devolution – of Nova Scotia's forests and forest policy, to which his amassed files, clippings and correspondence bear witness. He has put together a damning case of abdication of political responsibility.

"It's just fantastic that you could take an inventory, a fabulous amount of wealth, and you could squander it, to destroy so many jobs and the livelihood of so many people and end up with nothing."

Prest is one of the victims but feels that he got off easily. The big losers, he contends, are the forest itself, and the future generations that would have profited from proper management. Prest's personal troubles began in the early 1960s. He had private holdings of 14,000 acres (5,670 hectares), but selective cutting had depleted his reserves of mature sawlogs to the point that he could not keep up with demand. He refused to cut immature stands –

"You don't cut tomorrow's crop, it's not good business" – so that he was obliged to lease Crown land and to buy stumpage from Scott Paper, which had large freeholdings of its own in the area. For a few years, it proved a workable and amicable arrangement for all parties: "We cut the stuff and paid them for it, and everybody seemed to be happy."

However, Prest, like other lumbermen in the province, could not have foreseen the dramatic shift in government policy that took place in 1965, with the signing of the Scott Maritime Pulp Limited Agreement Act. Nova Scotia lumbermen bitterly resent the Act today, believing that it bargained their birthright with the giveaway of Crown land to the multinational corporation. It seemed to the lumbermen that their own government was turning its back on homegrown industry to please outsiders. The sense of betrayal cut deep.

THE SCOTT ACT WAS THE WELCOME MAT laid out for the Philadelphia-based multinational forestry giant by the new government of Premier Robert Stanfield. The benefits included a 20-year tax break on all forest land owned by or leased to the company as well as on the site of its new pulp mill at Abercrombie Point, Pictou County. The federal government contributed $5 million and an additional five-year income tax holiday. The 230,000 acres (93,080 hectares) in eastern Halifax County that Nova Scotia leased to Scott Maritime had some of the finest standing timber left in the province. And critically, for Prest, it was this very land that he had been leasing from the government and which he was counting on for a future assured source of sawlogs.

"We were kind of having a love affair with industry at any cost," explains Prest. "That's when we started looking for whatever we could give away to buy industry. The forest was one of the things."

Although the Scott takeover of the Crown land leases was a major factor in the eventual demise of Prest's mill, his lasting resentment toward government relates to its abandonment of protective legislation for the forest.

The same day that the Scott Act received royal assent, March 30, 1965, the existing Small Tree Act, which protected immature stands, was scrapped, to be replaced by the Forest Improvement Act. The Forest Improvement Act was acknowledged to be an enlightened piece of forest practice legislation, but it was not proclaimed until December 8, 1976, more than a decade later. And for the most part, it has never been enforced.

Prest has come to the conclusion that the Act's unfortunate political fate was no accident: "The Act was brought in as window dressing and to get clear of the Small Tree Act," he charges. "The pulp and paper industry wanted to get rid of the Small Tree Act, and the only way that they could do that was for government to bring in something that appeared better – people wanted protection for their forest."

As a native Nova Scotian, Prest has been appalled at successive governments' lack of will to enforce the Act and to protect the heritage of a naturally productive forest. He says that he feels like the Arab in his childhood school text, who was pushed out of his tent by the camel that wanted to get in out of the sand storm: "In business, it's fine to trust, but it's also wise to be a little practical. Let's put down the rules of the game first. You're welcome into my house, but these are the rules of common courtesy. And when you violate them – out you go. This was never done."

And there are still no house rules. With the scrapping of the Small Tree Act and the propping up in its place of what proved to be a straw man (the Forest Improvement Act), the stage was set for what Prest has characterized as "a full-scale blitzkrieg – twenty years of the most destructive methods of forest harvesting in Nova Scotia's history."

The granting of the tax moratorium, in the absence of protective legislation, proved an invitation to abuse. "I guess any of us would do it," Prest says magnanimously, "if we had a large investment and a five-year tax-free holiday. We would turn as much into money as fast as we could – and that's what happened. They plundered in the worst manner possible, as fast as they could."

Prest, the business man, pretends to understand the exploitation of immature stands. However, he refused to be party to such a policy, even when it was clearly to his financial advantage to do so. On September 16, 1966 (less than a year after the Scott Act was declared), Prest was called to Scott headquarters in Abercrombie for a meeting with Woodlands Manager Bob

Murray. Murray spelled out the company's change in policy. For Prest, it amounted to an ultimatum.

"They said we could start at Mooseland and work back as long as we clear-cut everything, or we could go into Lake Charlotte and work out as long as we cut everything. But if we left a tree four inches on the butt and eight feet long, a quarter of a mile over the hill, we had to go get it – she's all coming off.

"Well, that was a shocker, because I couldn't believe after twenty-five or thirty years of trying to save the country and promote it, that that was going to happen. I said that I wasn't buying that deal. In fact, I said, 'Look, if Christ himself came through that door and told me I had to do this, I wouldn't.'"

Prest came home and wrote down the conversation as a way of coping with his own disbelief and to have a record of his version of events for posterity. However, he had to face the reality of the new status quo: If the forest was going to be managed for pulpwood, then there was no future for the sawlog industry. It was just a matter of time. Prest reverted to cutting more on his own land but would not touch his immature stands. He also felt a responsibility to the half-dozen young people who expected to find steady work at his mill, build homes and stake their future in Mooseland: "There's no way I could let them invest, when I could see the end of the line." In 1974, Prest made the hard decision to close the mill. The young people left, and Prest went into retirement.

Prest did not drop from sight, however. He has maintained a high profile in the forestry industry, primarily as a member of the Forest Practices Improvement Board, an advisory body to the Minister of Lands and Forests. He spent his 10-year term, which ended in May 1983, vainly promoting the Forest Improvement Act. Though he no longer has voting privileges, he continues to argue his minority view of forest management in his official role as Acting Consultant to the board.

PREST PRESENTS A PARADOX: He is the establishment, and at the same time, he bucks it. A hard-nosed free enterpriser, he espouses the principles of ecological forest management that you expect to hear coming from a less pragmatic environmentalist. He admits to being a stockholder in a multinational company while accusing them of modern-day feudalism. He has been one of the most outspoken critics of the deal struck by the Stanfield Conservatives, and he heaps scorn on the present provincial Conservative administration, describing it as "the most unproductive era in the Department of Lands and Forests history," yet he unabashedly labels himself as "a lifetime Conservative."

Faced with this snakepit of contradictions, you have to keep in mind that, to Murray Prest, business sense and concern for the future forest are one and the same thing. And most important, his ultimate loyalty is not to any political party, movement or interest group, but to the forest itself. It has been good to him, now he wants to give it something in return.

"We owe the forest something. Somebody my age who has experience, who has studied the thing a lifetime, is duty bound to try to preserve it."

Prest says that his education in forestry began when he set his first rabbit snare and when he caught his first trout. "You might say I have an unfettered view," he quips. "If I'd gone to college, I wouldn't have been a free thinker. I'd have been moulded to that discipline, and it's a discipline that you damn well don't step over." The discipline that Prest is so bold to challenge is intensive forest management: the classic Canadian pattern of clear-cutting, followed, theoretically at least, by artificial reforestation. To Prest, it spells folly, for it ignores the potential of the natural Acadian forest that is Nova Scotia's rich heritage.

Prest has travelled from the Yukon to the Andes, from California to Europe, and his travels have only served to convince him that Nova Scotia's long-lived species – red spruce, white pine, yellow birch and rock maple – are as good as any trees grown anywhere.

The most lasting impression was made close to home, however. Prest considers himself privileged to have seen the last vestiges of the original Acadian Forest. In the 1950s, there were still 300-year-old stands that had escaped the axes of the original settlers and their successors in the isolated granite country around Mooseland. Because these stands had reached their natural life span and would have been lost to old age if not harvested, Prest cut them. But he never forgot the object lesson they held concerning Nova Scotia's natural forestry potential. "I've seen what can be done. I've seen the virgin hills of yellow birch, and I saw the last of our virgin spruce," Prest says with a zeal that makes you think it was only yesterday that he saw them and not thirty years ago. "Even these old stands that had taken years of beating from the weather and wind were magnificent."

The climax species of the Acadian Forest inspired early settlers to write of "vast cathedrals" and "shady groves of giants." Understandably, most contemporary Nova Scotians cannot think of these rapturous descriptions as anything but romantic hyperbole, or perhaps even fantasy. What they are usually confronted with is the legacy of generations of man's depredation of the forest. It has produced dwarf stands of balsam fir, white spruce and larch – what foresters contemptuously refer to as "sylvan junk."

Nova Scotia has the longest period of logging history in North America. Prest is able to read that history in the forest itself; to him, each stand of trees is a chapter in man's 400-year-long, unfolding story of interaction with the forest.

"I want to show you what they can do to the country," he says as we get into the car for the 15-mile (25-kilometre) drive to the coast.

Near Tangier on the Eastern Shore, a municipal dump sign marks the site of an old gold-mine works. The hill above it was repeatedly clear cut to feed the mine's steam boilers. Now, it is a mass of spindly balsam fir, 50,000 to 60,000 stems to the acre, few of which will ever reach harvestable size. Prest points out that this is the inevitable result of clear-cutting and, he predicts, a harbinger of tomorrow's forest, if current harvest practices are allowed to continue.

We also follow woods roads to present-day clear-cuts. A number come to a dead end at red spruce stands that, more than anything now, resemble a war scene. Only the stumps, debris of clear-cutting and scrubs remain: "If this is your scientific man-agement," Prest says, surveying the devastation, "it leaves quite a little bit to be desired."

WHAT BOTHERS PREST MOST is that the regeneration potential of the natural forest is being destroyed. His outrage applies particularly to the red spruce, which has always been the mainstay of the sawlog industry. He staunchly maintains that the species is also the hope for the future of both the pulp (it produces long fibre) and sawmill sectors: "If you manage a forest for sawlogs, everyone else's requirements are met in the process," is his dictum.

Red spruce can grow to a height of a hundred feet (30 metres) and remain vigorous for 250 years. Prest has been amazed at the tree's ability to resist disease, animal browsing and insect attack, withstand windstorms and adapt to site conditions. In the granite country, it grows literally on top of boulders, transforming into a sylvan scene an area that otherwise would look like the moonscape of Peggy's Cove. "We used to have a saying that red spruce isn't there because it's good soil, it's good soil because red spruce is there."

For all its virtues, red spruce is more vulnerable than most species to careless harvest techniques, for the simple reason that it reaches harvestable size – at least for pulpwood purposes – before it produces a seed crop. As a result, it is often harvested before it establishes a new generation on the ground. This was graphically illustrated, in one instance, where Scott land abutted Prest's holdings.

On one hand, there was a clear-cut: stumps, bleached grey tops and branches, a few raspberry canes trying to heal the wounds in the earth. But there were no young spruce on the denuded forest floor.

The property line was clearly delineated. Prest's land began where the straight stems of red spruce reached a height of sixty feet (20 metres). Under the forest canopy, it was cool. The shade had eliminated any competing hardwood vegetation. There was only the all-important moist seedbed of moss, where young spruce seedlings had established a crop for future generations.

Prest selectively cut this stand in 1969. Since then, it has more than doubled its volume, and it will continue to do so every decade, until the trees are at least 150 years old. "It's accumulating interest," the always practical Prest observes.

Prest has no doubt that red spruce stands, managed to ensure natural regeneration, hold out a long-term solution for possible wood shortages in Nova Scotia's future. In essence, that is what he told the provincially convened three-man Royal Commission on Forestry, now [1983] in its second year of deliberations on the best course for Nova Scotia's forestry future: "It becomes apparent that the best way to increase the annual growth of merchantable wood is to maintain a crop of trees ten inches and larger (on the butt), sixty years and older, by selective cutting and not by denuding the land through indiscriminate clear-cutting."

The multinational pulp companies certainly have no intention of switching to a 100-150 rotation. Neither do they need a high-quality tree. They simply want a fast-growing tree for one purpose only – fibre, and cheap fibre at that.

They argue that the best way to meet their industry's goal is through intensive forest management: clear-cutting and artificial reforestation, with the use of herbicides to suppress unwanted competition. The Department of Lands and Forests' reluctance to enforce its own Act seems to provide at least tacit support for this approach, and implementation of the Forest Improvement Act seems more remote all the time. In its brief to the Royal Commission, the department calls the Act "a conundrum" and suggests "review and updating in conjunction with other forestry legislation."

AS ELSEWHERE IN CANADA, the rate of reforestation is falling seriously behind the rate of cutting, and the Lands and Forests' brief confirms that about one-third of the 70,000 acres (28,500 hectares) of forest harvested annually in Nova Scotia does not regenerate naturally. To deal with the problem – which Prest maintains is avoidable in the first place, given disciplined forest practices – the province and the pulp industry have built new tree nurseries and expanded existing facilities. By the mid-1980s, they say, they will be producing 18 to 30 million seedlings annually, enough to reforest the 24,700 acres (10,000 hecatres) being laid bare by clear-cutting each year.

If, in fact, the province opts for the artificial reforestation route – which it seems poised to do – then Prest foresees tragic consequences for Nova Scotia's traditional relationship to the forest and for the creatures in the forest.

Prest also envisages forest farms encircled by wire fences. Inside the compound, chemicals have been applied to eliminate any animals that might browse the expensive and supposedly genetically superior seedlings. Outside, a guard has been posted to patrol the perimeter. For the first time in their 400-year history, Nova Scotians will not be free to travel their woods without fear of reprisals. What has been considered an inalienable right will have been lost. Prest has coined a term for this nightmarish scenario: *the interlocking process.* It proceeds by a frighteningly logical series of steps that, once set in motion, can only have one conclusion.

THE PROCESS BEGINS WITH CLEAR-CUTTING. Skidders remove the protective duff or moss layer, creating conditions for the establishment of cover species, such as raspberry and pin cherry. Herbicides are applied to suppress this unwanted competition for softwood – sometimes at the cost of killing valuable yellow birch or rock maple. Dead brush is bulldozed into piles and burned, eliminating niches for wildlife.

The next step is to reforest this man-made barrens artificially. Prest has worked out the costs per acre: site preparation $110, nursery seedlings $108, planting $120. Fertilizer may now have to be added as the natural source of nutrients has been removed by herbicides, bulldozing and fire. Add another $100. To this stage, the total cost is $438 per acre, and says Prest, you are a minimum of forty years from harvesting your first trees.

Even without calculating the interest on this capital investment over the 40-year growth period – which brings the cost to a staggering $2,900 per standing cord – Prest scoffs at the claim that the artificial forest can meet the pulp and paper industry's stated goal of "cheap fibre forever."

"If this kind of artificial reforestation were profitable in Nova Scotia, or even if it could be expected to produce wood fibre at a reasonable cost," he told the Commission, "industry would carry out a program of its own. It would not wait for government. Clearly, industry does not have enough faith in an artificial forestry program to consider it an acceptable investment."

With government investment, the link of financial bondage is clasped shut. "If you're going to spend $500 an acre to plant, you're going to guard it jealously," reasons Prest. You cannot afford to have animals browsing expensive seedlings or people inadvertently driving over plantations in snowmobiles.

The inevitable last step is the passage of legislation banning people and animals from the forest (the precedent exists in Scotland). The interlocking process is then complete: clear cut – herbicide – fire – pesticides – financial bondage – and restrictive legislation.

For a few cords of wood, the people of Nova Scotia will have lost a priceless part of their heritage – a consequence that is anathema to Prest, who has always viewed the forest as more than a place to procure logs.

There is a way out of this Kafkaesque bureaucratic cycle – if the fateful first step is not taken. Prest says that forest management must begin with disciplined harvest techniques that complement the natural regeneration of high-value species like red spruce and yellow birch. Otherwise, you are locked into a prohibitively expensive reforestation program. And people are locked out – in effect, disinherited.

Prest allows that artificial reforestation is justified where the natural potential of the forest to regenerate has been destroyed as in the case of fire barrens, but only then.

"I've always been amazed at the natural ability of the forest to regenerate and to adapt to different site conditions," Prest reflected, as we stood in one of his magnificent red spruce stands.

"If I ever had any doubt about my theories, all I had to do was go to the woods."

The Enemy Above

Millstream, New Brunswick

DARK NEW BRUNSWICK. I first heard that phrase years ago. It takes its meaning from the trees, the dark and brooding softwoods that are the province's economic mainstay. Many of those trees are now blackened and browned; for three decades they have been the fine fodder of the spruce budworm. In the past year [1982] I have made many excursions from my Nova Scotia home into neighbouring New Brunswick in an attempt to understand how this unnaturally persistent epidemic is affecting life there. As I drove across the vast flat expanse of the Tantramar Marsh, the land bridge between the two provinces, I imagined crossing over into another troubled country. The deeper I travelled into the realm of political intrigue and personal tragedy – as much the budworm's domain as the fir and spruce woods – the more the phrase Dark New Brunswick came to symbolize the very mood and fate of the New Brunswickers themselves.

There was hardly a person I encountered who had not been affected by the budworm infestation and the thirty years' war of chemical spraying that has tried to keep the insect down. It seems that the budworm outbreak, perversely perpetuated rather than eradicated by the spray, has fuelled a similar outbreak of social disease in the human population. Since Confederation – maybe earlier – Maritimers have cultivated a cynical hardiness in the face of the powers-that-be, a sceptical attitude toward political and corporate ends that I'm well acquainted with in my own community, just fifty kilometres away from the New Brunswick border. But I found that despair, anxiety, mistrust and fear cut a wide swath through the New Brunswick psyche. And it was not only individuals who had been brushed by the wings of the spray, but whole communities that exhibited a deep-seated set of troubled emotions.

Among the first people I went to see were Jimmy Singleton's parents, James and Joan Singleton, at their farmhouse near the northern milltown of Newcastle, at the mouth of the Miramichi River. It was one of those perfectly clear Indian summer days that seem overburdened with nostalgia – in this case not just remembrance of past times but of loss still suffered.

Jimmy Singleton died on the day after his tenth birthday, June 29, 1979. As of this writing [1982], he was the the most recent child to die of Reye's syndrome in New Brunswick – the last one diagnosed and reported, that is. Earlier I had met with Dr. Ken Rozee, who heads a team of researchers at Dalhousie University in Nova Scotia. They had verified, with blood samples from actual Reye's patients, that the syndrome is sparked by a viral-enhancing effect which they had previously linked to the petrochemical emulsifiers used in the spray.

For the Singletons, it had all started with a mild flu that gave Jimmy a sore stomach; within forty-eight hours his symptoms had escalated through nausea, confusion, delirium, convulsions and coma until he died due to massive intracranial pressure. Had he managed to survive he would have been severely brain-damaged. The Singletons remember every detail of his illness, including the last mad rush 140 kilometres to the Moncton Hospital at two in the morning.

Their son's convulsions were so strong that James had to ask for help to hold him; James is a big man, over six feet tall and heavily muscled from his labouring job at the Boise Cascade mill in Newcastle. Early diagnosis is crucial to the successful treatment of Reye's syndrome, which progresses so rapidly that drastic action, including cutting open two flaps of the skull to relieve the swelling of the brain, has to be taken. The Singletons remember every suspected cause: it might have been an allergic reaction to the prescription their doctor had already given Jimmy for his stomach. Had Joan forgotten to tell the doctors some crucial part of her son's medical history? Near the end, one of the Moncton doctors asked something that took the Singletons completely by surprise: "Did they spray in your area?"

"I just looked at him and he looked at me," Joan remembers. "I didn't know what they were talking about." She and her husband didn't find out until three weeks after Jimmy's funeral, when they read the cause of his death on the front page of *The Moncton Times.* It is hard to believe, considering the amount of ink and indignation that has flowed over the spray program in the past six years, but that was the first time James and Joan Singleton had heard of Reye's syndrome. Northern New Brunswick, the absolute heart of the province's forest and pulp and paper industries, is even "darker" than the rest.

GOVERNMENT AND PROVINCIAL pulp and paper companies have been spraying to control budworm in the New Brunswick forests since 1952. The only thing that has changed from year to year is the insecticide. From 1952 until 1968 DDT was the chemical used; when its long-term deleterious effects on the environment became clear in the mid-1960s, an organophosphate compound called phosphamidon was phased in. It was the predominate spray for the next decade, then it too was replaced by a supposedly safer organophosphate spray called fenitrothion. Fenitrothion is now the chemical of choice, although Matacil (a carbamate) was used on a wide scale in 1979 when fenitrothion temporarily fell from favour while the New Brunswick government ordered health tests on it. Like it or not, New Brunswickers are caught up in a fickle game of chemical chairs.

The names blur and are hard to pronounce, but one thing to remember is that both types of sprays used since 1968 (the organophosphates and the carbamates) are neurotoxins. They block the enzyme cholinesterase, which is essential to the transmission of nerve impulses in all organisms, from insects to humans. They work on the budworm by knocking the larvae off the trees – once on the ground they are unable to get back to the buds and new growth, so they starve. The sprays also "knock down" bees, wasps, spiders, birds and other natural predators of the budworm. Research on human beings exposed to chronic low levels of these kinds of insecticides shows that they suffer a higher than normal level of nervous disorders and a greater incidence of leucopenia (low white blood cell count) which makes them more susceptible to infectious diseases. No general health study of the province has ever been done, but the very least that can be said is that New Brunswickers are a population at risk.

In 1981 alone, 680,000 kilograms (1.5 million pounds) of fenitrothion (not counting the other chemical components of the spray, the solvents, and emulsifiers) were sprayed over 18,000 square kilometres of the province. A 1.6-kilometre setback zone (since modified to 305 metres) from human habitation was established in 1977 but it hardly provides adequate protection when a "good" spray is considered one in which half of the chemical arrives on target. The other half drifts in the wind and has been found in rainwater eighty kilometres from the nearest spray block. The best available data indicated that as little as 3 percent and sometimes more than double the dose can land within the target area.

Before 1976, the debate on the efficiency of the budworm spray program and its possible environmental and health effects was basically an insiders' argument between two camps promoting competing interpretations of "good" forest management. The corporate model, which was sponsored and spawned by big business, government and the Canadian Forestry Service, believed that the forest was a farm and should be treated as such. Level it in the cheapest and quickest way possible (clearcut with big machines), plant it (using herbicides to keep out the weed varieties and pesticides to keep insects away), let it grow for its forty years to maturity and then go in and harvest. Start again.

The other model, known as silviculture, called for selective cutting of mature trees and planting to get the forest back into a healthy semblance of its pre-20th-century self. It was labour intensive – prone to the chainsaw rather than the chemical approach to "control." In other words, to silviculturists the forest had to be treated like a forest.

Even the corporate woodsmen agreed that the object of spraying wasn't to get rid of the spruce budworm. There didn't seem to be a way to wipe the insect out, since spraying seemed to keep the insect at permanent semi-epidemic levels by preserving the mature trees for its food supply. The budworm would never starve. But with the attitude that the trees were a crop that the forestry industry had a right to harvest, the crop had to be protected; thus year after year of stopgap spraying, and ever increasing areas of budworm infestation.

Until 1976, the New Brunswick people were fairly acquiescent about spraying. The industry and government could take care of the industry because, after all, the industry took care of New Brunswickers. In 1982 there were 15,000 jobs directly involved, and another 20,000 indirectly. The forest industry contributed almost $1 billion a year to the provincial economy in a normal year. It represented more than two thirds of the province's exports in foreign markets, affecting its balance of payments. In short, it is a very critical foundation resource to the wellbeing of all New Brunswickers.

BUT IN 1976 SEVERAL EVENTS CONSPIRED to give birth to the first anti-spray protest group in New Brunswick and the first citizens' assault on the status quo. The first studies of the Dalhousie research team, establishing what was then only a probable link between Reye's syndrome and the spray, became public knowledge in the spring of '76, sparking the first intensive public scrutiny of the budworm war. Nova Scotia had never sprayed and had weathered two previous epidemics in the century, but was under extreme pressure from the forest industry to spray to control an epidemic then raging in the Cape Breton Highlands. With the added impetus of the revealed health hazards, a citizens' protest group in Cape Breton successfully countered every argument that the forest industry brought to bear, even the threat by Nova Scotia Forest Industries (NSFI), owned by the Swedish multinational Stora Kopparberg, that it would have to move right out of Nova Scotia in five years if spraying of its wood supply wasn't undertaken immediately. Since there was no legacy of spraying to counter, the Cape Bretoners could argue about economics first and possible health hazards later, so they were effective at meeting both industry and Gerald Regan's Liberal provincial government on businesslike ground. As the group's economic and supply forecasts predicted, six years later NSFI is still able to operate in Cape Breton and the budworm epidemic has collapsed on its own.

In New Brunswick the issue was much more visceral. At the same time as the Dalhousie research was making headlines, Forest Protection Limited (FPL), the government-and-industry-run company that handles the annual spray campaign, was gearing up for the largest spray ever – 3.8 million hectares (9.5 million acres) of New Brunswick forests. You didn't have to be in the fields or woods that spring to be at risk; planes seemed to spray with impunity, fighting the good fight over fields, lakes, houses and even schoolyards. One schoolyard was sprayed during recess in the small town of Hampton, near Saint John in southern New Brunswick, and over the next seven months three of the children developed meningoencephalitis. Two of the three subsequently died, with symptoms similar to those of Reye's syndrome. Simply and appropriately, the anti-spray group born in response to this incident was called Concerned Parents.

Concerned parents represented the beginnings of public opposition to the official sanction of the spray and they paid a personal price of character attacks for their views. "We have been quite hysterically accused of being irrational," quips Catherine Richards, researcher for the group since its inception and perhaps more responsible than any of its three hundred or so active members for its public credibility. "We're always accused of being emotional. I think it's because we called ourselves 'parents' and a lot of us are women so that the label was an easy one to apply."

Richards, a housewife and mother in her mid-thirties, is without question the most knowledgeable lay person on the budworm issue in New Brunswick, a kind of Stanley Knowles of the budworm world. The dining room of her suburban Fredericton house is her research centre. An office filing cabinet holds court, stuffed to overflowing with reprints of scientific papers touching on almost any aspect of the budworm question – in her cheerful and fastidious way she can lay her hands on any one you might want at a moment's notice.

Take this one for instance: In the spring of 1980 Richards got her hands on a hard-to-come-by translation of a Japanese study (conducted by Dr. Takashi Kawachi of the National Research Centre of Cancer in Japan) which showed that fenitrothion caused both mutations and chromosome aberrations. Of twenty-five chemicals ranked according to their strength in mutation and chromosome aberration tests, fenitrothion ranked second and sixth respectively. It produced significant chromosome breakage in rat bone marrow when administered to live rats, and also affected chromosomes in human embryo cells.

Concerned Parents thought these results particularly disturbing because the Sumitomo Chemical Company, a manufacturer of fenitrothion, has claimed that it is "completely devoid" of mutagenic activity. Richards also pointed out that fenitrothion is one of the one hundred suspect chemicals on the Industrial Biotest (IBT) list. In 1977 the U.S. company was found to have falsified tests, and as a result all of its testing (which the Canadian government depended on in its decisions to license chemicals) is currently under review in the U.S. and Canada. Two-thirds of the IBT studies reviewed so far have been found invalid.

This information disseminated by Concerned Parents takes on significance in light of cancer rates for New Brunswick released by Statistics Canada in 1981 (based on 1977 data). Richards publicized the figures, which show that New Brunswick's overall rate of new cases of cancer is greater than the Canadian average. And even though for all intents and purposes the two Maritime provinces share the same climate, landscape and genetic stock, New Brunswick's rate was one-third higher than Nova Scotia's. Health Minister Brenda Robertson's reaction to the cancer rate was to say that one can't be too simplistic when evaluating such statistics – perhaps the higher New Brunswick rates were due to better detection on the part of the province's doctors. When it was pointed out to her that a doctor in New Brunswick serves 922 patients on average while Nova Scotia doctors handle only 560, Robertson stood her ground: "It's very easy to say that they're spread more thinly, but I can't agree that their diagnosis is going to be less accurate. I would suggest that our doctors work a lot longer hours than if we had more doctors."

"It's kind of funny," Richards says. "It's the way politicians work – you say something and they twist it just a little bit and they answer what they twisted rather than what you really said."

Even so, Concerned Parents has had its victories: The acreage sprayed in 1977 was reduced by half from the record previous year, and the group can accept credit for that government concession. The now-wavering setback zone was also established in 1977, and because of Concerned Parents' loud protests the spray operators try as best as they can to avoid flying their loads of pesticide mist over private land in southern New Brunswick. But the group has been nowhere near as successful as its counterpart in Nova Scotia, and this is directly attributable to the fact that the pro-spraying forces in New Brunswick are an institutionalized part of the province's life. The departments of Natural Resources, Environment and Health, the Canadian Forestry Service's Maritime branch based in Fredericton, Forest Protection Limited and the pulp and paper companies, the Hatfield Conservative government which has held office eleven years – all are wrapped up in the warp and weft of a pro-spray forestry policy.

PERHAPS A LOOK AT FPL is the best way to explain how it all works. Formed in 1952 by the government in cooperation with the industry, FPL's board is still dominated by ministers of the Crown and executives of the pulp companies, including Bud Bird, Brenda Robertson and Gordon Baskerville, the new Assistant Deputy Minister of Natural Resources. H.J. (Bud) Irving, the former forest firefighter and pilot who is now managing director of FPL, sets out the flow chart: "Although it has a share structure, the shares are owned over 90 percent by the government through the Department of Natural Resources and less than 10 percent by the forest industry. We operate as a non-profit organization. . . .

"Approximately two-thirds of the funding comes from the province and one-third from the nine pulp and paper companies. The government at all times appoints the majority of the board of directors. So for all practical purposes we are controlled by the provincial government." The actual areas to be sprayed, Irving says, are figured out by the Department of Natural Resources, in consultation with the Canadian Forestry Service (which does the egg-mass counts on the budworm) and industry. The status quo is very interdependent, and in essence controlled by the elected representatives of the people.

Concerned Parents has tried the litigation route against FPL and discovered through a protracted and expensive court action that the laws of the land seem constituted to provide better protection to animals and fishes than to people. In March 1977, they laid thity-one separate charges against FPL arising from the 1976 spray season, under both Federal Fisheries Act and the Pest Control Products Act (PCP). FPL responded by arguing before the Supreme Court of New Brunswick that it was an agent of the Crown and thus immune from such charges.

The Supreme Court ruled that FPL was not an agent of the Crown and turned the case back to the local magistrates for the trial. FPL appealed and won half its point – the Appeal Court ruled in May 1979 that the Fisheries Act does bind FPL but that the Pest Control Products does not. Both FPL and Concerned Parents sought leave to appeal that decision to the Supreme Count of Canada, but leave was denied both of them.

FPL has one more maneuvre up its sleeve. It sought a stay of proceedings with respect to the charges it still faced under the Fisheries Act. The stay was granted in May 1980. Concerned Parents might have pressed ahead against that last decision, but decided it wasn't worth the effort or the money. Instead they are lobbying hard for an amendment that has been given first reading in the House of Commons that would make the PCP Act binding on the Crown.

It is naive of Concerned Parents to be indignant about this three-year, wear-you-down legal battle – that's how these kinds of things are fought. But Clark Phillips, a woodlot owner and organic farmer who chaired Concerned Parents' legal committee, is bitter about the outcome and worried about the consequences: "This is supposed to be a society of law, with democratic input into the structure of law. When one piece of society, this consortium of pulp companies held together with the government glue called FPL, develops for itself a position of absolute power, it can prompt a kind of desperate individual action."

Reasonable individual action is certainly hard to take, and confined to the few New Brunswickers who can afford it. In 1976, Abram Friesen, a University of New Brunswick professor who lives on a farm thirteen kilometres from Fredericton, did win a shortlived moral victory when he successfully sued FPL for trespass, nuisance and negligence. He and his family had been enjoying one of the New Brunswick rites of spring, picking fiddleheads on their property, when another of those rites passed over their heads and soused them with fenitrothion. Abe and his wife, Marie-Luise, developed acute symptoms of pesticide poisoning and the next day their 11-year-old son suffered a severe asthma attack. All three required medical attention. The Friesens were outraged, especially because they had requested and received written assurance from FPL that their property would be exempt from the spray area.

After a year of hearings the Friesens were awarded $1,328 in damages. It had cost them twenty-five times that much to prove their case – $32,000. Even with the court costs awarded to them they are still out $10,000, a financial burden that the average New Brunswicker could not consider incurring. And what's worse is that their successful day in court had the long-term effect of further diminishing the rights of the individual to challenge FPL's practices.

The New Brunswick government responded to the Friesen precedent by immediately proposing a special bill which would have given FPL powers to spray anywhere in the province – including private property and in spite of owner's wishes. It also advocated removal of the landowner's right to lay claim to damages. The measure proved too Draconian even for the New Brunswick political climate, and the government was forced to introduce an amendment which allowed actions against FPL for trespass – but only when damages to property could be proven. That is something which, Clark Phillips points out, is very hard to do. "We received a New Brunswick kind of justice," says Abe Friesen.

Most New Brunswickers are not in a position to speak out for others. Many do not even have the option of defending themselves. A character in a book by New Brunswick writer Alden Nowlan, himself the son of a pulp cutter, uttered the survivor's creed of the lower-class Maritimer: "You keep you mouth shut and your ass close to the ground." And look what happens when you trespass against that creed, even in southern New Brunswick where public activism has made inroads.

DON MORRIS HAS LIVED ALL his twenty-seven years in New Brunswick and spring isn't spring to him without spraying. He remembers as a child the planes flying low over the farmyard and his father wiping DDT from the windshield of the car. He inherited his father's 50-hectare farm, much of which is woodlot, in Ford Mills, Kent County, an economically depressed area in the southeastern part of the province. Don does as his father did before him, cuts pulp in the winter and keeps a few animals. If he lived elsewhere he might be called a homesteader but here that is definitely an outsider's term.

Don's own woodlot is budworm damaged ("It doesn't matter what size fir I cut, the heart is rotten"), but he is not complacent about the thought of being sprayed: "I've heard of woodsworkers in the Salmon River area getting sprayed but they don't seem to mind, like they're big tough lumbermen or something. They take the government's word – they trust these people." What happened to his 25-year-old wife Pamela last summer as she worked planting trees for the government is proof enough for Don that any trust is misplaced.

Most of the treeplanters in the area are women. Though lugging trays of three hundred seedlings while you plant is heavy work, competition for the jobs is keen. Pam, who held the job the summer before, felt pretty lucky to be rehired for 1981 on the basis of her good reputation – even though her crew was told by District Ranger Ed Parkhill that there was a possibility they would be sprayed because the planting area, along the Salmon River Road, was within the spray area. If they were worried, said Parkhill, they could call the Zenith number of FPL for the daily spraying schedule and stay home for a day without pay.

Pam did stay home on June 3rd to be out of harm's way when the planes went over. On June 4th, she finished her day's work by 11:30 a.m.

and was waiting for others in the crew, including her sister Johanne Amyotte, to walk back along the woods road with her to the cars. She looked up at the sound of engines and saw two planes flying low over the treeline toward the open planting areas. One of them still had its spray nozzles open. Planter Debbie Agnew, working right under the flightline, was drenched in the chemical mist. "They should have seen us," admitted duty ranger Dave Clark. "There were four cars along the treeline and my service truck – they should have seen that at least."

Pam Morris was so upset that she headed for the cars in tears, and Clark told her that to reassure herself she should give his boss Ed Parkhill a call. Parkhill was surprised by the accident, and told Pam to see a doctor if she wished. Pam also called a friend for advice, and perhaps wishes now she hadn't. The friend was connected to the anti-spray network, and got in touch immediately with Concerned Parents. The accident was reported on radio that afternoon and Pam Morris unintentionally became the leading figure in the breaking story.

Official reaction was swift. A directive came from the regional office of the Department of Natural Resources requiring that all those on the plantation that morning go for a specific kind of blood test (plasma pseudocholinesterase testing) considered reliable at detecting fenitrothion exposure. Pam and five co-workers went to the Rexton Medical Centre that evening to have samples taken by the public health nurse. The nurse could not get enough of a sample from Debbie Agnew, the one who had been doused, so she went to a doctor in Moncton the next morning where a sample was taken. Pam Morris and her sister, just to be on the safe side – because after all you never can tell – got a second set of blood samples taken at Rexton the next morning. In all, three sets of blood samples were taken – two done in Rexton and one in Moncton, where the Regional Laboratory is located.

Three weeks passed before a letter dated June 25 arrived from Dr. Albert Fraser of the regional lab to say that the samples had been "discarded by mistake prior to analysis. If required, please send another sample." Debbie Agnew re-members, "Pam called me and said hers was lost. The next morning I got a phone call that the sample I had done in Moncton had been misplaced. When I found out all the ones from Rexton were lost too I thought it was kind of funny."

Spokesmen for the Department of Health and Moncton Hospital, which houses the regional lab, thought it kind of funny too, but the only explanation I got from them when researching this story was "An error was made" – until I made it clear to Fred Rayworth, public relations officer for the hospital, that not just one set of samples but three separate batches had been lost. He got in touch with Albert Fraser of the lab, who quickly got in touch with me. Fraser said that all the samples had been batched and placed in the lab freezer (a common practice for infrequently done tests) so that they could be analyzed at the same time when the lab's senior technologist got back from vacation. Fraser didn't know how they came to be discarded, just that when the technologist got back on the job they were nowhere to be found.

The lab processes approximately 100,000 tests a month and understandably a few are lost or broken. But it only processes forty to fifty cholinesterase tests a year, and this was the first time the lab had lost any. Fraser told me that at least two other samples, from greenhouse workers in Hillsborough, had been tossed out with the Rexton batch: "This proves that there was no conspiracy to deliberately discard the Rexton samples."

For Pamela Morris, who did or didn't do what and when seems purely academic now. Shy and thin, with a redhead's pale complexion, she was obviously depressed the last time I talked with her, speaking in even shyer halting tones. It seems that the Department of Natural Resources had fired her a month after the incident for failing two regular department inspections of her work in the category of "firmness." (Foreman Doris Scott told me: "I'm up and down between the rows all the time. Anytime I inspected her work it was all right. She was a real good planter. I was surprised when she failed, really surprised, especially the second time.") Two strikes and she was out, but a third was sent her way. She had just found out that she was pregnant with her second child, due in February of 1982 - meaning that the baby might have been conceived before she was sprayed.

Things in general are not easy with the Morrises. The loss of Pam's job jeopardizes their financial security – it has been nearly two years since Don held a paying job off the farm. There is little hope of her being rehired as a planter on her "good" reputation this year, and she has resigned herself to it: "That's the situation we're in. A lot of people have put up with being sprayed." The unspoken thought is that if they don't, they suffer more than just the consequences of the spray.

JOHN LABOSSIERE, A NEIGHBOUR of Pam and Don Morris, lives a few kilometres away in Bass River, where he is trying to get a farm going, and substitute teaches in Rexton to make ends meet. In 1980, LaBossiere stepped down after four years as leader of the provincial NDP party, the most thankless job in New Brunswick politics, for at the time, the NDP had yet to secure a single seat. But it gave LaBossiere a podium from which to broadcast his opposition to the spray.

Of the three major New Brunswick political parties, the NDP under LaBossiere was alone in its anti-spray policy. LaBossiere thinks that his former political colleagues don't share his views simply because they are misinformed: "My impression of politicians in New Brunswick is that there are only a few who do their own research and that a great number of them rely on existing sources to tell them about the forest industry." He lists those sources as the chemical manufacturers, and even the five English-language daily papers, some radio stations and the CBC-TV affiliate in Saint John, which are owned by the powerful K.C. Irving empire, whose forestry holdings are the largest in the province. All, he points out, have a considerable vested interest in the spray program.

So LaBossiere can understand the average New Brunswicker's quiet acceptance of the status quo: "What can you expect of people in a poor province whose economic wellbeing is controlled by a small number of people? Obviously you are going to be reluctant to speak out in public because your entire future can be jeopardized by what you say."

Any cruise of the power grid in New Brunswick would be incomplete without a stop to consider the inscrutable and reclusive Irving family. There is K.C. himself, who caused a certain amount of provincial indignation by retiring right out of the province and into a life in the Bahamas in 1971. And there is his trio of middle-aged executive sons, James, Arthur and John, who between them control vast interests in every sector of the provincial economy. Nobody has yet succeeded in compiling a corporate flow chart; it is simply true that in New Brunswick K.C. Irving's interests matter most.

J.D. IRVING LTD. IS THE FORESTRY SECTOR, reputedly the largest such company in the world, with holdings covering an estimated half million hectares of New Brunswick. They are so big that although they are part of the industrial group contributing to FPL they also run their own spray operation, Forest Patrol Limited, easy to confuse with the government operation because it shares the same initials. Forest Patrol Limited sprays each year for budworm – after it finds out what FPL plans to cover – but it hasn't used the viral-enhancing emulsifiers with its fenitrothion for six years. David Oxley, woodlands manager for J.D. Irving Ltd., says, "We feel we are moving in the right direction being able to drop the emulsifier component, which was becoming controversial."

But 10 percent of their spray program involves applying broadleaf herbicide to J.D. Irving's $10-million annual reforestation program – and controversy is where they are headed. In 1980 Forest Patrol Limited sprayed 7,230 hectares of New Brunswick with 2,4,5-T when it had a permit from the Department of Environment to treat only 5,000 hectares. "We were definitely concerned," says Kenneth Browne, head of Environment's Toxic Substances Branch. "We found out where those acres were and checked to see that they met conditions of setback from habitation and water courses. But, as the company explained, they didn't anticipate that they would need to treat all the acres that they did.

"It was probably a violation," Browne admits. "They acknowledge it, but there is no way of taking them to court because we didn't witness it." Browne says the situation has been corrected. In future the company simply will "overestimate" the number of hecatres it wants to treat. So it's more or less all up to J.D. Irving – which hardly reflects a cautious approach on the part of the government to the use of a chemical that has been banned in a number of European countries (Norway, Sweden, Italy, the Netherlands) and has been severely restricted in the U.S. following an Oregon study which connected miscarriages to its use as a forest spray. In fact, some of the 2,4,5-T in question was purchased by Irving from Ontario Hydro after the chemical had been banned in that province.

The Department of Environment did successfully prosecute Forest Patrol Limited in May 1981 for "flagrantly" disregarding Section 16 of the provincial Pesticides Act, by spraying Roundup – a new and relatively untested herbicide – without a permit. In fining the company $200 (maximum sentence would have been $1,000 or 100 days in jail), Provincial Court Judge Donald Allen said: "'To flagrantly disregard the section of the Pesticides Act would be to use the chemical without knowledge of its effects. They knew what they were doing but it was too late to obtain a permit." It seems that the public interest in these matters is being constantly entrusted to the discretion of J.D. Irving Ltd. And J.D. Irving is certainly aware that it needs to inspire this trust.

The illegal spraying of Roundup took place in Dubee Settlement, southern New Brunswick, one and a half kilometres from the head of Millstream. It is hard to say where Millstream begins and ends, just that for several miles from the head to a place called Berwick Corner houses are strung like beads along the river. Pastureland slopes up to wooded hills and cows graze: this is the centre of Sussex farmland well known throughout the Maritimes for its dairy products. It is appealingly pastoral, beautiful, calm, but Millstream is both a repository of all the common fears of New Brunswickers about the chemical management of their forests and the source of some of the most outspoken anti-spray protest.

Paul and Madeline Taylor moved to Millstream in 1975 after Paul, a United Church minister, accepted charge of the circuit of local churches. Their first spring, spray planes flew close to their house. The manse was not plastered with fenitrothion as were some of the neighbouring homes, but inside the manse were the Taylors' five children. "I thought, I can't be a good mother if I don't fight this thing," says Madeline. She soon joined the fledgling Concerned Parents Group. Commitment to her children led to commitment to a cause – last spring she was elected president.

Madeline is a nurse. Her part-time shifts at Sussex Hospital and her involvement in local church work brought her face to face with what she sees as a phenomenon of ill health in her pretty little community. "I have never lived in a place that discussed health so much," she told me. "It seems there's always something to do with sickness or death. You can just go down the road," she said with a sweep of her arm as we sat on the manse verandah looking out on summer fields, and she began to list the illnesses which had touched each neighbouring house: women who suffered a rare blood disease, brain cancer, a mastectomy; a young man with cancer of the testes; a young girl with lung cysts.

Her gesture has extended further. She has searched the local church records and discovered that since 1969, of forty-one deaths not attributable to old age, fourteen were due to cancer and four were stillbirths. At a United Church Women's meeting one evening she looked around the room and realized that out of twelve women present four had been treated for breast cancer. Another member had died recently of breast cancer and still another of intestinal cancer. She knows that there is not enough comparable information about the health of the general population in New Brunswick or the rest of Canada for her informal surveying to be significant scientifically, but she firmly believes her friends and neighbours have been victims of their environment, saturated with three decades of chemical spraying. As a result, she has dedicated herself to overcoming the persistent air of fatalism within the community of Millstream.

She has had some success. Madeline Taylor's lobbying within her own profession, with help from another Concerned Parents member, physiotherapist Peggy Land, resulted in the Sussex medical community becoming the first in New Brunswick to officially state its opposition to the spray. In February 1981, sixty-nine health care workers, including seven doctors, signed a petition calling on government to discontinue the spray program because "its questionable effectiveness does not justify the risks to human health."

That may not seem like much of a radical move, but it has in effect isolated medical workers in Sussex from their provincial colleagues. Despite the fact that in 1976 the Nova Scotia Medical Society decided that there was enough proof of harmful effects on health to come out strongly against aerial spraying, the New Brunswick Medical Society has not yet uttered a peep. When asked if the Rozee human tissue research into Reye's might change medical minds, spokesperson Dr. John Bennett said that the society is waiting for Rozee's study to be validated, presumably by the government-appointed panel headed by McGill pharmacologist Dr. Donald Ecobichon, since the society has no funds for such work: "When it is validated I think people will have something on which to make a decision. But as long as there are pros and cons being put forward it is very difficult to be dogmatic as to what is right or wrong."

Dr. Sol Khederi, one of the Sussex doctors to sign the petition, defends the stand he took: "We felt that until you could prove something is safe you don't use it. They say the chemicals haven't been shown to be harmful – that's basically a negative argument. They haven't been checked to any extent. . . . It surprises me that things like 2,4,5-T that have been banned elsewhere are readily used here. It seems that in New Brunswick, we have become a dumping ground." A rider on the Sussex medical petition called for an immediate ban on the use of herbicides such as 2,4,5-T that contain dioxin.

HERBICIDES HAVE NOTHING TO DO WITH the budworm spray program and everything to do with large scale industrial forest management. Herbicides have become another issue in this environmental war. Madeline Taylor heard that J.D. Irving Ltd. had applied to spray sixty hectares at the head of Millstream with 2,4,5-T in June and she quickly circulated a petition. Widespread community support brought the Sussex Town Council on side – and not only drew a retraction of the Irving plans but brought James, K.C.'s eldest son and head of the forestry sector, out to Millstream on a hot July morning, something unheard of in the annals of reclusive Irvingdom.

I happened to be in luck. I had got to Clark Phillips' the evening before (and stayed up half the night while Clark reviewed the history of Concerned Parents' court battles for me) and was there at 7:30 on July 23 when Madeline called with the news that James Irving was flying in for a meeting.

I got to Berwick Corner in half an hour. It was already hot and I was glad to slip into the cool rooms of the manse, where Madeline was busy tidying up in preparation for her guest. Two other Millstream women arrived: Peggy Land and Ursula Becker, a local farmer. We went out on the verandah where we chatted until we heard the concussive beating of the helicopter blades. Madeline crossed the yard to the abandoned pastures where the helicopter set down. None of us could quite believe that this was happening, and everyone seemed as much amused as intimidated by the spectacle.

Jim Irving came back across the field following Madeline. A tall, heavyset man dressed casually in short rain jacket, grey flannels, blue shirt and garish paisley tie, the first thing he said after introductions had been made was almost maudlin: "I'm interested in growing trees."

He then proceeded to give us a short course in reforestation. He needed sprays like 2,4,5-T to kill broadleaf growth in stands of young fir and spruce so that the hardwoods would not smother out the seedlings. Herbicides were indispensable to his company's reforestation programs. In fact J.D. Irving has been using broadleaf herbicides (2,4-D and 2,4,5-T formulations) since the late 1950s. In 1981, 13,760 hectares were treated. Irving ended his lecture rhetorically: "You really believe that these chemicals are dangerous?"

Peggy Land replied that dioxin, a contaminant in 2,4,5-T, was considered by some scientists as the most deadly chemical known to man. Irving deferred graciously: "I see that you know more about this than we do. If we've done something wrong we want to change it." However, Irving had not come to concede that his company practices were hazardous, nor to offer his apologies for any wrongdoing. He had a proposition to make: His company would fund a study of the health hazards of 2,4,5-T. He appealed to the women to keep an open mind, and asked that if his study demonstrated that the herbicide was safe, they would publicly acknowledge their mistake.

After the helicopter lifted off, I stood in the manse yard with Ursula Becker. She was sceptical: "I think that Irving already knows that there is something wrong, that there may come a time that people say 'We are hurt.' He needs something to protect him. He wants to have it in black and white that he did everything right. It cost a lot of money. It must be worth something to him." The next day I read in papers owned by Irving that Concerned Parents had agreed to cooperate with the company on a safety study of herbicides.

The next time I saw Ursula was in November. I drove with her and Madeline Taylor to the source of the Shack Brook, which spills from the high wooded ground behind the Becker farm into their pasture and is the sole source of water for their 125-head Holstein herd. Below the Becker property it runs into Millstream. The brook was the Beckers' private symbol for the pristine character of their adopted country when they moved to New Brunswick from West Germany in November 1975. Lothar Becker chose the location of the farm because there was no one living upstream of the spring-fed water source: "I thought, it's nice, no one's peeing in my brook."

Ursula steered the half-ton truck through the tight turns of the rain-soaked and deeply rutted woods road. Several miles in back of the Becker farm we came upon a clearcut area – Irving ground. Forty hectares, give or take a few, had been levelled. Since it was November, I had expected to see the broadleaf vegetation wilted, but the women explained that the young saplings were black even in mid-summer. The only green was of new-growth softwoods emerging from the tangle of rotted vegetation and uproot-ed deadwood.

Ursula took a branch road to the right and parked the truck on a ridge. Below us was the Shack Brook, bisecting the herbicide treated plantation. A stone's throw from where it crossed the road was its source among the only mature trees left standing in this virtual wasteland. The land sloped toward the brook from both sides and it was obvious that any run-off would find its way into the brook. "I believe that the problems we saw this year are due to the fact that J.D. Irving sprayed Roundup there," Ursula said. "They sprayed here since 1952 with fenitrothion but for herbicide spray it was the first year, last year."

Since May 1981 the Becker herd has produced seven sets of twins and eleven of these calves have been stillborn. "It makes me bankrupt, you know," Lothar told me. "If you have seven sets of twins in one year that would be all right. But if they come backwards and they're stuck – we're just lucky that we get the cows through all right." Besides the high rate of twinning and stillbirths, the Holsteins have also had infertility and abortion problems of late. Two cows aborted in midterm in July 1981; in September a hairless calf was born prematurely at six months. Many cows have not been conceiving when bred either by artificial insemination or by bull. Lothar has no explanation – the feeding and breeding regimens are the same as in previous years. Neither does veterinarian Dr. Ian Leask, who says that tests have turned up no infectious cause for the abortions. "For now," he says, "I put the twinning down to stats. I'm not saying that these herbicides couldn't be causing it, but I would be going out on a limb if I said they were."

A long limb indeed, because no one is sure of the possible health effects of Roundup. In fact Agriculture Canada, which licenses all experimental permits for chemicals like these, stopped okaying experimental permits for Roundup in 1981. They hand out permits for two reasons: first to test the efficacy of the chemical – does it work? – and, second, to test health and safety. Enough permits had been granted to prove Roundup effective at killing broadleaf vegetation, but none had been granted to test for effects on health so Agriculture Canada said to pause a while. In 1980, under experimental permits, nearly 4,100 hectares were sprayed with Roundup in New Brunswick and the permits allowed spraying within 80 metres of habitation. The Monsanto Chemical Company claims that Roundup (glyphosate) is "relatively non-persistent." But the U.S. Environmental Protection Agency (EPA) has asked that all studies on Roundup be repeated. Monsanto in turn has sued the EPA to prevent release of registration data on the chemical to the public. Its toxicity is definitely in question, and it is one of the names on the suspected chemical list of Industrial Biotest.

The Beckers' health problems have not only been with their cattle. Here is a list of recent family ailments: Since July 1980, their son Martin has been hospitalized three times. He has suffered convulsions and lost consciousness briefly during the last episode. No diagnosis has been made though food poisoning has been suggested. "They don't know what it is," Ursula says. "He runs a high fever and vomits. It seems to me that he is sensitive to something and we don't know what it is." Ursula herself has undergone exploratory surgery for a gall-bladder ailment of unknown etiology. In all, members of the family have been hospitalized six times within a year. Before coming to Canada they were healthy.

The events of last year [1981] prompted Ursula, already active in Concerned Parents, to go out into her community to conduct a health survey. She has interviewed all of her neighbours within a three-mile radius. At first people were reluctant to cooperate: "People have shame about sickness.

They want to appear healthy and happy," says Ursula. But the ideal community image was far more real. She tabulated a distressing number of complaints – seventy described by sufferers as serious out of a population of 170. Lung problems, including asthma, emphysema and persistent colds, predominated. Ursula's scribbler delivered another count: five birth defects, one stillbirth, four miscarriages and three premature births.

What Ursula Becker and Madeline Taylor perceive as a phenomenon of illness in their community is unsubstantiated. But the insidious fear shared by many in Millstream that three decades of spraying is now taking its toll is tragic in itself. People in Millstream think that they have a right to know whether their health is being endangered by government policy. And they also know that not knowing what is undermining their health – Is it in their heads? Is it really happening? Is it the same anywhere else? – can sometimes be worse than being faced with a definite diagnosis.

NEWCASTLE, BATHURST, CAMPBELLTON, and Dalhousie: all northern New Brunswick milltowns, and very little in between except the forests that feed the mills. As I drove north from Newcastle where I had visited Jimmy Singleton's parents, the arguments concerning the economic imperatives of spraying became more nagging. I wondered whether the proponents of the spray might at least be partially justified in saying that "southerners can afford their doom-saying."

The settlements interspersed between the milltowns are poor; their reason for being is not readily apparent. Occasionally I saw a log skidder parked in a back yard, but realized that the owner probably contracted for multinational pulp companies. The small sawmills are dying: four of the six in the Miramichi River area have closed. Unemployment is almost palpable as you pass through the villages of this economic outback. Dalhousie is as far north as you can get in New Brunswick. There's no question that it is a milltown. The New Brunswick International Paper Company (NBIP) – formerly Canadian International Paper, the instigator of the spray program back in 1952 – takes up one whole side of the main street. There is a mountain of pulp constantly in the making as a river of barked logs spills from a mammoth conveyor. In the background are the silhouettes of the Quebec mountains that hem in the Baie des Chaleurs.

Len Clifford grew up in Dalhousie and like many native sons went to work in the NBIP mill after high school. In the early '70s he headed out west to work for a few years, but he and his wife Marsha (also Dalhousie-born) always wanted to return to New Brunswick to raise their family – Natasha, 9, Crystal Dawn, 7, and Lenwood, 2. In 1976, they came home to build a bungalow on a farm in St. Maure, a little community twenty-five kilometres inland from Dalhousie. And in 1980, after four years of knocking on the door, Len got his old job back at the mill. Things seemed to be working out for the Cliffords, until this spring when a close encounter with the spray shook their confidence in their future in New Brunswick.

The incident is like most of the others. Len had requested that his property be exempt from the spray and had received a letter of confirmation when he was awakened by the sound of planes flying near his house. He headed off to the local airport and after some trouble found out that the nearest spray zone to his house was three kilometres away. But when he got home that night: "The planes were spraying right in my back yard. So we took off and went to a hotel for the evening. The next day we came back and the children got sick."

So they took off again, this time to the Quebec side of the Baie des Chaleurs for a few days but when they came back home the baby, Lenwood, got sick and this time had to be hospitalized. "The doctor couldn't say for sure it wasn't the spray, but he couldn't say it was. It was just sort of mysterious to him," says Marsha. "But it was an awful coincidence for it to recur when we got home. Would the flu do that?"

The Cliffords decided that maybe they should get their well water checked for fenitrothion, and the Department of Health sent an inspector from Campbellton, but he came equipped to test for bacteria only. "He told us the water was potable," Len said with a chuckle. Then their inquiries got bounced from the Department of the Environment to Natural Resources and back, and it was only when Len applied to MLA Allen Maher for help (and Maher raised the incident in the legislature) that Environment began to monitor the water in the Clifford's well.

Five tests have all indicated traces of fenitrothion in the family's tap water, and the latest, performed in January this year, registered the highest reading – 0.9 parts per billion (still well below the Canadian drinking water standard of 100 ppb). But Lenwood continues to be sick. Two weeks after my visit he was hospitalized again in Moncton for tests due to suspected pressure on the brain. Those tests showed no gross neurological damage, but Lenwood still suffers from headaches and his doctor is keeping him under close observation. Meanwhile, his father is looking for jobs out of the province.

"Working at the mill is like a marriage. You're punished for being unfaithful." That's the common attitude in Dalhousie, one millworker told me. The NBIP mill has been a good provider for the community, paying salaries of up to $30,000 to senior employees. But not all employees accept the company's practices without question. One of the dissenters is John McEwen, forty years old, native to the north and proud of it: "You're sort of on your own up here, and of course it makes a better breed of people."

He has worked twenty-two years, all his adult life, at the NBIP mill and is currently serving a term as vice-president of the New Brunswick Federation of Labour. He is concerned about the clearcutting that the company has been practising for two decades in the drainage area of Southeast Upsalquitch, which is where the budworm epidemic was first detected. And he believes his concern about the future wood supply is shared by his fellow workers. "People here are not that removed from when we didn't do these things. We practised selective cutting when we had all sawmills. When you're a sawmill worker, you make damn sure you have a good tree next year. People know it's not being done properly now." He worries that real forest management will not be adopted in New Brunswick "as long as their mentality is entrenched in the 1940s perspective of things – you just go out and chuck something on the forest."

McEwen also has reservations about the spruce budworm spray program, not only because of health risks but because he believes it has failed even within the limited expectations of "crop protection." Defoliation is up 130 percent in New Brunswick (compared to a 50 percent drop in Nova Scotia where the epidemic has died). This could lead one to believe that spraying is ineffectual in curbing defoliation, which is the only government argument for keeping it. McEwen doesn't think his view makes him "unfaithful" to his industry: "I work in the paper mill. I want to continue to work there and I want it to continue to operate in the community. I think the one I work for is a good corporate citizen. But I want the wood supply to still be there. I'm convinced from what I've read and from talking to other people that there are better ways to manage a forest."

MAYBE IT WAS THE melodramatic effect of driving around in the dark forests of New Brunswick, but I kept cycling on the classic image of Prometheus manacled to a mountain where nightly a vulture devoured his liver. Each day the liver regenerated and each night the grisly vivisection was repeated. Spraying seems a similarly ugly forever proposition in New Brunswick. Hercules was finally able to unbind Prome-theus from his mountain torture rack with a typically Herculean show of strength. It will take an equally forceful act of political will to unbind the budworm.

The consequences of not doing so are found in that man-made mountain of pulp in Dalhousie. The seemingly numberless logs spilling from the conveyer are in fact calculable. They are integers that can be slotted into the gross provincial product or the pulp and paper mills' year-end dividends or the bureaucrats' cost-benefit ratios. They are useful to those whom we hold accountable. The costs of the program to the environment and the human population are less amenable to empirical methods. They are so subtle it may take a long time for their numbers to come up. But when they do we may find ourselves powerless to express our collective loss.

V. Legacy

The Life and Tides of Fundy

TWICE DAILY THE GREAT TIDES of Fundy – world renowned for their 16-metre height – meandered along the umbilical loops of the marsh-fringed Chebogue River at the mouth of the Bay of Fundy and inched into the salt-water farm creek where I grew up. In season, a stream of living things moved with the tides. In April, smelt crowded so thickly into the creek mouth that I could snag them barehanded. Soon after, sea trout slipped from salt to fresh water and lay tantalizingly off the end of hook-and-line in the shaded spawning pools of Brook Farm. Each summer, willet scolded me when, crossing over the raspy carpet of chord grass, I ventured too close to their salt marsh nests. Blue herons were prompt as biological clocks, at daybreak flying in to work their riverine feeding grounds and at dusk seeming to ferry night itself within their gangly silhouettes as they returned to an island heronry. Striped bass worked the shallows, and juvenile "tinker" mackerel shot upriver in late summer; shorebirds and ducks trailed the parade until freeze-up. Looking back I see that the tidal river, like a great saltwater heart filling and emptying, first brought me close to the riches and rhythms of nature, and of the Bay of Fundy in particular.

Where there is natural abundance, there is also human greed. I learned this unnatural lesson as a fresh-faced biology student working in the regional fisheries inspection lab in Yarmouth, Nova Scotia, in the late 1960s. Daily I analyzed the protein content of the greenish slurry excreted from herring meal plants – ten foulsmelling factories grinding hundreds of thousands of tons of perfectly edible herring into fish meal. By summer's end, the grinders and coolers were silently rusting and the 60-strong herring seiner fleet was tied up. The stocks of this vital species feed stock for fish, whales, and seabirds had been decimated; some populations, like those on Georges Bank, have never recovered.

It would be another decade, this time at the farthest reaches of the Bay of Fundy, before I would face up to another threat to this uncommonly productive body of water. With the OPEC oil embargo fresh in their minds, politicians in New Brunswick, Nova Scotia, New York, and the New England States revived the perennial dream of exploiting the tidal energies of the Bay of Fundy. Nearly half a century earlier, the U.S. Army Corps of Engineers, under the direction of Franklin Delano Roosevelt, had first studied the feasibility of large-scale tidal power plants in Passamaquoddy Bay, near the President's summer residence on Campobello Island. The tidal power dream has risen phoenix-like every decade since, and in 1978 seemed more imminent than ever before.

The schemes called for the erection of massive dams to block one or both of the inner arms of the Bay of Fundy – the Minas Basin and Cumberland Basin. The impact of shortening the length of the Bay would be felt as far south as Boston, where high tide levels were expected to rise as much as fifteen centimetres, and in the vicinity of the dam, where productive salt marshes would be drowned and sensitive bottom sediments disturbed. I was living near Joggins, the earmarked Nova Scotia terminus of the Cumberland Basin dam. Suddenly I had to contemplate what a wholesale habitat change might mean for the productivity of my beloved Bay.

My education, both formal and informal, had coincided with the rise of environmentalism. Now, at least, megaprojects such as Fundy tidal power could no longer be undertaken without an environmental review. Regional scientists moved quickly to address a host of questions about the Bay of Fundy which, though in their backyard, had remained largely unexplored from an ecological viewpoint. I joined the quest. For the next ten years I followed scientists, naturalists, and fishermen from one end of the Bay to the other, from the Tantramar Marshes, the great maritime prairie that bridges the Maritime provinces of Nova Scotia and New Brunswick, to the seabird sanctuary of Machias Seal Island that straddles the invisible marine boundary between the Bay of Fundy and the Gulf of Maine.

One of the first revelations came from the computers at the Bedford Institute of Oceanography in Dartmouth, Nova Scotia. Numerical models showed that the Bay of Fundy and Gulf of Maine formed a single oceanographic system, a perfect bathtub in which Fundy's conspicuous tides sloshed back and forth harmoniously – a phenomenon known as resonance, or more simply "the bathtub effect."

The study of Fundy as a living system put its high productivity into perspective. Graham Daborn, founder of the Acadia Centre for Estuarine Research, has dubbed the Bay of Fundy "a system with a biological pump at both ends." In the lower Bay, strong tides pump nutrients from the seafloor up into the light, which sets in motion the marine food chain: phytoplankton, copepods, herring, seabirds, and whales. In the shallower upper Bay, huge expanses of mudflat and salt marsh act as biological factories. At low tide slicks of single-celled algae and fields of marsh grass collect solar energy, then distribute it to the marine system at high tide as a nutrient soup for bottom dwellers, fish, and birds. This vast marine smorgasbord attracts migratory species from far hemispheres.

In short, scientists concluded that the real power of the tides rested in their ability to promote and sustain biological productivity.

But it was only in the field – among the pageantry of whales spouting, seabirds gorging on red rivers of krill, shorebirds unfurling in poetic flight patterns – that I found the truth of this generalization took on vivid meaning.

TO THE UNINITIATED the muddy waters of the inner reaches of the Bay of Fundy might look like a watery desert. Closer inspection proves they are far from barren.

Several years ago, I stood on the high marsh, watching as the brown tide inexorably transformed the mud-walled, dry-bottomed Allen Creek into a navigable channel. Marven Snowden, of Wood Point, New Brunswick, quickly powered his boat into the open waters of the Cumberland Basin where four generations of his family had fished for American shad, the largest, and most succulent, member of the herring family.

Marven had seen many changes in the fisheries of the upper Bay of Fundy. His grandfather fished during the heyday of the shad fishery at the turn of the century. Then, hundreds of thousands of kilograms were salted in barrels for export to the Eastern Seaboard. During his father's time, the fishery had collapsed suddenly. In recent years, Marven had seen the shad making a comeback.

The burly fisherman steered toward the Nova Scotia side of the basin. He knew that shad move with the strongest currents. "You try to get in the strongest stream and work toward the slack water," he explained as his son and another crewmember set the two kilometres of gill net.

We cut power and drifted on the tide. Marven freely shared his local wisdom. There are three distinct runs of shad in the upper Bay, he told me; and fish come here to feed, not to spawn.

In recent times, science has often ignored local data gatherers – the fishermen. Fortunately, Dr. Michael Dadswell, then a federal fisheries research scientist, sta-tioned in St. Andrew's, New Brunswick, was willing to listen to Marven Snowden. Though he says that his first meeting with Marven in 1978 was a case of serendipity, Dadswell deserves credit for piecing together the information into a workable hypothesis.

Science sometimes advances in leaps, like salmon or poetry. Dadswell had a hunch that the increase in Fundy shad might be related to the restoration of major shad spawning rivers in the United States, such as the Susquehannah, Delaware, and Hudson. As anadromous fish, shad spawn in fresh water and then return to the salt water. It was a long standing mystery in fishery science, however, just where the shad went after returning to the sea.

Dadswell asked Marven to help him tag shad in the Bay of Fundy. The next spring the florescent dorsal fin tags began returning with southern postmarks. Eventually, he received tags from every river with a known spawning shad population, from Florida north to Labrador. He now believes that every shad comes to the Bay of Fundy at least once during its life history.

Other species return annually to rich feeding grounds spread out by the ebb and flow of Fundy's tides. No migration is more spectacular than of the sandpipers, or "peeps" as Fundy denizens affectionately call them. The peeps flock to special places along the upper Fundy shoreline to feed and, it seems, to perform their aerial ballet.

HUNDREDS, THOUSANDS, tens of thousands of sandpipers spiral from the mudflats like snow devils, then string sinuous banners of flight. The play of light on their dark backs and buff breasts as the flock banks in perfect synchrony, is designed to foil a raptor's strike. But to the appreciative observer, the birds' flight seems nothing less than joyful expression, like a musical chord or brush stroke.

Much of the sandpipers' time, however, is spent on the flats in more pedestrian fashion, doggedly bobbing up and down in pursuit of the "mud shrimp." These fatty, translucent morsels are tucked into the fine tenements of mud in astronomical numbers – 20,000 to 60,000 per square metre. On this side of the Atlantic, they are found only in the Bay of Fundy and Gulf of Maine, and then only in great enough numbers at several sites to attract major shorebird flocks.

One of these mud shrimp hotspots is Mary's Point, New Brunswick. From a sandpiper's view, it has everything: the fertile muds of Ha Ha Bay on one side, the salt marshes of Shepody on another, and, in between, a crescent sandspit for roosting.

Sandpipers arrive here unerringly, on or about July 18, from their Arctic breeding grounds. For them it is a fuel stop, or as one ornithologist remarked, "a fat station." In two weeks, they will double their weight, becoming winged butterballs. That envelope of fat will carry them on a non-stop flight over the Atlantic to their wintering grounds on the north coast of South America.

It has been known since Audubon's time that the inner Bay of Fundy is an important staging area for shorebirds. But it was not until the late 1970s that biologists came to appreciate that it is the most important shorebird site in eastern North America, annually hosting some 1.5 million shorebirds of thirty-four species. By far the most numerous are the semipalmated sandpipers. In a given year, one-half to three-quarters of the world population stops to feed on the intertidal offerings of Fundy's mud flats.

There to greet them for the last two decades has been one of the Maritime's extraordinary naturalists, Mary Majka. Mary's restored farmhouse and beachside cottage stand vigil over Mary's Point and its migrants. "We know from history that many species have been extinguished because they couldn't be as flexible as human beings," Mary once observed as we sat on the beach next to a roost of 30,000 sandpipers. "And I think that certain species are very much more dependent on special environments, and those birds definitely are. They certainly cannot survive without the Bay, its tides, and its beautiful mud."

The truth of Mary's words received official sanction in 1987 when Mary's Point was dedicated as the first Western Hemispheric Shorebird Reserve in Canada – a critical link in the migratory chain.

NATURALISTS, conservationists, ecologists, environmentalists. By whatever name we choose to be called, all take it upon ourselves to understand, describe, and ultimately conserve communities of life – that is, ecosystems. In my experience, there is another kind of environmentally friendly individual who does not necessarily articulate "green" principles, but whose very life is an unselfconscious object lesson in how to merge economy and ecology.

Let me introduce one such person.

In the ice-free months, April to October, Clayton Eagles of Five Islands, Nova Scotia, can be found on the intertidal prairie exposed at low tide in the Minas Basin; one of 200 Breughel-like figures bent at the waist, arms outstretched in the shape of a human tripod.

In the 1940s, when Clayton started clamming, diggers took only the larger clams because the smaller ones were uneconomical to shuck. Clayton can't break himself of the habit. On every dig, he still plucks out only the choice, mature clams and leaves the rest. This traditional conservation technique seems to have been abandoned by the new generation of clammers forced onto the flats by hard times in the 1980s. This unchecked exploitation of the resource haunts Clayton.

"They think I'm crazy, I don't like diggin' everything. I don't know, clams got to have somewhere to start," he told me on a discouragingly poor digging day. "Years ago, there used to be breeding beds, we'd call them. We never used to dig them at all. They started diggin' them out. I think it made a difference. I just can't see it. You dig everything out, what's going to be left to grow?"

In Fundy, the great tides dominate all living things – from the microscopic glass house of the benthic diatom to the 70-foot leviathan, the fin whale. Survival here depends on the ability to adapt to tidal range and rhythm. I have found that this principle can hold as true for people as it does for plants and animals that live by and under the Bay's waters. And no person I met along the Bayshore lived more in tune with the tides than Five Islands' weir man Gerald Lewis.

For forty years, he drove his horse and wagon over the bottom of the sea, his movements mirroring the ebb and flow of his tidally ruled environment. His V-shaped, two-and-a-half-kilometre-long brush weir was a giant fish basket woven of spruce boughs, saplings, and twine. It gathered passively, sometimes only enough flounder for table fare, other times enough herring and shad for salting, and occasionally a rare catch, such as a tuna, which Gerald cut into steaks for his neighbors. The weir was a permeable dam that was moderate in its catching power. And it was impermanent, as each winter ice carried the 1,500 hand-driven weir stakes to sea. How unlike a tidal dam, I thought. It would be permanent, and immoderate both in scale and in its impact on the environment: disturbing clam beds, burying mud shrimp, and chopping shad to bits.

I can only hope that when the dream of tidal power undergoes its inevitable revival the lessons of the last fifteen years are not forgotten: the true power of the tides is in their ability to do biological work. Said another way, tidal life *is* tidal power. It took this native born, Fundy boy – adrift among tide pools, marsh hay, and mudflats – three decades to express that simple thought.

Mother Miramichi

New Brunswick

THE LONG CEDAR-STRIP CANOE knifes through the frigid water before being exhaled from the river's face. Through the morning mist, the water reflects the first flares of fall from the hardwood-covered ridges that usher the river's seaward journey. At the back of the canoe sits Charlie Rose, fishing guide at The Old River Lodge. In crumpled hat and dark, practical clothes, he might be Yeats' wise fisher with "his sun-freckled face."

Other anglers are also out early, working a pool downriver, and they have company: red-breasted mergansers, with their jaunty caps, and a blue heron whose beak in silhouette looks like a pipe resolutely clamped in a fly-fisher's teeth. Startled, the mergansers beat the river with their wings, throwing off sun-spangled beads of water; the heron, too, reluctantly leaves its fishing spot as our canoe bears down. We glide above the river's golden gravel and under the shadows of dark hemlock, where two men work a long, swift run with their rhythmic casts. Like the feathered fishers upriver, their quarry is the Atlantic salmon, specifically adult *Salmo salar*. Every year, 2-to-18-kilogram salmon return from the sea to spawn in this, the river of their birth. Theirs is no ordinary river, but the greatest producer of Atlantic salmon in the world. Pulsing beneath the canvas skin of our eight-metre canoe is the mighty Miramichi.

To the fly-rod-in-hand salmon fisher, the musical word "Miramichi" is known the world over. As native son and novelist Wayne Curtis notes in his book *Fishing the Miramichi*: "It is probably better known internationally than the province it courses through. When we think of Brazil, we think of the Amazon; Egypt, the Nile; Germany, the Rhine. And when we think of New Brunswick, we think of the Miramichi. No wonder: its waters, including some major tributaries, fan out arterially to drain one-third of the Maritime province's hinterland."

The Miramichi is so fractured by its own watery fission that not even the 53,000-odd people who call it home can know it fully. Those who visit, like me, usually come to catch a salmon. In trying to get to know the Miramichi, I decided to let the salmon be my guide. Like the salmon, I stuck my nose upstream and followed the Main Southwest River, from salt water at Miramichi City to spring-fed headwater at Juniper, a distance of 400 kilometres.

Along the way, I met aboriginal peoples, outfitters, river guides, camp cooks, wardens, woodsmen, and come-from-aways like me, whom Miramichiers call "sports." All of them think of the Miramichi as home waters, but what binds them all into a loose confederation is not just the river, but the salmon that move through it. They are what people revere, gossip about, fight over, covet, curse, poach, and protect. It has always been so.

UNTIL I FOLLOWED THE SALMON'S upriver urge, I knew the Miramichi only by reputation. Throughout the region's history, it has been the river that nurtured life. When Europeans first came to the area in the seventeenth century, explorer Nicolas Denys wrote: "So large a quantity of them [salmon] enters into this river that at night one is unable to sleep, so great is the noise they make in falling upon the water after having thrown or darted themselves into the air." In the eighteenth and nineteenth centuries, the river yielded legendary bounties of salmon, which were shipped overseas to feed Europe. Virgin stands of white pine along its length provided British warships with sturdy masts. When the Great Miramichi Fire of 1825 consumed one-quarter of the province's forests, the river was, quite literally, the people's salvation, as they stood up to their necks in the cooling waters.

My firsthand knowledge of the Miramichi was scant, however. I knew it largely as a fictional landscape, vividly re-created in the sinuous prose of the region's laureate, David Adams Richards. Richards' richness of language and compassionate portraits of working-class life in the river's woods, mills, mines, and waters have earned him comparison to William Faulkner. His Miramichi is a Mississippi of the North, a natural force that has created a confluence of cultures, with predictable tensions.

Like many Canadians, I also knew the Miramichi from media reports of the all-too-real violence of recent years. In 1989, there was the deadly rampage of convicted killer Allan Legere, who, after a daring escape from prison, held his native Miramichi in a state of siege, killing four persons – three women and a priest – before being hunted down. And I knew the Miramichi of lore, enlivened by stories spun out at lumber camps and music swirling from Acadia and the Celtic roots of Scottish and Irish settlers. The river culture also has fashioned a distinctive idiom. Old men and boys alike are addressed as "lads"; when they curse, you hear "geesley." And, not surprisingly, there is the vernacular of the river itself. Backwaters are "bogans," a cross channel is a "quagus." The origin of the river's lyrical name remains a mystery, though some claim that it is a Montagnais word meaning "Mi'kmaq Land." What is beyond dispute is that the Mi'kmaq were the first Miramichiers, and they are still very much here. On a crisp fall morning, I drove out of the mill town of Newcastle (now part of Miramichi City), the self-appointed Salmon Capital of the World. Moving upriver, I passed piles of pulp waiting to be fed into the maw of one of the world's largest pulp-and-paper mills.

I left the Main Southwest briefly, following the Northwest Miramichi to the Red Bank First Nation reserve, the longest continually inhabited community in New Brunswick. In the mid-1970s, archaeologists unearthed 2,500-year-old middens pitched on glacial terraces high above the modern river. The Augustine Mound, named for Red Bank resident Joseph Augustine who discovered it, was packed with fish bones from sturgeon and, of course, salmon. Though the spawning grounds of the bottom-dwelling sturgeon were smothered by bark from nineteenth-century logdrives, the community is still economically and culturally dependent on the salmon.

THERE HAS ALWAYS BEEN a Mi'kmaq food fishery, and in 1990, the Supreme Court of Canada reaffirmed the right of aboriginals to fish salmon for food and ceremonial purposes, subject only to conservation requirements. Non-native groups worried aloud that the native fishery would imperil the rebuilding salmon stocks. Their worries, it appears, were unfounded. In 1994, the Red Bank reserve became the first on the Miramichi to voluntarily pull its gill nets from the river in favour of trap nets, which allow live capture of fish and the return of large spawners to the river.

Toni Paul, a young woman working in the nontraditional female role of fisheries officer for the Red Bank First Nation, engineered the community's conversion to the use of trap nets, an action that earned it a conservation award from the National Audubon Society. Conservation, Paul insists, is not a new concept for her people. "It's our way of life," she said earnestly, sitting in the band office. "We were brought up with respect for the food that allowed us to live. We were practising conservation centuries ago, and now they [non-natives] are playing catch-up."

Under the Aboriginal Fisheries Strategy, a federally funded salmon enhancement program worth $397,000 to the band, Red Bank is allowed an annual quota of 4,000 grilse, small adult salmon that have spent one year at sea. In keeping with the communal tradition of resource sharing, the fishers distribute their catch to the elders, the unemployed, and finally to all other families on a rotating basis. They also harvest a small number of large salmon for ceremonial purposes, such as the annual powwow and weddings.

Their trap nets are two elegant structures poised like giant water spiders on the glassy-smooth waters where the Little Southwest and the Northwest Miramichi meet. The nets are tended by community elders. Early in the day, Ron Ward, a former Red Bank chief who just recently passed away, greeted me. His reddish hair stuck out from under a baseball cap as he invited me to climb into one of two flat-bottomed, blunt-nosed boats, which he called Miramichi scows.

"Miramichi never fails," said Ward as we motored out the shallow channel, carefully avoiding the sandbars that lurked just below the surface. "There's a good run of fish now. In the past, we really depended on the salmon. We smoked them and salted them. At one time, if you didn't have a barrel of salmon, you thought you weren't going to survive the winter."

We pulled up beside the net, and an elder planted his feet on the gunwales of our teetering boat and began hauling up the heavy cotton twine. Salmon boiled the water and slapped their tails before being measured and tagged. "*Dosaga*," Ward yelled to young Brian Tenass, who was holding up a grilse of borderline size: "Throw him back."

The voluntary conservation practised by the Red Bank First Nation and the nearby Eel Ground First Nation has done much to quiet the historical scapegoating of natives, which on occasion has threatened to erupt into outright violence. In the summer of 1995, a group calling itself the Mi'kmaq Warrior Society – most from outside the Miramichi region – blockaded the Northwest Miramichi, claiming the federal fisheries department had no jurisdiction over native fishing rights. The two-month standoff resulted in fifty-four charges.

Such flareups are the inevitable consequence of a depleted resource. Once, Miramichiers had the river to themselves. Today, they must stand nearly shoulder-to-shoulder with fellow New Brunswickers and foreign anglers – 17,000 in all – doing what has come to be called the Miramichi shuffle: step-and-cast, step-and-cast. The routine is performed on so-called public waters. On the Miramichi, a landowner doesn't necessarily own adjacent riparian rights, which would give him exclusive access and fishing rights from the mean high-water mark to the centre of the river. They, too, must be purchased and taxes paid on them just as one does for terrestrial real estate. As a result, half of the 1,200 kilometres of salmon waters in the Miramichi system are privately controlled, or freehold, and many of the best areas are controlled by foreign and elite corporate interests.

Because of a quirk of natural history, there is a further twist to salmon economics. The fish don't rush headlong upriver to their spawning grounds, or redds. They stop and rest in pools, where the river deepens. It is in these pools that an angler is most likely to hook a salmon. Such pools are bought, sold, leased, and traded by outfitters, who offer L.L. Bean-fashioned anglers exclusive rights to fish them for upwards of $400 a day.

I bypassed the public waters of the lower river and drove by Quarryville, above which most waters are privately owned, stopping in Blackville to look up a writer-friend, Wayne Curtis. I found him at his riverside log cabin, dubbed Oriole Lodge for his favourite fly. A woodsy-looking man with a grizzled beard, Curtis is a self-confessed river rat. When he was a child, he spent summers watching the salmon runs pass underneath bridges and boats. Later, he fished with Miramichi aficionados such as baseball great Ted Williams, who owed a camp on the river, and the late fly-fishing legend, Lee Wulff. Now he is a guide for Americans and Europeans.

Entranced by the water's mesmerism, I stood on the banks of the Curtises' home pool. "Private waters have been good for the river," he mused. "It prevented a lot of abuse. But," he added, "a deed on a piece of paper in New York doesn't give them the river. We're here."

The Curtises have been on the Miramichi for four generations, ever since Wayne's grandfather canoed upriver to reclaim Aunt Sally's place, with the dining room table balanced on the craft's gunwales. "I feel privileged to have a river like the Miramichi as my home stream," Curtis said as we sat on the veranda, watching the river flash brightly between the dark silhouettes of conifers. "The Miramichi is more than a river, it's a state of mind."

That state of mind is not always as tranquil and soothing as it was that night. The fact that tragic events such as the Legere murders colour the outside view of the Miramichi grieves native sons such as Curtis. "Look, it's a liberal place to live, very liberal," he said. "This river's not constipated. One of the prices you have to pay for liberalism is the extremes that we've suffered, with the extreme criminals and extreme preachers who save souls on the other end. Freedom creates both."

Such freedom can incite behaviour that might be comical if it wasn't so sad. Curtis recalled an incident in the 1950s when a man was convicted of poaching after shooting a salmon as it humped its back out of water. And just a week earlier, two locals engaged in a high-speed car chase, which ended for one in the Renous River, a tributary that enters the Main Southwest.

Unfazed, people merely fished around the abandoned Monarch as if it were a glacial erratic.

In the morning, our minds turned to salmon and where the fish were lying these days. Such confidences pass along the river like insider trading tips on the stock market. A call to a friend led us to the Renous. As we stood streamside, Curtis "read" the water for me. I floated a Bomber, a dry fly tied with deer body hair, and hooked a 4.5-kilogram salmon just where Curtis said a fish was lying. After a 10-minute tussle, I tailed the silvery fish with my hand and released it to meet its upriver destiny.

I, TOO, MOVED UPRIVER, to the very heart of Miramichi salmon-fishing water, at Doaktown, home of the Atlantic Salmon Museum. To take the pulse of the river, one need only drop into W.W. Doak, a fine colonial-style building on Main Street. It is the river's clearinghouse: fishers come here daily to discuss water levels, pools that are producing, and especially fly patterns – which are "fishing" and which not.

Wallace Doak built his business on the egalitarian principle that customers, rich or poor, were all simply fishers when they walked through his door. His son Jerry, himself a classic flytyer, adheres to the down-home values of his late father but has added a successful mail-order business, which now keeps three other flytiers busy full-time.

I found Jerry Doak in the back room, surrounded by the incongruous tools of his trade – a deer hide to provide hair for the flies and a computer on his desk. A student of philosophy in university, he took over the family business in 1977. He has become something of a streamside philosopher since, given to waxing eloquent about his beloved river.

In Doak's mind – as in his business – river, fish, and people are inextricably intertwined. "I have a wonderful opportunity to view the river through other people's eyes," he said. "People who come originally for the angling, they make absolutely no bones [about the fact] that there are other places where you can catch fish, but there's something more here. They fall in love with the river and, in a lot of cases, with the people. You can see it in the respect for the people who have been guiding here for thirty years – the friendship a CEO will have with a guy who hasn't finished grade four."

That point was made clear to me after I headed downriver from Doaktown to The Old River Lodge, a rustic main building and a collection of log cabins tucked into a stand of birch. There, I chatted with "sport" Bruce Klein, a business executive from New York on his fourteenth return visit to the Miramichi. During the midday break, he sat absent-mindedly whittling a figure as he looked out upon the bright waters. "When I started coming up here, I was an executive," he said, for the moment putting aside his woodwork. "About the third year, it dawned on me why it's such a great trip: for a whole week, the only decision I have to make is what fly do I use. All the other crap you have to deal with in life gets washed away. And then you come up here after lunch and watch the river go by – it's really, really relaxing. Occasionally, you even get lucky and catch a salmon."

When that happens, the fish often has to be given back to the river. Only fish under sixty-four centimetres, known as grilse, can be kept. Female grilse produce only one quarter of the eggs of larger salmon, which stay at sea two years before seeking out their natal river to spawn. Hard as it was for some fishers to accept, catch-and-release was one conservation measure needed to halt a precipitous slide in salmon stock, in a river capable of producing one million fish every year. The nadir was 1983, when only about 35,000 salmon reached their spawning redds. At that point, Jerry Doak declared the river "terminally ill." Accepting the grim diagnosis, the federal government grudgingly banned commercial netting at the mouth of the river in 1984. Subsequently, the high-seas Greenland and Newfoundland fisheries, which intercepted salmon on their winter feeding grounds, were closed. In the past decade, the Miramichi has made a steady climb back to health, with an average of 120,000 salmon returning annually in recent years.

The greening of the Miramichi saved the outfitters. But despite the local economic benefits of healthy salmon stocks, poachers remain a perennial concern. Big Hole Brook in Doaktown, one of the best pools on the river, has its own caretaker to deter those who would jig or net fish. This being New Brunswick, Big Hole Brook is owned by the mighty Irving empire, which flies in clients to the camp for fishing weekends.

Perched on a sedimentary promontory, the camp offers an eagle's-eye view of the holding pool. Caretaker-cum-warden Frank Storey shook his head as he told me how a few years ago, before Irving bought the lodge, poachers occasionally used the high ground to stone federal fisheries wardens trying to police the waters. "If this pool was public," said Storey, "there'd be no fish. People would come in here at night and jig. Ruining a pool like this would affect the whole river."

The fact that there is restricted access to much of the river is perhaps one of the reasons salmon still return to the Miramichi in such numbers. And the river itself flows freely, unobstructed by dams, untenanted, and even unseen for much of its length.

THE LAST LEG OF MY JOURNEY UPRIVER was a long, sometimes dusty drive through the province's woodsy interior. Until the 1950s, young men born in the upper Miramichi followed a seasonal cycle: cutting wood in winter, driving logs downstream in spring, and either guiding or working in the sawmills in summer. The log drives are long gone, and much of the river above Boisetown has passed into the hands of corporate cliques. Unemployment now hovers around 20 percent.

It was not until I nearly reached Juniper that I again saw the river. At the Forks, where the North Branch meets the Main Southwest, I found Freddie Grant, lifelong guide and woodsman, once described to me as "the slickest [person] poling the river I ever seen."

Poling a canoe is a refined, but fast disappearing, Miramichi art. Standing at the back of the canoe, the navigator works the shallow depths with a three-metre-long pole, usually made of black spruce. A generation ago, everyone poled the river by necessity. Now outboard motors, forestry roads, and ATVs have made nearly every wilderness sector of the watershed accessible.

I hoped that Freddie would pole me downriver along the still pristine Half Moon to Boisetown section. But he informed me, with a shake of his head, "The water is barely as high as a mouse's knees." Instead, he invited me inside, where the woodstove was driving off the first chill of autumn. He proudly showed me the hazelnuts he had been gathering and the elegantly curved, white ash canoe seats that he had hand-fashioned. In a few days, he would guide for the fall moose hunt; in spring, he would cure black bear hides, and then, as summer turned, he would await the return of the salmon. Here, I thought, was a man thoroughly at home in his river environment, a Miramichier to his marrow. The river was still his highway and livelihood. He enjoyed the freedom that many along its banks haggled over, paid dearly for, and jealously guarded, or only eulogized. Like the salmon, he followed the river's way in season. As the salmon would in spring, I, too, now turned and moved downstream toward the sea from whence I had come.

The Cod Comeback
Newfoundland

FOG AND RAIN had leached all the colour from the land and the water except for the Day-Glo orange of a net buoy bobbing on the chop of the Northwest Arm of Trinty Bay, Newfoundland. On the buoy was written "Rhonda Cora" in memory of Gilbert and Fern Penney's daughter who died in infancy more than two decades ago. The scene might have invoked melancholy in the uninitiated, but that bright September day, the first of the reopened Newfoundland cod fishery, the atmosphere was anything but funereal.

Gilbert Penney's face beamed from the front of his 8-metre boat as he controlled the winch that pulled his gill net from the North Atlantic. Cod were coming over the side fast and furious – mature, deep-bellied cod whose glistening, freckled flanks shone with a gold and amber light.

"We're happy, we're happy," Fern chanted as she picked cod from the net's mesh. "It's a great feeling," she said. We might have been down, but we were never out."

When the net was reset and the boat was speeding up the sound to pull in the remaining two nets, Gilbert and Fern tried to express their feeling about the fishery, open now for the first time since July 1992, when the calamitous collapse of the once bountiful cod stocks forced a moratorium on the activity that defined Newfoundland as a province and a culture. "Fishing is a noble profession," Gilbert said. "When the moratorium came, it was almost like a death in the family, and when the fishery was reopened, it was like being handed a newborn child."

The health of that newborn child is still in some doubt, however. There are two cod fisheries in Newfoundland: the inshore fishery in the numerous bays and nearshore waters surrounding the island, and the offshore fishery that takes place farther from home. The fishery was reopened because of the apparent return of cod to inshore waters, and though the spirits of outport Newfoundlanders like the Penneys have revived, the Department of Fisheries and Oceans (DFO) stock assessments, issued annually since the moratorium, still show that offshore stocks are at historic low levels, with spawning biomass about 1 percent of what it was a decade ago. Furthermore, there is little recruitment of young fish, especially on the offshore banks – including the legendary Grand Bank, once the spawning grounds of the greatest cod stock on the planet.

In Renews, south of St. John's on the Avalon Peninsula, fisher Paul Kane is involved in the sentinel fishery, a DFO-run program in which inshore fishers have acted as data collectors since 1995. Kane has not found an abundance of cod. "There's a few fish, but nothing like there used to be here," he says. "This was the home of the cod, by Jesus, b'y, and I've never seen them this scarce."

Given this divided outlook, this see-sawing from bay to bay, between hope and despair, it's no wonder the limited reopening of the northern cod fishery in September was rife with controversy. When The Atlantic Groundfish Strategy – the $1.9 billion federal program known as TAGS initiated in 1994 – was phased out in 1999, fishers' groups lobbied hard for a limited reopening. TAGS was designed to retrain, buy out, or tide over Atlantic Canada's 40,000 fishers and fish-plant workers until the cod recovered. "Without TAGS, we had to have cod," Gilbert says, "or we couldn't survive."

With the reopening, fishers like the Penneys were given individual boat quotas of 3,400 kilograms of cod. In total, fishers in northeastern Newfoundland were allocated 9,000 tonnes round or whole (as opposed to HOG which means head-on-gutted), a substantial amount of cod but still a far cry from the total allowable catch, or TAC, of the 1980s, which peaked at 266,000 tonnes. The fishery was restricted to the inshore, where fishers were reporting large numbers of cod in the bays. The Fisheries Resource Conservation Council (FRCC), an independent watchdog group established to advise the federal DFO minister on conservation measures, admitted that "the setting of a TAC for this stock cannot be done in a defensible, scientific manner." Any estimate was a complete stab in the dark.

"No doubt about it, we were gambling," says FRCC chair Fred Woodman. The FRCC thought that 9,000 tonnes would not significantly affect the status of the stock and might give them much needed information "to make a more science-based recommendation for the year 2000."

In the absence of a fishery, scientists have had to rely on annual trawls and the sentinel fishery to estimate cod numbers. They have confirmed that very few young fish are being produced in offshore waters, and even those are dying off at incredibly high rates. And scientists do not understand why. One theory has it that seal predation is retarding recovery; another holds that the recovery rate is to be expected, given the few mature fish left offshore when the moratorium was declared. And there is this vexing new paradox to ponder: Why are there apparently so many cod in some bays, fewer in other bays, and virtually none on the offshore banks?

At the time of the moratorium, DFO held that the collapse of the northern cod stocks was sudden and largely unforeseen. The department pointed to environmental causes – in particular, to unusually cold water temperatures, which, it said, could have resulted in high adult mortality and low survival of juveniles to replace them. Official fingers also pointed at the burgeoning harp seal population numbering 5.15 million animals.

Although most scientists, both within and independent of DFO, acknowledge that environment always plays a role in natural population fluctuations, there is now almost universal acceptance that overfishing was the major, and possibly the only, cause of the disaster. The consensus was reached amid much acrimony. Some DFO scientists testifying before a 1997 parliamentary committee on DFO policies and practices claimed they had been muzzled, that politicians and the top brass in the DFO bureaucracy "gruesomely mangled" and misused their results. Among the department's most vocal critics were two of its former employees, Jeffrey Hutchings and Ransom Myers, both now at Dalhousie University in Halifax.

"Suddenly, everyone thinks that fishing was the primary cause," says Hutchings ruefully. "It did not always used to be the case. I can certainly tell you it wasn't always so."

Shortly after the moratorium was imposed, Hutchings and Myers analyzed reams of data dating back more than a century in an attempt to sort out the relative contributions of environment and human activity – fishing – to the cod collapse. In a landmark paper published in the *Canadian Journal of Fisheries and Aquatic Sciences*, they systematically dismantled the hypothesis that the collapse was due to natural causes. None of the evidence that they looked at supported a link between cod abundance and water temperature. If water temperature was the cause, they reasoned, the crash should have happened before. They found that water temperatures were colder throughout the 19th century, up until the 1920s, when the fishery harvest was as large as or larger than that of the 1980s. In the more recent past, they looked at five years in which the water was particularly cold (1972, 1973, 1974, 1984, and 1985) and found no consistent relationship between temperature and the recruitment of young fish to the adult stocks. In two of those years, in fact, recruitment was greater than average.

Furthermore, they showed that the collapse had begun in the north, where trawlers dragged up tens of thousands of tonnes of fish as they formed dense spawning schools, and worked its way south, a pattern they called "fishing down," until the predictable end came.

Neither did their findings support the seal predation theory. Seals eat primarily one- and two-year-old cod, and the number of three-year-old cod did not decline in the 1980s, as would have been expected. The two former DFO scientists could only conclude that the cod collapse was due primarily to overexploitation.

A related theory, known as the shift hypothesis, has been put forward by George Rose, senior chair of fisheries conservation at the Fisheries and Marine Institute of Memorial University of Newfoundland. Between 1990 and 1992, Rose (then with DFO) tracked a huge "mob of fish" as they migrated across the continental shelf along a deepwater trench known as the Bonavista Corridor. Estimated at 500,000 tonnes, it was probably the last great aggregation of northern cod in history. Rose believes the fish were concentrating in the southern part of their range to follow their prime prey, capelin. Unfortunately, their travels led them straight into the waiting nets not only of the Canadian fishing fleet, both inshore and offshore, but also of a huge foreign fleet, for in 1990, the Spanish arrived on the Nose of the Bank with fifty big trawlers.

"In a nutshell," Rose says, "you had this natural phenomenon, this aggregation process going on, and they became vulnerable, and we just killed them with fishing. That's the only explanation that makes sense to me as to how that stock could have collapsed so quickly."

Like Hutchings and Myers, Rose rejects DFO's theory that the collapse was due to natural mortality caused by cold water or seals. However, he does believe that cold northern waters may have caused the capelin to move southward, drawing the cod stocks after them. Hutchings and Myers discount this shift hypothesis, contending that the distribution changes of cod were solely the reflection of fishing down and that the process was gradual and therefore predictable. Whichever theory is more accurate, it was inshore fishers who first sounded the alarm – to no avail – in the mid-1980s, as they saw their catches sharply decline.

All of which points to the unsettling fact that the most shocking lesson to be learned from the collapse of the fishery was how little is actually known about the basic biology and ecology of this cornerstone species. No one knew, for instance, exactly how and where cod spawned or their degree of dependence on other species, such as capelin. In the past, DFO research had concentrated on counting fish from experimental trawls in order to set harvest rates. Even at that, overestimation of stock size in 1986 contributed to the setting of a disastrously high TAC, a miscalculation that was not recognized until 1989, after the stocks had been irreparably damaged. What was known was that northern cod spawned during winter throughout the continental shelf, from Hamilton Bank, off Labrador, south to the Grand Bank. They then undertook spring feeding migrations to inshore waters in pursuit of capelin, a smelt-like species that spawns, or "rolls," on the beaches. The cod then moved offshore again in autumn and began forming dense prespawning and spawning aggregations. That was pretty much the sum total of knowledge from five hundred years of observation and exploitation.

THE SECOND MORNING OF THE FISHERY, I went to the wharf at Lower Lance Cove, on the Smith Sound side of Random Island, where I found Jack Marsh splitting cod at his stage, the traditional low, weathered shed built over the water on pylons. He had just landed the morning's catch – more than 300 kilograms per net. In the past, he said, fifty kilograms per net was considered an excellent haul. He looked up from his cleaning table, his eyes gleaming. "I'll tell you something," he said. "There's never been as many fish in these waters since John Cabot was here."

In a way, he wasn't far wrong, for in 1995, a huge aggregation of spawning cod had been discovered in Smith Sound. According to George Rose, echograms from acoustic surveys showed "that the whole sound is like a coffee cup – it's full to the top." As late as last January, Rose estimated there were 11.5 million cod overwintering in the deep, inshore waters.

Outport fishers such as Marsh have always claimed that there were bay stocks of cod – stocks that spawned inshore and stayed there over winter – in addition to the offshore stocks that spawned offshore in winter and migrated inshore in summer to feed on capelin. Scientists have been slow to recognize the existence of these bay stocks, even though there are records of overwintering inshore cod dating back more than a century and similar inshore stocks are known from Greenland and Norway. In the past, they may have been lost in the huge inshore migration of fish from offshore, which formed the mainstay of the Newfoundland fishery. With the disappearance of the offshore stocks, however, the bay stocks have become far more important. Saving these once poor cousins of the offshore cod stock may be the key to the recovery of the northern cod.

However it got there, Rose is hoping that the production in Smith Sound will stabilize and spread. "We hope those fish will go elsewhere in some numbers. Eventually there's got to be too many of them to fit into one small area. There's a lot of precedent for that in fisheries ecology." In fact, Rose believes that the process may already have begun. Cod are much more widespread in Trinity Bay than they were even a few years ago, and Rose feels that areas to the north, in Bonavista and Notre Dame bays, may have been "reseeded" as well.

Meanwhile, tagging work carried out by research scientist John Brattey and his colleagues at DFO's science branch shows a great deal of movement of cod between bays, including summer feeding migrations from southern areas such as Placentia Bay into inshore areas along the east and northeast coast. On the other hand, DNA analysis has revealed that inshore cod are genetically different from offshore stocks. "So far," says Brattey, "the genetic work is telling us that there are enough differences between the inshore fish on the northeast coast and the offshore [fish] to suggest there's very little interbreeding between the two. Although they mix during the summer, they don't seem to interbreed."

Ultimately, only the offshore habitat is productive enough and, at 300,000 square kilometres, large enough to sustain northern cod populations at historic levels. But if the offshore stocks are to recover, they might well have to depend on the inshore cod eventually moving into offshore habitat and breeding there. As the 1999 DFO stock status report states, recovery based on the few fish now there is "dismal in both the short and long term." The process of building up the stocks is likely to take decades.

"The evidence so far is not very reassuring," Rose admits, "but I think it's far too early in the game to make any kind of conclusions." On the plus side, he cites improving ecological conditions, rising ocean temperatures around Newfoundland, and the fact that capelin are reclaiming their northern range. Rose believes that capelin may lure inshore cod to offshore waters. "If the capelin move back in there, we may see some very dramatic and quick changes in that ecosystem," he says.

"Cod are a very successful species," Rose observes. "It never ceases to amaze me how much abuse they have taken over the last five hundred years and yet still survive at all. They're survivors."

THE SAME MAY BE SAID OF NEWFOUNDLANDERS. Since the moratorium, survival for fishers such as the Penneys and Paul Kane has meant diversifying. The Penneys now fish herring in early spring, lobster from April to July, snow crab and capelin in summer, and squid in late fall. Kane took a TAGS-supported diving course and fishes for sea urchins and has opened a meat shop where he makes fat-free sausages and butchers the moose and caribou his neighbours hunt on the nearby Trepassey Barrens.

Even if the cod do make a comeback, few fishers want to see a return to the wasteful practices of the past, such as discarding undersized fish and misreportings of landings. Kane wants a wholesale return to a traditional, baited hook-and-line fishery; gill nets, he says, which often cannot be tended daily, "are wasteful of fish."

Gilbert does not want a return to the free-for-all fishery that existed before the moratorium, with fishers competing to catch fish before their neighbour does, a syndrome known in environmental literature as "the tragedy of the commons." Boat quotas circumvent such competition but create a new problem whereby fishers from fish-poor areas pile into sectors where fish are abundant. To stop this, the DFO recommended Smith Sound be restricted to local residents. If inshore stocks are to be conserved, such local management will have to replace the existing large regional fishing zones established by the North Atlantic Fisheries Organization, says Rose.

For his part, Jeffrey Hutchings has recommended that an offshore fishing ban be imposed between January and May, when cod form dense spawning schools. (Recent work at his Dalhousie laboratory has shown that cod spawning behaviour is highly ritualized, not the random process it was once thought to be, and is therefore likely to be seriously disrupted by dragging activity.) In effect, this would re-establish refuges for northern cod that existed prior to the 1950s, when trawlers arrived on the scene.

Even with more conservation-wise practices in place, though, it is doubtful that the cod fishery will ever again play the role it once did in outport Newfoundland.

But for a few glorious days in September, there was a familiar and joyful sight in Trinity Bay, as for the first time in seven years, boats returned to port with cod iced in their holds.

"Hickman's Harbour was a gloomy town, and people looked down on us," said Fern Penney. "But as I said, we were down but not out."

Near dusk, followed by a cloud of gulls and three bald eagles, Gilbert turned the bow of his boat back up Northwest Arm to land a handsome haul of 375 kilograms, which will fetch $1.70 per kilogram, compared with 27 cents when the moratorium was declared.

"It's been a very productive day," said Fern, glancing astern at her husband's smiling face. "A wonderful day."

Island Legacy

Bon Portage Island, Nova Scotia

IT IS TO VISIT BON PORTAGE Island that I find myself driving along the southwestern shore of Nova Scotia. I follow the jigsaw pattern of the coast, past snugly cut harbours. The road winds between the great glacial boulders that litter the landscape, rivalling, in some cases, the bulk of the fishers' houses. Offshore, like pieces of a puzzle waiting to be snapped into place, are the islands to which I am heading, dark, low-lying silhouettes jaggedly outlined by wind-shorn evergreens.

Except for Cape Sable Island (which is joined to the mainland by a causeway), these islands are no longer inhabited year round. Once, however, it was a different story. In the days of sail, they were home to many fishers and their families. The motorboat, however, made the rich offshore fishing grounds easily accessible from the mainland, and over the years the fishers moved their homes there, abandoning the islands to the sheep and the lighthouse keepers. Today, even the lighthouse keepers have gone, their presence made unnecessary by technology.

Duck hunters, Irish-moss gatherers, lobster trappers, picnickers, sheepshearers and birdwatchers still visit the islands on occasion. And each summer Bon Portage plays host to a number of university students and teachers, for it is here that Nova Scotia's Acadia University runs a biological field station and offers a summer course in natural history and field biology.

But it is not the field station alone that sets the island apart from the others. Bon Portage was once home to one of Nova Scotia's best-loved writers, Evelyn Richardson, who, with her lightkeeper husband, Morrill, bought the island, save for the government land on which the lighthouse sat. Their thirty-five years on the island instilled such a deep love for its natural history that they wished to conserve it for future generations to enjoy. When they retired to the mainland in 1964, Acadia University – with financial help from friends of the Richardsons – acquired the land for its fledgling program in ecology and wildlife management. Today, the Evelyn and Morrill Richardson Field Station in Biology is a valuable research resource. As well, it helps hundreds of students gain an understanding of nature such as they could never gain on a university campus.

We Keep a Light, Evelyn Richardson's touching but unsentimental record of her years on the island, is a literary landmark. Her first book, it won the Governor General's Award for Creative Nonfiction in 1945 and has subsequently been published in both the United States and Britain. Today, more than half a century later, it is still in print.

"So here I am," Evelyn wrote, "a light-keeper's wife on a small island three miles from the mainland, isolated much of the year, and living under conditions that most of the country outgrew fifty years or more ago."

It was a hard life of self-sufficiency in which the Richardsons had to juggle the around-the-clock duties of light-keeping, raising a family and tending a farm. "Morrill was tremendously busy, with new tasks and demands for time and efforts facing him every time he turned around," wrote Evelyn. "For my part, I learned to make bread, to churn and make butter, care for milk pails and separator, fill and clean oil-lamps, and do the many extra things that never enter housekeeping in a town or city.

"I learned, too, to clean and fill and care for the Light, in case Morrill should be detained or absent at lighting time."

But *We Keep a Light is* much more than a record of a bygone way of life, anticipating as it does the back-to-the-land and environmental movements of the late 1960s. "I'm really glad my mother wrote the book, because

I think it helped people to understand that you didn't have to live in suburbia or downtown to enjoy life," says the Richardsons' youngest daughter, Betty June Smith, who, as an adult, kept a light with her husband, Sidney, on nearby Cape Sable. The book also served as an inspiration to other women, including female writers striving in the 1950s for a more independent lifestyle.

If independent, Evelyn's life was unstintingly busy. Despite duties as mother, teacher, homemaker and, often, lighthouse keeper, she managed to write eight books, including an award-winning historical novel, *Desired Haven*, and a celebration of the island's natural history, *Living Island*. *Where My Roots Go Deep: The Collected Writings of Evelyn Richardson* appeared posthumously in 1996. In each work, the joy of a life shared with loved ones and her beloved birds shines through.

FROM THE SHAG HARBOUR wharf, the saddleback shape of Bon Portage, known locally as Outer Island, dominates the western horizon. My 12-year-old daughter, Meaghan, and I see the fishtail wake of a boat closing the distance between the island and ourselves. At its helm is Dr. Peter Smith, a professor of biology at Acadia University and director of the field station.

Minutes later, Smith neatly maneuvres the bow of the boat into the lee of a rough timber-and-rock-wharf. Only on a dead calm day such as this is it possible to scramble dry-footed onto the well-named "slip," a 40-metre-long wooden ramp that climbs the natural sea wall of beach stone at a steep angle.

Once ashore, I discover that to explore Bon Portage is to encounter a literary landscape: everywhere I am reminded of Richardson's words. On the back of an all-terrain vehicle, the kilometre-long road to the field station is a rough introduction to what she called Bon Portage's "unexpected share of island charm." The road cuts through dense thickets of fir before opening to a prospect of the ocean.

The shore is a rag-and-bone shop of everything lost at sea. On our arrival, there is a particularly rich collection of flotsam and jetsam, the legacy of tropical storm Felix, which had swept the coast the week before. The mangled green wire cages of modern lobster traps lie beside the weathered laths of the traditional traps.

Hurled above the tide line, on the landward side of the beach-stone road, is an arresting monument to the sea's treachery and power – the skull of a fin whale. This 20-metre-long giant was washed ashore in 1993. The great head bone, with its projecting rostrum, looks like a giant sundial. It is surrounded by an aromatic wreath of bayberry and wild rose bushes, diminishing its melancholy look. As Richardson observed in *Living Island*, "When the island wears summer's rich caparison, its brave opposition looks not altogether hopeless, for then many deep wounds are hidden under green leaves and bright blossoms."

We continue on our way beside the sea to the light station, which stands at the island's south end. The view from here is limitless, the Atlantic rolling away to New England.

ALTHOUGH THE VIEW IS unchanged, little else remains from the Richardsons' time. At low tide, however, two wondrously preserved artefacts, the boilers of the Clydeside-built steamer *Express*, are exposed at the foot of the lighthouse. "Steadfast and undaunted," as Richardson wrote, they are all that survive of the steamship that went aground here in September 1898 – fortunately, with no loss of life. Today they serve as powerful reminders of the lighthouse's enduring purpose of warning mariners of the treacherous currents and shoals that surround the island.

The original lighthouse, a tapered wooden tower with an attached dwelling, has been replaced by a spartan square tower with a flatroofed addition to house the generators. Nearby stand a radio tower and two lightkeepers' houses. Neither has been occupied full time since 1984, when the light was "destaffed," to use the dehumanizing bureaucratese. In summer, however, they serve as the residence and laboratory for the Acadia staff and students.

Dr. Harrison Lewis, the first chief of the Canadian Wildlife Service, was a "treasured friend" of the Richardsons. He introduced Evelyn to the joys of bird-watching and was the first person to recognize Bon Portage's potential as a biological study site. Lying off the southernmost tip of Nova Scotia, the island attracts unusual numbers of birds on their migratory flights. "The trees and bushes seemed alive with birds, the bright coats of the Yellow Warblers predominating over the more sober hues of the others . . . ," Richardson wrote of her early days on the island. "I had never seen so many birds in so small a space, and the numerous birds on the Island have continued to be one of our chief joys."

The seasonal flush of feathered visitors to Bon Portage is the basis for an ambitious banding program and the postgraduate research of students like Andrew Davis, who, as part of his work, strings mist nets along lanes cut through the dense forest. I follow him one early morning, helping to band a northern water thrush.

"As soon as I set foot on the island, I wanted to spend a lot of time here," says Davis, who, when collecting data on the nesting and feeding habits and the age and sex ratios of the migrating bird populations, spends weeks alone at a rustic cabin in the woods.

For two decades, the island has also been the centre of the field station director's ongoing investigation of one of the sea's most mysterious creatures, the Leach's storm petrel. Birds of the open ocean, they come to land only at night and only in breeding season, announcing their arrival with unearthly calls. Each spring some 50,000 of them come to Bon Portage, where their young spend their early weeks in burrows excavated in the shallow turf carpeting the forest floor.

The island is, in Peter Smith's words, "the perfect outdoor laboratory." The sea makes a show of her marine riches quite casually to the island visitor. Daily, from the field station doorstep, we see seals returning our curious gazes, gannets diving for herring and porpoises spouting.

"At university, the only time you ever saw animals was in the lab. Every day you see them here, even if you only walk back and forth to the field station," marvelled Peter Lawrance last summer, when he took Acadia University's summer course on Bon Portage.

During the intensive, dawn-to-dark course, Lawrance and his eighteen fellow students explored all facets of island life. They live-trapped meadow voles, identified plants, birds and insects, collected beach debris, and learnt the techniques of radiotelemetry (the tracking of radio-tagged birds and animals).

"There's a different thinking involved in this course. For the most part, it's how to apply what you already know," said Lawrance. "You're forced to think about problems and solutions. It's very practical."

PETER SMITH'S ASSOCIATION with Bon Portage began at an early age. As a child he visited the island with his father, the late Chalmers Smith, who was also a biology professor at Acadia. "As a kid it was just marvellous being here," he recalls. "It really fired me. I hadn't decided what I wanted to do at that point. But after that one visit, just one day on and off, I was a biologist."

A boat tour around the island reveals Smith's inspiration. A wonderful diversity of shorebirds – sandpipers, sanderlings, plovers and dowitchers are working the food-rich wrack at the tide line. Grey seals cruise by the boat with the grace of synchronized swimmers.

Whereas island wildlife is, and always has been, abundant, evidence of the long human presence on Bon Portage is now scant. The first European contact with the island was made in 1604 by the French explorer Samuel de Champlain, who called it "Iles aux Cormorant" for the nesting seabirds, known locally as shags (thus Shag Harbour). He collected wild duck and gull eggs on the island and then moved on to establish New France's first settlement at Port Royal. The island was named Bon Portage sometime later, although the rationale for the name remains obscure. It was not until about 1840 that the first families settled on the island.

I observe that Smith is as sensitive to and protective of the island's human culture as he is of its ecology. When walking around the island, he is always aware of what he calls its "living history."

"Half the people who come on the islands walk these beaches and think it's the first time that they have been walked," he says with incredulity. "But, my God, no. There have been births and deaths here and livings made for many, many years.

"Part of what I try to do with the students is get them not only to look at the island's natural history but to think about its historical and human aspects."

Smith welcomes the use of the island for traditional purposes. As in the Richardsons' time, local people are still welcome to come ashore to hunt ducks, salvage wrecked lobster traps or have a picnic. Smith's generosity is returned. There are always mainlanders willing to lend a helping hand with projects, such as wharf repair, or to respond to an emergency. Says Anthony Smith, a local fisher: "Peter knows that no matter what time of day or kind of weather, I'll be there if he needs me."

"We couldn't have a field station here," admits Smith, "unless we had the full cooperation of the local people."

Ironically, fears and superstitions about island ghosts made it difficult for the Richardsons to hire local people for any duration. Smith, who has spent long periods alone on the island, admits that he has had experiences on Bon Portage that have been almost mystical. "There are times when I'm out at night on the petrel paths or walking on the beach and I sense the Richardsons or a presence of some sort – I really do."

The storm petrels themselves are a ghostly presence. Richardson called them "queer black birds . . . that walk the watery waste." This illusory behaviour has earned them their common name, petrels, from St. Peter, who also is reputed to have walked on water.

After dark, the petrels' eerie calls electrify the damp air of Bon Portage. The woods resonate with their excited discourse – like the babble of a synthesizer or the animated chattering of a rainforest. Our last night on the island, Meaghan and I follow Ian Paterson, a graduate student, as he monitors the elbow-deep burrows dug into the island's mossy turf. Attracted to our flashlight beams, the sooty-coloured birds flutter harmlessly against our chests as they zigzag through the dense underbrush.

At 2:00 a.m., Meaghan and I walk back to the field station through the salt-charged dark, our way intermittently lit by the sweep of three lights – those of Bon Portage, Cape Sable Island to the southeast and distant Seal Island to the southwest – crossing and recrossing one another. These "friendly smiles of comrades in the struggle against sea and wind" reassured Richardson throughout her years of isolation on Bon Portage. Though now un-watched by lighthouse keepers, they still shine for mariners and, on this moonless night, for us.

EVELYN RICHARDSON'S "LITERARY LIGHTHOUSE" also continues to cast its sure light. Looking back, I can see that her views on nature did indeed anticipate by a half century an environmental ethic that is only now gaining wider acceptance: "The chain of human life unrolls as limitless as the waves in the sea that laps all shores.... The spots of earth we call our own, as we take our place in the life continuity, never actually belong to any of us; what are really ours are the eyes and the ears to see and hear, and the soul to love and understand the beauties around us. Though Morrill holds a title to the Island of Bon Portage, who could sell or buy the sea among the rocks, the winds rippling the fields of grass, the moon's lustrous path across the surging water, or the star-studded bowl of the night sky? They are without price, and priceless, and will be here for those who follow us. Then the work of our hands, those insignificant scratches on the face of the earth, may serve to remind others of our passing...."

Acknowledgements

I am sincerely grateful to Lesley Choyce for his belief in the value of collecting this body of work about the region – adopted and native – that we love. As well, I am in debt to Peggy Amirault for her help in collating, copy-editing and, in some cases, updating the articles. I also wish to thank the editors of the magazines which first published these articles, some of which appear here is slightly revised form.

Atlantic Insight:
   "Mining a Thin Seam Wasn't God's Idea," June 1979.
   "End of the Trail," September 1983 (appeared as "Advocate, N.S.").

Audubon:
   "The Devil's Work is an Ark of Sand," March 1989.

Canadian Geographic:
   "Island Pastoral," June/July 1990.
   "The Last Lighthouse Keeper," March/April 1992.

enRoute:
   "A Memory of the Wind," August 1996.

Equinox:
   "Outport Renaissance," December 1981.
   "Storming the Sand Castles," September/October 1984.
   "After the Bump," September/October 1984.
   "The Glory and the Grit," November/December, 1985.
   "Bottom Line," July/August 1987.
   "Mother Miramichi," August/September 1997.
   "The Cod Comeback," February/March 2000.

Harrowsmith:
   "The Fat of The Land," February 1981.
   "The Enemy Above," April/May 1982.
   "Prest's Last Stand," August/September 1983.
   "Of Cabbages and Kings," November/December 1986.

Imperial Oil Review:
   "The Magic of Wooden Boats," Autumn 1996
         (appeared as "The Wooden Boats of Nova Scotia").
   "Island Legacy," Spring 1997.

Island Journal: The Annual Publication of the Island Insitute
   "The Life and Tides of Fundy," volume 10.